T0407819

HEALTH AND HUMAN DEVELOPMENT

# TEXTBOOK ON EVIDENCE-BASED HOLISTIC MIND-BODY MEDICINE

## HEALING THE MIND IN TRADITIONAL HIPPOCRATIC MEDICINE

# HEALTH AND HUMAN DEVELOPMENT

***JOAV MERRICK - SERIES EDITOR***

NATIONAL INSTITUTE OF CHILD HEALTH
AND HUMAN DEVELOPMENT,
MINISTRY OF SOCIAL AFFAIRS, JERUSALEM

**Adolescent Behavior Research: International Perspectives**
*Joav Merrick and Hatim A. Omar (Editors)*
2007. ISBN: 1-60021-649-8

**Complementary Medicine Systems: Comparison and Integration**
*Karl W. Kratky*
2008. ISBN: 978-1-60456-475-4 (Hardcover)
2008. ISBN: 978-1-61122-433-7 (E-book)

**Pain in Children and Youth**
*Patricia Schofield and Joav Merrick (Editors)*
2008. ISBN: 978-1-60456-951-3 (Hardcover)
2008. ISBN: 978-1-61470-496-6 (E-book)

**Alcohol-Related Cognitive Disorders: Research and Clinical Perspectives**
*Leo Sher, Isack Kandel and Joav Merrick (Editors)*
2009. ISBN: 978-1-60741-730-9 (Hardcover)
2009. ISBN: 978-1-60876-623-9 (E-book)

**Challenges in Adolescent Health: An Australian Perspective**
*David Bennett, Susan Towns, Elizabeth Elliott and Joav Merrick (Editors)*
2009. ISBN: 978-1-60741-616-6 (Hardcover)
2009. ISBN: 978-1-61668-240-8 (E-book)

**Children and Pain**
*Patricia Schofield and Joav Merrick (Editors)*
2009. ISBN: 978-1-60876-020-6 (Hardcover)
2009. ISBN: 978-1-61728-183-9 (E-book)

**Living on the Edge: The Mythical, Spiritual, and Philosophical Roots of Social Marginality**
*Joseph Goodbread*
2009. ISBN: 978-1-60741-162-8 (Hardcover)
2013. ISBN: 978-1-61122-986-8 (Softcover)
2011. ISBN: 978-1-61470-192-7 (E-book)

**Obesity and Adolescence: A Public Health Concern**
*Hatim A. Omar, Donald E. Greydanus, Dilip R. Patel and Joav Merrick (Editors)*
2009. ISBN: 978-1-60692-821-9 (Hardcover)
2009. ISBN: 978-1-61470-465-2 (E-book)

**Poverty and Children: A Public Health Concern**
*Alexis Lieberman and Joav Merrick (Editors)*
2009. ISBN: 978-1-60741-140-6 (Hardcover)
2009. ISBN: 978-1-61470-601-4 (E-book)

**Bone and Brain Metastases: Advances in Research and Treatment**
*Arjun Sahgal, Edward Chow and Joav Merrick (Editors)*
2010. ISBN: 978-1-61668-365-8 (Hardcover)
2010. ISBN: 978-1-61728-085-6 (E-book)

**Chance Action and Therapy: The Playful Way of Changing**
*Uri Wernik*
2010. ISBN: 978-1-60876-393-1 (Hardcover)
2011. ISBN: 978-1-61122-987-5 (Softcover)
2011. ISBN: 978-1-61209-874-6 (E-book)

**Advanced Cancer Pain and Quality of Life**
*Edward Chow and Joav Merrick (Editors)*
2011. ISBN: 978-1-61668-207-1 (Hardcover)
2010. ISBN: 978-1-61668-400-6 (E-book)

**Advances in Environmental Health Effects of Toxigenic Mold and Mycotoxins**
*Ebere Cyril Anyanwu*
2011. ISBN: 978-1-60741-953-2

**Alternative Medicine Yearbook 2009**
*Joav Merrick (Editor)*
2011. ISBN: 978-1-61668-910-0 (Hardcover)
2011. ISBN: 978-1-62081-710-0 (E-book)

**Behavioral Pediatrics, 3rd Edition**
*Donald E. Greydanus, Dilip R. Patel, Helen D. Pratt and Joseph L. Calles, Jr. (Editors)*
2011. ISBN: 978-1-60692-702-1 (Hardcover)
2009. ISBN: 978-1-60876-630-7 (E-book)

**Child Health and Human Development Yearbook 2009**
*Joav Merrick (Editor)*
2011. ISBN: 978-1-61668-912-4

**Climate Change and Rural Child Health**
*Erica Bell, Bastian M. Seidel and Joav Merrick (Editors)*
2011. ISBN: 978-1-61122-640-9 (Hardcover)
2011. ISBN: 978-1-61209-014-6 (E-book)

**Clinical Aspects of Psychopharmacology in Childhood and Adolescence**
*Donald E. Greydanus, Joseph L. Calles, Jr., Dilip P. Patel, Ahsan Nazeer and Joav Merrick (Editors)*
2011. ISBN: 978-1-61122-135-0 (Hardcover)
2011. ISBN: 978-1-61122-715-4 (E-book)

**Drug Abuse in Hong Kong: Development and Evaluation of a Prevention Program**
*Daniel T.L. Shek, Rachel C.F. Sun and Joav Merrick (Editors)*
2011. ISBN: 978-1-61324-491-3 (Hardcover)
2011. ISBN: 978-1-62257-232-8 (E-book)

**Environment, Mood Disorders and Suicide**
*Teodor T. Postolache and Joav Merrick (Editors)*
2011. ISBN: 978-1-61668-505-8 (Hardcover)
2011. ISBN: 978-1-62618-340-7 (E-book)

**International Aspects of Child Abuse and Neglect**
*Howard Dubowitz and Joav Merrick (Editors)*
2011. ISBN: 978-1-60876-703-8 (Hardcover)
2010. ISBN: 978-1-61122-049-0 (Softcover)
2010. ISBN: 978-1-61122-403-0 (E-book)

**Narratives and Meanings of Migration**
*Julia Mirsky*
2011. ISBN: 978-1-61761-103-2 (Hardcover)
2010. ISBN: 978-1-61761-519-1 (E-book)

**Positive Youth Development: Evaluation and Future Directions in a Chinese Context**
*Daniel T.L. Shek, Hing Keung Ma and Joav Merrick (Editors)*
2011. ISBN: 978-1-60876-830-1 (Hardcover)
2011. ISBN: 978-1-62100-175-1 (Softcover)
2010. ISBN: 978-1-61209-091-7 (E-book)

**Positive Youth Development: Implementation of a Youth Program in a Chinese Context**
*Daniel T.L Shek, Hing Keung Ma and Joav Merrick (Editors)*
2011. ISBN: 978-1-61668-230-9 (Hardcover)

**Principles of Holistic Psychiatry: A Textbook on Holistic Medicine for Mental Disorders**
*Soren Ventegodt and Joav Merrick*
2011. ISBN: 978-1-61761-940-3 (Hardcover)
2011. ISBN: 978-1-61122-263-0 (E-book)

**Public Health Yearbook 2009**
*Joav Merrick (Editor)*
2011. ISBN: 978-1-61668-911-7 (Hardcover)
2011. ISBN: 978-1-62417-365-3 (E-book)

**Rural Child Health: International Aspects**
*Erica Bell and Joav Merrick (Editors)*
2011. ISBN: 978-1-60876-357-3 (Hardcover)
2011. ISBN: 978-1-61324-005-2 (E-book)

**Rural Medical Education: Practical Strategies**
*Erica Bell, Craig Zimitat and Joav Merrick (Editors)*
2011. ISBN: 978-1-61122-649-2 (Hardcover)
2011. ISBN: 978-1-61209-476-2 (E-book)

**Self-Management and the Health Care Consumer**
*Peter William Harvey*
2011. ISBN: 978-1-61761-796-6 (Hardcover)
2011. ISBN: 978-1-61122-214-2 (E-book)

**Sexology from a Holistic Point of View**
*Soren Ventegodt and Joav Merrick*
2011. ISBN: 978-1-61761-859-8 (Hardcover)
2011. ISBN: 978-1-61122-262-3 (E-book)

**Social and Cultural Psychiatry Experience from the Caribbean Region**
*Hari D. Maharajh and Joav Merrick (Editors)*
2011. ISBN: 978-1-61668-506-5 (Hardcover)
2010. ISBN: 978-1-61728-088-7 (E-book)

**The Dance of Sleeping and Eating among Adolescents: Normal and Pathological Perspectives**
*Yael Latzer and Orna Tzischinsky (Editors)*
2011. ISBN: 978-1-61209-710-7 (Hardcover)
2011. ISBN: 978-1-62417-366-0 (E-book)

**Understanding Eating Disorders: Integrating Culture, Psychology and Biology**
*Yael Latzer, Joav Merrick and Daniel Stein (Editors)*
2011. ISBN: 978-1-61728-298-0 (Hardcover)
2011. ISBN: 978-1-61470-976-3 (Softcover)
2011. ISBN: 978-1-61942-054-0 (E-book)

**Adolescence and Chronic Illness. A Public Health Concern**
*Hatim Omar, Donald E. Greydanus, Dilip R. Patel and Joav Merrick (Editors)*
2012. ISBN: 978-1-60876-628-4 (Hardcover)
2010. ISBN: 978-1-61761-482-8 (E-book)

**AIDS and Tuberculosis: Public Health Aspects**
*Daniel Chemtob and Joav Merrick (Editors)*
2012. ISBN: 978-1-62081-382-9 (Softcover)
2012. ISBN: 978-1-62081-406-2 (E-book)

**Alternative Medicine Yearbook 2010**
*Joav Merrick (Editor)*
2012. ISBN: 978-1-62100-132-4 (Hardcover)
2011. ISBN: 978-1-62100-210-9 (E-book)

**Alternative Medicine Research Yearbook 2011**
*Joav Merrick (Editor)*
2012. ISBN: 978-1-62081-476-5 (Hardcover)
2012. ISBN: 978-1-62081-477-2 (E-book)

**Applied Public Health: Examining Multifaceted Social or Ecological Problems and Child Maltreatment**
*John R. Lutzker and Joav Merrick (Editors)*
2012. ISBN: 978-1-62081-356-0 (Hardcover)
2012. ISBN: 978-1-62081-388-1 (E-book)

**Building Community Capacity: Minority and Immigrant Populations**
*Rosemary M Caron and Joav Merrick (Editors)*
2012. ISBN: 978-1-62081-022-4 (Hardcover)
2012. ISBN: 978-1-62081-032-3 (E-book)

**Building Community Capacity: Skills and Principles**
*Rosemary M Caron and Joav Merrick (Editors)*
2012. ISBN: 978-1-61209-331-4 (Hardcover)
2012. ISBN: 978-1-62257-238-0 (E-book)

**Child and Adolescent Health Yearbook 2009**
*Joav Merrick (Editor)*
2012. ISBN: 978-1-61668-913-1 (Hardcover)
2012. ISBN: 978-1-62257-095-9 (E-book)

**Child and Adolescent Health Yearbook 2010**
*Joav Merrick (Editor)*
2012. ISBN: 978-1-61209-788-6 (Hardcover)
2012. ISBN: 978-1-62417-046-1 (E-book)

**Child Health and Human Development Yearbook 2010**
*Joav Merrick (Editor)*
2012. ISBN: 978-1-61209-789-3 (Hardcover)
2012. ISBN: 978-1-62081-721-6 (E-book)

**Health Risk Communication**
*Marijke Lemal and Joav Merrick (Editors)*
2012. ISBN: 978-1-62257-544-2 (Hardcover)
2012. ISBN: 978-1-62257-552-7 (E-book)

**Human Immunodeficiency Virus (HIV) Research: Social Science Aspects**
*Hugh Klein and Joav Merrick (Editors)*
2012. ISBN: 978-1-62081-293-8 (Hardcover)
2012. ISBN: 978-1-62081-346-1 (E-book)

**Our Search for Meaning in Life: Quality of Life Philosophy**
*Søren Ventegodt and Joav Merrick*
2012. ISBN: 978-1-61470-494-2 (Hardcover)
2011. ISBN: 978-1-61470-519-2 (E-book)

**Public Health Yearbook 2010**
*Joav Merrick (Editor)*
2012. ISBN: 978-1-61209-971-2 (Hardcover)
2012. ISBN: 978-1-62417-863-4 (E-book)

**Public Health Yearbook 2011**
*Joav Merrick (Editor)*
2012. ISBN: 978-1-62081-433-8 (Hardcover)
2012. ISBN: 978-1-62081-434-5 (E-book)

**Randomized Clinical Trials and Placebo: Can You Trust the Drugs are Working and Safe?**
*Søren Ventegodt and Joav Merrick*
2012. ISBN: 978-1-61470-067-8

**Textbook on Evidence-Based Holistic Mind-Body Medicine: Basic Philosophy and Ethics of Traditional Hippocratic Medicine**
*Søren Ventegodt and Joav Merrick*
2012. ISBN: 978-1-62257-052-2 (Hardcover)
2013. ISBN: 978-1-62257-707-1 (E-book)

**Textbook on Evidence-Based Holistic Mind-Body Medicine: Basic Principles of Healing in Traditional Hippocratic Medicine**
*Søren Ventegodt and Joav Merrick*
2012. ISBN: 978-1-62257-094-2 (Hardcover)
2012. ISBN: 978-1-62257-172-7 (E-book)

**Textbook on Evidence-Based Holistic Mind-Body Medicine: Healing the Mind in Traditional Hippocratic Medicine**
*Søren Ventegodt and Joav Merrick*
2012. ISBN: 978-1-62257-112-3 (Hardcover)
2012. ISBN: 978-1-62257-175-8 (E-book)

**Textbook on Evidence-Based Holistic Mind-Body Medicine: Holistic Practice of Traditional Hippocratic Medicine**
*Søren Ventegodt and Joav Merrick*
2012. ISBN: 978-1-62257-105-5 (Hardcover)
2012. ISBN: 978-1-62257-174-1 (E-book)

**Textbook on Evidence-Based Holistic Mind-Body Medicine: Research, Philosophy, Economy and Politics of Traditional Hippocratic Medicine**
*Søren Ventegodt and Joav Merrick*
2012. ISBN: 978-1-62257-140-6 (Hardcover)
2012. ISBN: 978-1-62257-171-0 (E-book)

**Textbook on Evidence-Based Holistic Mind-Body Medicine: Sexology and Traditional Hippocratic Medicine**
*Søren Ventegodt and Joav Merrick*
2012. ISBN: 978-1-62257-130-7 (Hardcover)
2012. ISBN: 978-1-62257-176-5 (E-book)

**The Astonishing Brain and Holistic Conciousness: Neuroscience and Vedanta Perspectives**
*Vinod D. Deshmukh*
2012. ISBN: 978-1-61324-295-7

**Translational Research for Primary Healthcare**
*Erica Bell, Gert. P. Westert and Joav Merrick (Editors)*
2012. ISBN: 978-1-61324-647-4 (Hardcover)
2012. ISBN: 978-1-62417-409-4 (E-book)

**Treatment and Recovery of Eating Disorders**
*Daniel Stein and Yael Latzer (Editors)*
2012. ISBN: 978-1-61470-259-7

**Adolescence and Sports**
*Dilip R. Patel, Donald E. Greydanus, Hatim Omar and Joav Merrick (Editors)*
2013. ISBN: 978-1-60876-702-1 (Hardcover)
2010. ISBN: 978-1-61761-483-5 (E-book)

**Building Community Capacity: Case Examples from Around the World**
*Rosemary M Caron and Joav Merrick (Editors)*
2013. ISBN: 978-1-62417-175-8 (Hardcover)
2013. ISBN: 978-1-62417-176-5 (E-book)

**Bullying: A Public Health Concern**
*Jorge C. Srabstein and Joav Merrick (Editors)*
2013. ISBN: 978-1-62618-564-7 (Hardcover)
2013. ISBN: 978-1-62618-588-3 (E-book)

**Conceptualizing Behavior in Health and Social Research: A Practical Guide to Data Analysis**
*Said Shahtahmasebi and Damon Berridge*
2013. ISBN: 978-1-60876-383-2

**Health and Happiness from Meaningful Work: Research in Quality of Working Life**
*Søren Ventegodt and Joav Merrick (Editors)*
2013. ISBN: 978-1-60692-820-2 (Hardcover)
2009. ISBN: 978-1-61324-981-9 (E-book)

**Human Development: Biology from a Holistic Point of View**
*Søren Ventegodt, Tyge Dahl Hermansen and Joav Merrick*
2013. ISBN: 978-1-61470-441-6 (Hardcover)
2011. ISBN: 978-1-61470-541-3 (E-book)

**Managed Care in a Public Setting**
*Richard Evan Steele*
2013. ISBN: 978-1-62417-970-9 (Softcover)
2013. ISBN: 978-1-62417-863-4 (E-book)

**Pediatric and Adolescent Sexuality and Gynecology: Principles for the Primary Care Clinician**
*Hatim A. Omar, Donald E. Greydanus, Artemis K. Tsitsika, Dilip R. Patel and Joav Merrick (Editors)*
2013. ISBN: 978-1-60876-735-9 (Softcover)

HEALTH AND HUMAN DEVELOPMENT

# TEXTBOOK ON EVIDENCE-BASED HOLISTIC MIND-BODY MEDICINE

# HEALING THE MIND IN TRADITIONAL HIPPOCRATIC MEDICINE

SØREN VENTEGODT
AND
JOAV MERRICK

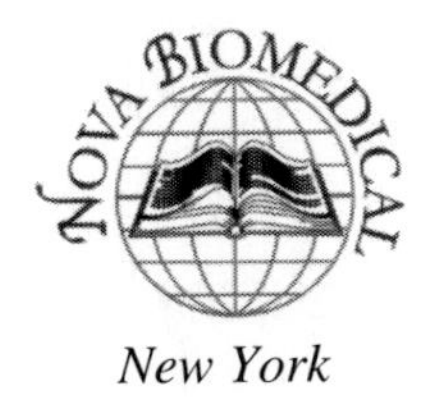


*New York*

For permission to use material from this book please contact us:
Telephone 631-231-7269; Fax 631-231-8175
Web Site: http://www.novapublishers.com



**Library of Congress Cataloging-in-Publication Data**

ISBN: 978-1-62257-112-3

Library of Congress Control Number: 2012939747

*Published by Nova Science Publishers, Inc. † New York*

# Contents

# Preface

Holistic medicine, or quality of life as medicine, as we often call it, is basically a strategy for improving the patients quality of life, through mobilizing of inner resources. This can never harm and will almost always benefit the patient's wellbeing and often also help him or her to fight back the disease. The cure is very much the same for all patients: Help to know yourself better and to step into character and be more yourself, and more in tune with the universe. So it can be started right away, also without a specific diagnosis. Is modern, holistic medicine powerful? Oh yes, very much so. Holistic medicine is a truly powerful medicine, in spite of nobody really understanding the deepest structures of consciousness, the connection between mind and body, and the way holistic medicine works. But just because our scientific understanding admittedly still is limited we should not stop doing what we know works. In this book the authors cover the basic principles of healing and ethics of traditional Hippocratic medicine from a new and modern scientific approach.

# Introduction

*Søren Ventegodt and Joav Merrick*

The mind is thoughts. The thoughts cannot be wrong in the sense that all thought are just that – thoughts. They are not true or truths that you can patent; they are made by words, which are fairly relative in meaning and significance. There is nothing wrong with a thought in itself. The problem comes when we believe in the thoughts, because we then believe or project them into experiential existence.

This is the power of consciousness that we can do that. If we believe a girl is our girlfriend, this becomes our experience. If she is not, we are facing a real problem, and lots of suffering comes out of that. In general suffering comes from thought we believe in, when we should not. To see that and to let go of all attachment to thoughts is therefore the gate to mental health and freedom.

In this book (the fourth mind-body book) we focus on the mental nature of the human being. There have been many models explaining the constitutions of the human being and the structure of talent and human character (1). What have been most difficult to understand are the concepts of good or evil. Freud believed that man had two basic instincts, the constructive Eros and the destructive Thanatos, and many philosophers of life have had similar concepts.

The simplest way to understand the most severe diseases like schizophrenia is that the sexual energy unconsciously is channelized into the belief of all kinds of strange thoughts, which then becomes the weird and idiosyncratic experience of the mentally ill person, like harmful voices only heard by him or her. When this dynamic is clearly understood by both the ill person and the therapist, the sexual energy can be channelized into useful and appropriate patterns by the therapy, and the illness almost always heals. This is in short the project of psychoanalysis as well of all modern psychodynamic psychotherapy. When a therapist has this understanding he or she can then work with the patient, even in a psychotic stage, without use of any drugs.

We are not here to judge our patients, but to set them free. We are healers so we come from love and understanding, not from judgment and punishment. The patients can freely admit all their misdeeds to us. And they can share all the misdeeds done to them by others.

Only when you have reached a certain point of development will you realize that both good and evil are divine. Everything comes from the same source, our life. Only when you understand this fully can you help a patient tormented by evil done to him or her and by him or her. Violent and sexual abuse, fail and neglect and all kinds of misery has been the patient's life. To heal mind and existence is to step beyond the evil. To integrate the human shadow. To see everything as a necessary part of life, a necessary part of the journey of the spirit.

In this book we search for the deepest understanding we can get of the human existence. Not to justify the evil. But to be able to understand, forgive and heal.

## Reference

[1] Ventegodt S, Kromann M, Andersen NJ, Merrick J. The life mission theory VI. A theory for the human character: Healing with holistic medicine through recovery of character and purpose of life. ScientificWorldJournal 2004;4:859-80.

# Section 1. Healing the mind

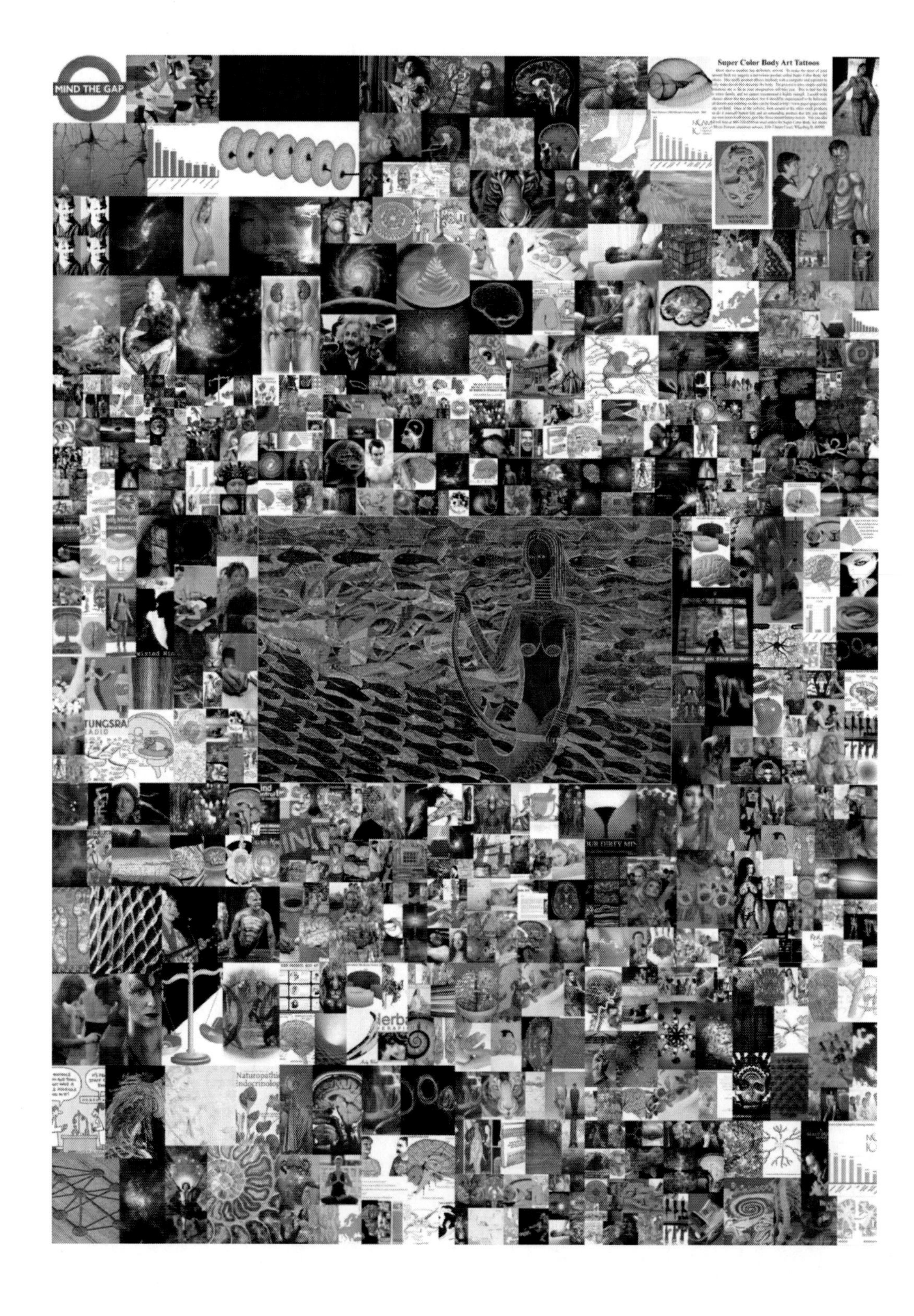
MIND THE GAP
Super Color Body Art Tattoos

*Chapter I*

# Human brain and consciousness

"The hard problem" is the difficulty in neuro-philosophy about how mind and matter interact. It seems like matter and consciousness exist on two fundamentally different levels. We know that we can turn the level of awareness up or down with drugs like cocaine and chloroform; we also know that the state of consciousness can be changed by drugs like LSD and psilocybin (magic mushrooms) (1-3).

But the content of human consciousness seems to be completely unaffected by such drugs. The activity of the brain has something to do with human consciousness, but seemingly only on a quantitative level. The brain is necessary for verbal and mental consciousness, but it does not determine the content of consciousness. The body does that, especially what is connected to sexuality, at least according to Freud, Jung, Reich, Searles and hundreds of psychodynamic researchers from the last century.

The problem has not been solved (4-10). We shall not claim that we have solved it either. It remains a true mystery.

In this section we look into the hardwiring of the human brain and try to map human consciousness. We model a world seemingly induced from sensory input, but for a more thorough analysis the whole world is an interpretation based on our purpose of life. The life mission theory thus seem to be better in order to explain the fundamental structure of human consciousness and unconsciousness that even the best biological description of the human brain is unable to do today.

At the core of the life-mission theory is the idea that we can convert thought into experiential existence. Many eastern philosophies have been talking about that, and our series of theories about the human existence are not at all as profound and wise as they appear. But hopefully a little easier to understand.

## References


[1] Grof S. LSD psychotherapy: Exploring the frontiers of the hidden mind. Alameda, CA: Hunter House, 1980.

[2] Grof S. Implications of modern consciousness research for psychology: Holotropic experiences and their healing and heuristic potential. Humanistic Psychol 2003;31(2-3):50-85.

[3] Goleman D. Healing emotions: Conversations with the Dalai Lama on the mindfulness, emotions, and health. Boston, MA: Mind Life Inst, 1997.
[4] Kelso JAS. Dynamic patterns: The self-organization of brain and behavior. Cambridge, MA: MIT Press, 1995.
[5] Kelso JAS, Engstrom DA. The complementary nature. Cambridge, MA: MIT Press, 2006.
[6] Wolfram S. A new kind of science. Champaign, IL: Wolfram Media, 2002.
[7] Penrose R. Shadows of the mind. Oxford: Oxford Univ Press, 1996.
[8] Hofstadter DR. I am a strange loop. New York: Basic Books, 2007.
[9] Kandel ER, Schwartz JH. Principles of neural science. Amsterdam: Elsevier, 2000.
[10] Hermansen TD, Ventegodt S, Merrick J. Human development X: Explanation of macroevolution— top-down evolution materializes consciousness. The origin of metamorphosis. ScientificWorldJournal 2006;6:1656-66.

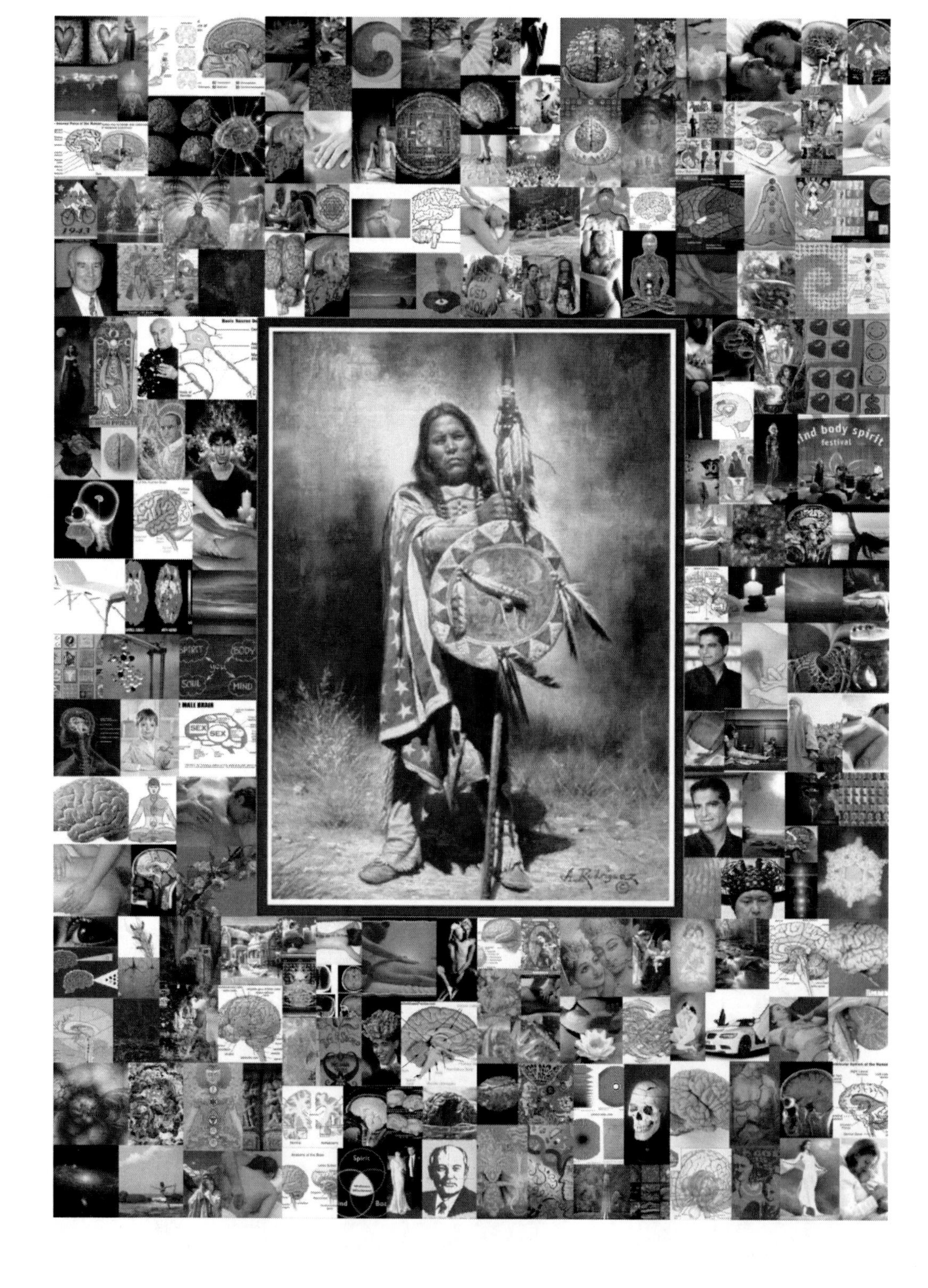

1943
ind body spirit
festival
SPIRIT
BODY
SOUL
MIND
MALE BRAIN
SEX
SEX
Spirit

*Chapter II*

# Human existence

The deeper we look into human existence the less we seem to understand, until the day we realize the nature of our true Self through personal experience. We take a theoretical look into the fundamental dimensions of human existence that were introduced in section three. We shall also look into the healing crisis that almost always is connected with holistic healing – a crisis that often is mistaken for a transient psychosis, or even a mental disorder caused by the therapy.

The strangest concept we shall meet in this section is the concept of human metamorphosis. This is a concept that is as old as holistic medicine itself. The analogy is the metamorphosis of the larvae into the butterfly or the tadpole into the frog. It is a complete and almost immediate reorganization of form, behaviour and basic intent, that most, higher life forms seems able of. Human beings have a series of genes known to be involved in metamorphosis if frogs.

We believe that small children are able to go through a process of metamorphosis where they change, if not their physical appearance, then their energy, character and purpose of life in order to take a form that please their parents more so they are more able to survive even a rough childhood. We believe this, because we often see dramatic processes that look like this process being reversed after so many years with the person finally returning to his or her true self. We have called this dramatic almost instant process of human transformation for “adult human metamorphosis” in spite of the fact that the scientifically correct concept should be “adult human re-metamorphosis”. We simply found the concept complicated enough as it was.

The problem of this section is that some of its theory is not very likely to be true. The theories are too farfetched. On the other hand, we need theories of this level of complexity to fully understand what is going on. Needless to say, we need much more research in this problematic research area of human existence.

If you want to understand our thoughts in it full depth we need to refer you to our series of papers on “human development” (1-10) and to our previous books on holistic medicine (11-14). We hope and pray that the complexity of the concepts that makes the basis of the three chapters we have included in this section will not totally de-motivate our readers.

# References


[1] Hermansen TD, Ventegodt S, Rald E, Clausen B, Nielsen ML, Merrick J. Human development I: twenty fundamental problems of biology, medicine, and neuro-psychology related to biological information. ScientificWorldJournal 2006;6:747-59.

[2] Ventegodt S, Hermansen TD, Nielsen ML, Clausen B, Merrick J. Human development II: we need an integrated theory for matter, life and consciousness to understand life and healing. ScientificWorldJournal 2006;6:760-6.

[3] Ventegodt S, Hermansen TD, Rald E, Flensborg-Madsen T, Nielsen ML, Clausen B, Merrick J. Human development III: bridging brain-mind and body-mind. Introduction to "deep" (fractal, poly-ray) cosmology. ScientificWorldJournal 2006;6:767-76.

[4] Ventegodt S, Hermansen TD, Flensborg-Madsen T, Nielsen ML, Clausen B, Merrick J. Human development IV: the living cell has information-directed self-organisation. ScientificWorldJournal 2006;6:1132-8.

[5] Ventegodt S, Hermansen TD, Flensborg-Madsen T, Nielsen ML, Clausen B, Merrick J. Human development V: biochemistry unable to explain the emergence of biological form (morphogenesis) and therefore a new principle as source of biological information is needed. ScientificWorldJournal 2006;6:1359-67.

[6] Ventegodt S, Hermansen TD, Flensborg-Madsen T, Nielsen M, Merrick J. Human development VI: Supracellular morphogenesis. The origin of biological and cellular order. ScientificWorldJournal 2006;6:1424-33.

[7] Ventegodt S, Hermansen TD, Flensborg-Madsen T, Rald E, Nielsen ML, Merrick J. Human development VII: A spiral fractal model of fine structure of physical energy could explain central aspects of biological information, biological organization and biological creativity. ScientificWorldJournal 2006;6:1434-40.

[8] Ventegodt S, Hermansen TD, Flensborg-Madsen T, Nielsen ML, Merrick J. Human development VIII: A theory of "deep" quantum chemistry and cell consciousness: Quantum chemistry controls genes and biochemistry to give cells and higher organisms consciousness and complex behavior. ScientificWorldJournal 2006;6:1441-53.

[9] Ventegodt S, Hermansen TD, Flensborg-Madsen T, Rald E, Nielsen ML, Merrick J. Human development IX: A model of the wholeness of man, his consciousness and collective consciousness. ScientificWorldJournal 2006;6:1454-9.

[10] Hermansen TD, Ventegodt S, Merrick J. Human development X: Explanation of macroevolution — top-down evolution materializes consciousness. The origin of metamorphosis. ScientificWorldJournal 2006;6:1656-66.

[11] Ventegodt S, Kandel I, Merrick J. Principles of holistic medicine. Philosophy behind quality of life. Victoria, BC: Trafford, 2005.

[12] Ventegodt S, Kandel I, Merrick J. Principles of holistic medicine. Quality of life and health. New York: Hippocrates Sci Publ, 2005.

[13] Ventegodt S, Kandel I, Merrick J. Principles of holistic medicine. Global quality of life.Theory, research and methodology. New York: Hippocrates Sci Publ, 2006.

[14] Ventegodt S, Merrick J. Sexology from a holistic point of view. A textbook of classic and modern sexology. New York: Nova Science, 2010.

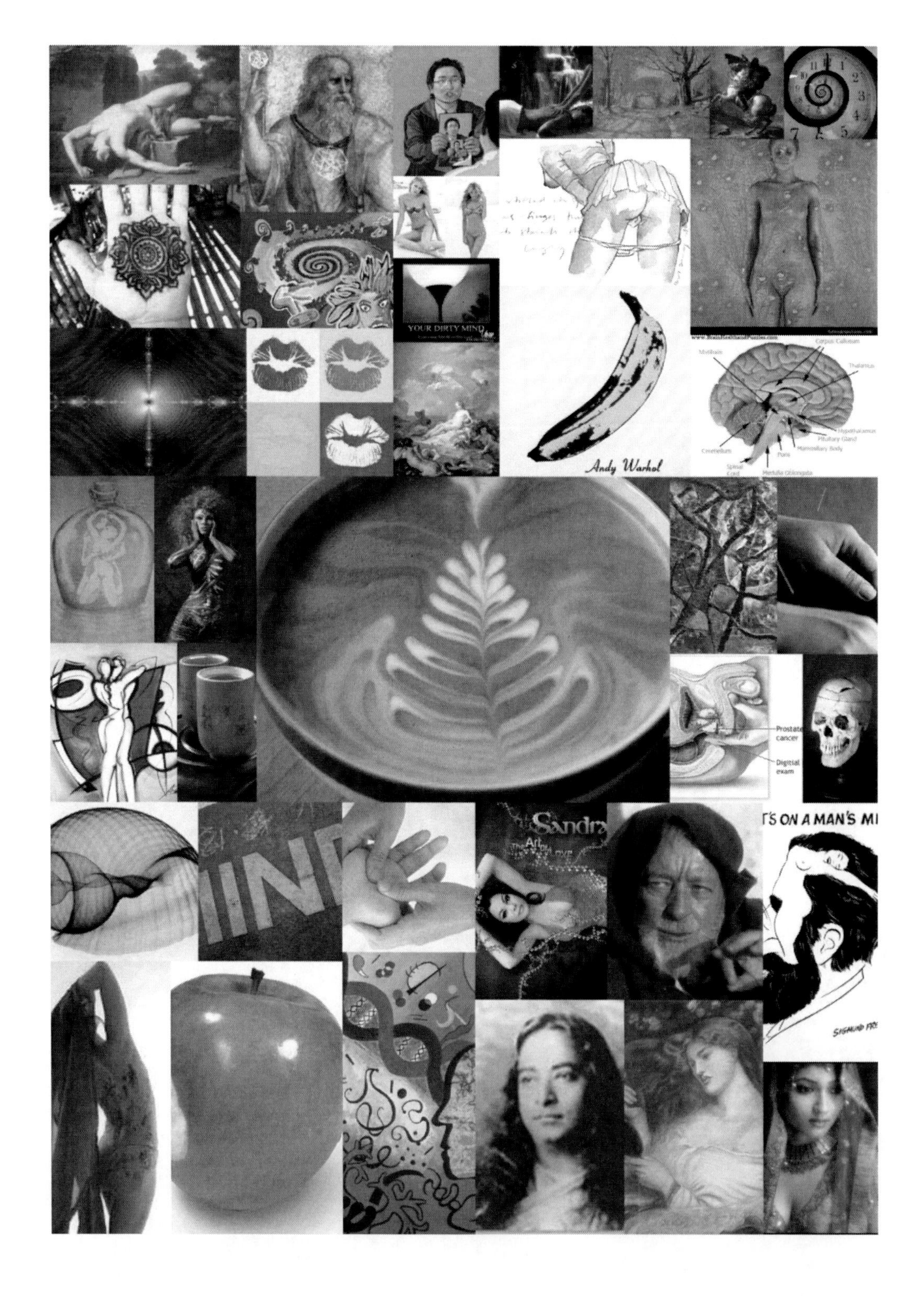

YOUR DIRTY MIND
Andy Warhol
Corpus Callosum
Thalamus
Hypothalamus
Pituitary Gland
Pons
Medulla Oblongata
Prostate cancer
Digital exam
MIND
Sandra
'S ON A MAN'S MI

*Chapter III*

# Concept of self in holistic medicine

René Descartes, Sigmund Freud and Anna Freud have among others developed the concept of self with a focus on ego development and self-interpretation. These concepts have also been used in counselling, where self-consistency has been seen as a primary motivating force in human behaviour and psychotherapy can be seen as basically a process of altering the ways that individuals see themselves.

In holistic medicine it is generally believed that there is an ego connected to the brain-mind and a deeper self, connected to the wholeness of the person (the soul), but we have yet another self connected to the body mind taking care of our sexuality. So this three-some of selves (ego, the body and the soul) must function and this is done best under the leadership of our wholeness, the deep self. This chapter with a few case stories illustrates the holistic medicine mind-set concerned with the concept of self.

## Introduction

Philosophically the self has always been problematic. Millions of Buddhists believe in the concept on "anata" meaning no-self and many more scientist and physicians of today believe that we are only chemical machines making the concept of consciousness and the self a matter of mere self-illusion. In psychoanalysis and related systems we have the ego, the super ego and the id, in most psychology we have a self that is the person's self-reference, his interpretation of own personified existence (1-4).

In holistic medicine we normally have an ego connected to the brain- mind, and a deeper self, connected to the wholeness of the person (often in religion and philosophy called the "soul") (5-19). We have yet another self connected to the body mind taking care of our sexuality (20). So this three-some of selves must function, and this is done best under the leadership of our wholeness, the deep self. To call it deep is really strange, because when you come from this self, you are not really coming from any depth, but only from yourself. The term is appropriate in education as most students are familiar to some extend with their ego, and to some extent with their sexual bodily self, but not with their totality. To discover this vast hall of existence in oneself often gives a feeling of revelation, of realizing that we are divine creates. The soul is close to God in our inner experience, and many religious experiences (21) thus come after discovering this existential layer in one self. What is interesting for medicine is that many people experience a dramatic improvement in their quality of life, general ability and their health when they break through to this dimension of "higher self", as it can be called (5-19). The term "higher" might be justified from the reference to the person's wholeness, higher then signifying "the top of the hierarchy of entities of this person".

## Purpose of life: The essence of self

In the scientific holistic medicine we intent to improve QOL, health and ability, all in one process (22,23). The only way to do this is by re-establishing the patient's existential coherence (19,24,25). This is often done in the holistic clinic by the rehabilitation of the patient in the three dimensions of love, consciousness and sexuality (15). The most important being love. To rehabilitate the patient's ability to love is done by helping the patient to acknowledge his existential depth, that is his wholeness, and what we call "the essence of the soul" or the purpose of life. The purpose of life, or life mission (13) is the primary talent of the person and when this talent is taken into use, the person can contribute in a constructive and valuable way to other people and society. Realizing this value to other people is often making the person very happy, which will facilitate the person to go to the next level of unconditional love. Happiness comes when a person realizes that the meaning of life is to give to other people, from the bottom of his soul, what he himself has been gifted with. This person can now give without wanting or needing anything in return. He has become a source of love, a source of value for his family and environment. Living the purpose of life is an experience as being in the state of existence that we were originally meant to be in. This is realizing our self (27). So love is only realized though the wholeness, the deep self or the soul. When we come from love we give from the core of our soul, and we give from our essence. On doing this, all human talents can be recruited to support this key intension of manifesting love, expressing our purpose of life (14).

Quite surprisingly this means that almost everybody contains huge hidden resources that can be mobilized. The experience of becoming oneself and finding the ability to love seems to be the biggest resource a patient can find. Often this is the initiation of an intense self-healing process (28,29). The background for the life mission theory (13) can be found in table 1.

**Table 1. The life mission theory (13)**

| | |
|---|---|
| The phases listed below chart the life and disease history of an individual (II-VII). At the outset, let us assume that a human being begins his or her existence with a plan or an ambition for a good and healthy life. We may put this assumption of a primordial plan in quite abstract terms (I): | |
| I. | *Life Mission*. Let us assume that at the moment of conception all the joy, energy and wisdom that our lives are capable of supporting are expressed in a "decision" as to the purpose of our lives. This first "decision" is quite abstract and all-encompassing and holds the intentions of the entire life for that individual. It may be called the personal mission or the life mission. |

This mission is the meaning of life for that individual. It is always constructive and sides with life itself.

II. *Life pain.* The greatest and most fundamental pain in our lives derives from the frustrations encountered, when we try to achieve our personal mission, be they frustrated attempts to satisfy basic needs or the failure to obtain desired psychological states.

III. *Denial.* When the pain becomes intolerable we can deny our life mission by making a counter-decision, which is then lodged in the body and the mind, partially or entirely cancelling the life mission.

IV. *Repair.* One or several new life intentions, more specific than the original life mission, may now be chosen relative to what is possible henceforth. They replace the original life mission and enable the person to move forward again. They can, in turn, be modified, when they encounter new pains experienced as unbearable. (Example: Mission #1: "I am good." Denial #1: "I am not good enough." Mission #2: "I will become good," which implies I am not).

V. *Repression and loss of responsibility.* The new life intention, which corresponds to a new perspective on life at a lower level of responsibility, is based on an effective repression of both the old life mission and the counter-decision that antagonizes and denies it. Such a repression causes the person to split in a conscious and one or more unconscious/subconscious parts. The end result is that we deny and repress parts of ourselves. Our new life intention must always be consistent with what is left undenied.

VI. *Loss of physical health.* Human consciousness is coupled to the wholeness of the organism through the information systems that bind all the cells of the body into a unity. Disturbances in consciousness may thus disturb the organism's information systems, resulting in the cells being less perfectly informed as to what they are to do where. Disruptions in the necessary flow of information to the cells of the organism and tissues hamper the ability of the cells to function properly. Loss of cellular functionality may eventually result in disease and suffering.

VII. *Loss of quality of life and mental health.* In psychological and spiritual terms, people who deny their personal mission gradually lose their fundamental sense that life has meaning, direction and coherence. They may find that their joy of life, energy to do important things and intuitive wisdom are slowly petering out. The quality of their lives is diminished and their mental health impaired.

VIII. *Loss of functionality.* When we decide against our life mission we invalidate our very existence. This shows up as reduced self-worth and self-confidence. Thus, the counter-decisions compromise not only our health and quality of life, but also our basic powers to function physically, psychologically, socially, at work, sexually, etc.

## The self and healing

When the patient enters the process of existential healing, we find what is important is the three steps that integrates old traumas and develops a positive philosophy of life: 1) to feel, 2) to understand and 3) to let go of negative beliefs and decisions (which has been formulated in "the holistic process theory of healing") (22). What this process does to a person is a rather peculiar thing: first the negative emotions from old traumas appear in the consciousness; second the repressed and forgotten contexts appear in the mind, where hidden and neurotic patterns are confronted and seen, and finally the many negative beliefs and attitudes collected though live failures are dismissed to reveal a natural and positive philosophy of life. The negative attitudes are really what give the brain-mind ego its lack of transparency. A sound ego is transcendent and allows the deep wishes of the soul (the wholeness) to be manifested in the mind and fulfilled by the person using all of the rich possibilities in this world. In the same way the self of the body-mind will become visible and present when shame, guild and other feelings attended to sexuality and the body are processed and the old traumatic life events integrated in holistic existential therapy (30-32).

So the three selves of a person, the ego, the body and the soul are closely related in the sound person. In the sick person these are often widely apart (33-35). Sexuality is repressed and the body's urges distorted and perverted, the soul and the true direction of the person is left out of the persons reach, and the mind is occupied with sheer survival.

Rehabilitation of existence is really rehabilitation of the soul, mind and body. The mind ego must become transparent (see table 2). The body's self must become free and happy. The soul must come into power to manifest its love and be a coherent part of the universe[36].

**Table 2. The process of healing and the ego (14)**

| The ego is our description of self in the brain-mind. It is important to notice that personal development is a plan not for the elimination of the ego, but for its cultivation. An existentially sound person will always have an operative mental ego, but it is centered on the optimal verbal expression of the life mission. Such an ego is not in conflict with one's true self, but supports the life and wholeness of the person, although in an invisible and seamless way. The more developed the person, the more talents are taken into use. So, although the core of existence remains the same throughout life, the healthy person continues to grow. As the number of talents we can call upon is unlimited, the journey ends only at death. |
|---|

## Case story 1

A female, aged 42 years with tinnitus, migraine, herpes simplex 1 and 2, low back pain, treatment-resistant genital warts, sun allergy and depression. Despite her age, Mia was already in a very poor condition, physically and mentally. But she possessed something special, an alertness and interest in the spiritual world. She wanted to develop as a person and that meant that she was ready to assume responsibility and take the rather bitter, holistic medicine offered her. We met in a good and sincere way. Processing her painful personal history took her directly to her life purpose. Following this acknowledgement her art began to flourish and grow like never before. Suddenly, she could do things that she had not even come close to doing before, and her art expressed her new state of acceptance and understanding of good and evil, beautiful and ugly, muck and mire and sky and light. Having acknowledged her life purpose, Mia largely became able to manage on her own. She could now develop further without our help. My work (SV) of guiding her through the pain that made her ill and blocked her enjoyment of life and self-expression is now finished. Her body and soul have largely healed, her tinnitus is almost gone and most of the time she cannot hear it at all. Obviously, this patient may become physically ill again, but her resistance and inner equilibrium appeared to be much greater than before, so next time she is likely to recover much faster.

This woman seemed to have almost all her diseases caused by inner conflicts between her ego and her true self. When the conflicts were solved in the holistic therapy, the most of her seemingly incurable diseases disappeared at the same time.

## Case story 2

The next case story was written by a Rosen Body Work practitioner at the Quality of Life Research Center. It is instructive as it shows an important aspect of how the conflict of the ego versus the true self is related to the subjective problems of a male with heart problems.

*Male, aged 55 years with the question if he had heart problems.* This patient was a family man and manager of a private firm. He seemed a happy and extrovert man with a good grip on things. However, his body was heavy and his muscles very hard. Shortly before he started at the clinic, he had been in hospital with a blood clot in his heart and was taking medication for hypertension. Most of the times, when he was on the couch, he fell into a deep sleep that was frequently interrupted by some very violent jerks throughout the body. He called these jerks his "electric shocks". Several times during the period when he came to our clinic he was admitted to the hospital with extreme cardiac pain and angina. Eventually he started medication for these symptoms and on the waiting list for bypass surgery. During some of his private sessions he became aware of some of the things that had greatly influenced his life, including an alcoholic father, who had been violent towards his mother. As a very young he received electroconvulsive therapy for severe depression. After he had realized this, the jerks that used to wake up both him and his wife ceased or diminished. It also became apparent that he was taking strong antidepressants and had done so for years. He chooses to reduce dosage so that he was far below the daily dose, and he was doing well without the excessive medication. Throughout the therapy he had some major problems with his staff and he felt they had taken a dislike to him. I (SV) had other clients from that workplace, and it turned out that others shared his belief. The patient mobilized all his strength to give notice and start again from scratch in another firm, where he is working today. At some point he was again admitted to the hospital with extreme pain and angina that was considered to be life threatening, so he was transferred to a cardiology ward for surgery at the earliest opportunity. However, when the cardiologists examined him thoroughly they could not find any disorder or defect in the heart or surrounding blood vessels, so they discharged him again. During the last private session with the patient he was truly happy about life, and full of vigour to devote to his family and friends. His jerks and cardiac problems had vanished completely, and he was enjoying his new job.

What happened here according to the theory of the ego presented in this chapter is, that the man finally let go of his cold and frozen-hearted ego, which was suppressing his feelings and emotions. It was also beneficial for his subjective experience of his heart, his quality of life, working life and ability of functioning in general.

The method of Marion Rosen Body Work (37) and other body therapies that make the patient note the feelings located in the body are effective tools in holistic medicine. Sometimes the patient can verbalize his feelings and let go of the limiting beliefs that keep them bound to the narrow world of the ego. For many middle-aged men, their Achilles heel is allowing themselves to feel. Often, it is extremely unpleasant for a grown-up man in a managerial position to register the old feelings from his childhood of being small, frightened or helpless. It is quite simply an insult to his ego, that he is still harbouring such feelings. To release them seemingly relieved his angina.

## Conclusion

René Descartes (1596-1650) wrote in 1644 the book "Principles of philosophy" (38) perceived as a milestone in reflection on the non-physical inner self. He proposed that doubt was a principal tool of disciplined examination, but he could not doubt that he doubted. He rationalized that if he doubted, he was thinking and therefore must exist and therefore existence depended upon perception. Concept of self was also part of the writings of Sigmund Freud (1856-1939) (1,39), who developed further and new understanding of the importance of internal mental processes. Freud hesitated to make self-concept a primary psychological unit in his theories, but his daughter Anna Freud (1895-1982) (40) focused on ego development and self-interpretation.

In counselling the psychologist Prescott Lecky (1892-1941) created a personality theory, but was never able to collect his writing into a completed form until his former Columbia University students in 1945 published a small posthumous volume (41), where self-consistency was seen as a primary motivating force in human behaviour. Others (42) have used the self-concept in counselling interviews and argued that psychotherapy is basically a process of altering the ways that individuals see themselves.

In holistic medicine we believe that there is an ego connected to the brain-mind and a deeper self, connected to the wholeness of the person (the soul), but we have yet another self connected to the body mind taking care of our sexuality (20). So this three-some of selves (ego, the body and the soul) must function and this is done best under the leadership of our wholeness, the deep self.

This chapter with a few case stories illustrates the holistic medicine mind-set concerned with the concept of self.

## References

[1] Freud S. Mourning and melancholia. London: Penguin, 1984.
[2] Jung CG. Man and his symbols. New York: Anchor Press, 1964.
[3] Sulivan HS. Interpersonal theory and psychotherapy, London: Routledge, 1996.
[4] Horney K. Our inner conflicts: A constructive theory of neurosis. London: WW Norton, 1948.
[5] Ventegodt S, Andersen NJ, Merrick J. Quality of life philosophy: when life sparkles or can we make wisdom a science? ScientificWorldJournal 2003;3:1160-3.
[6] Ventegodt S, Andersen NJ, Merrick J. QOL philosophy I: Quality of life, happiness, and meaning of life. ScientificWorldJournal 2003;3:1164-75.
[7] Ventegodt S, Andersen NJ, Kromann M, Merrick J. QOL philosophy II: What is a human being? ScientificWorldJournal 2003;3:1176-85.
[8] Ventegodt S, Merrick J, Andersen NJ. QOL philosophy III: Towards a new biology. ScientificWorldJournal 2003;3:1186-98.

[9] Ventegodt S, Andersen NJ, Merrick J. QOL philosophy IV: The brain and consciousness. ScientificWorldJournal 2003;3:1199-1209.

[10] Ventegodt S, Andersen NJ, Merrick J. QOL philosophy V: Seizing the meaning of life and getting well again. ScientificWorldJournal 2003;3:1210-29.

[11] Ventegodt S, Andersen NJ, Merrick J. QOL philosophy VI: The concepts. ScientificWorldJournal 2003;3:1230-40.

[12] Ventegodt S, Andersen NJ, Merrick J. Editorial: Five theories of human existence. ScientificWorldJournal 2003;3:1272-76.

[13] Ventegodt S. The life mission theory: A theory for a consciousness-based medicine. Int J Adolesc Med Health 2003;15(1):89-91.

[14] Ventegodt S, Andersen NJ, Merrick J. The life mission theory II: The structure of the life purpose and the ego. ScientificWorldJournal 2003;3:1277-85.

[15] Ventegodt S, Andersen NJ, Merrick J. The life mission theory III: Theory of talent. ScientificWorldJournal 2003;3:1286-93.

[16] Ventegodt S, Merrick J. The life mission theory IV. Theory of child development. ScientificWorldJournal 2003;3:1294-1301.

[17] Ventegodt S, Andersen NJ, Merrick J. The life mission theory V. A theory of the anti-self and explaining the evil side of man. ScientificWorldJournal 2003;3:1302-13.

[18] Ventegodt S, Andersen NJ, Merrick J. The life mission theory VI: A theory for the human character. ScientificWorldJournal 2004;4:859-80.

[19] Ventegodt S, Flensborg-Madsen T, Andersen NJ, Merrick J. Life Mission Theory VII: Theory of existential (Antonovsky) coherence: a theory of quality of life, health and ability for use in holistic medicine. ScientificWorldJournal 2005;5:377-89.

[20] Ventegodt S, Vardi G, Merrick J. Holistic adolescent sexology: How to counsel and treat young people to alleviate and prevent sexual problems. BMJ Rapid Response 2005 Jan 15.

[21] Buber M. I and thou. New York: Charles Scribner, 1970.

[22] Ventegodt S, Andersen NJ, Merrick J. Holistic Medicine III: The holistic process theory of healing. ScientificWorldJournal 2003;3:1138-46.

[23] Ventegodt S, Andersen NJ, Merrick J. Holistic Medicine IV: Principles of existential holistic group therapy and the holistic process of healing in a group setting. ScientificWorldJournal 2003;3:1388-1400.

[24] Antonovsky A. Health, stress and coping. London: Jossey-Bass,1985.

[25] Antonovsky A. Unravelling the mystery of health. How people manage stress and stay well. San Francisco: Jossey-Bass, 1987.

[26] Fromm E. The art of loving. New York: Harper Collins, 2000.

[27] Maslow AH. Toward a psychology of being, New York: Van Nostrand, 1962.

[28] Spiegel D, Bloom JR, Kraemer HC, Gottheil, E. Effect of psychosocial treatment on survival of patients with metastatic breast cancer. Lancet 1989;2(8668), 888-91.

[29] Ventegodt S, Morad M, Merrick J. Clinical holistic medicine: Induction of spontaneous remission of cancer by recovery of the human character and the purpose of life (the life mission). ScientificWorldJournal 2004;4:362-77.

[30] Ventegodt S, Merrick J. Clinical holistic medicine: Applied consciousness-based medicine. ScientificWorldJournal 2004;4:96-9.

[31] Ventegodt S, Morad M, Merrick J. Clinical holistic medicine: Classic art of healing or the therapeutic touch. ScientificWorldJournal 2004;4:134-47.

[32] Ventegodt S, Morad M, Merrick J. Clinical holistic medicine: The "new medicine", the multi-paradigmatic physician and the medical record. ScientificWorldJournal 2004;4:273-85.

[33] Ventegodt S, Merrick J, Andersen NJ. Quality of life theory I. The IQOL theory:An integrative theory of the global quality of life concept. ScientificWorldJournal 2003;3:1030-40.

[34] Ventegodt S, Merrick J, Andersen NJ. Quality of life theory II. Quality of life as the realization of life potential: A biological theory of human being. ScientificWorldJournal 2003;3:1041-9.

[35] Ventegodt S, Merrick J, Andersen NJ. Quality of life theory III. Maslow revisited. ScientificWorldJournal 2003;3:1050-7.

[36] Ventegodt S, Flensborg-Madsen T, Andersen NJ, Nielsen M, Morad M, Merrick J. Global quality of life (QOL), health and ability are primarily determined by our consciousness. Research findings from Denmark 1991-2004. Soc Indicator Res 2005;71:87-122.
[37] Rosen M, Brenner S. Rosen method bodywork. Accesing the unconscious through touch. Berkeley, CA: North Atlantic Books, 2003.
[38] Descartes R. Principles of philosophy. Dordrecht: D Reidel, 1983.
[39] Freud S. The interpretation of dreams. In the complete psychological works of Sigmund Freud. London: Hogarth Press, 1962.
[40] Freud A. The ego and the mechanisms of defense: The writings of Anna Freud. Guilford, CT: Int Univ Press,1967.
[41] Lecky P. Self-consistency: A theory of personality. New York: Island Press, 1945.
[42] Raimy VC. Self-reference in counseling interviews. J Consult Psychol 1948;12:153-63.

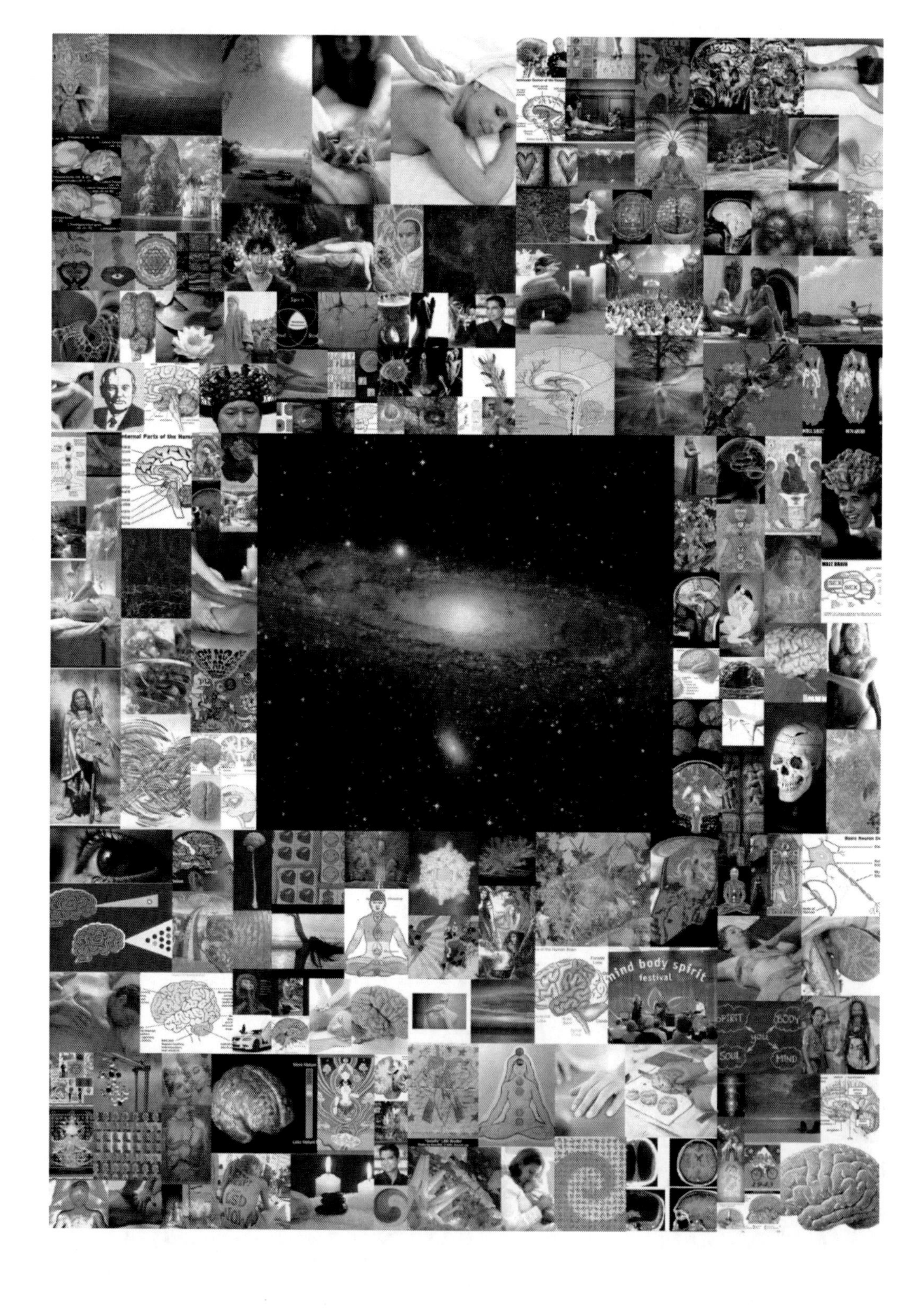

mind body spirit
festival
SPIRIT
BODY
SOUL
MIND

*Chapter IV*

# The therapist as the tool

In the following section we describe the tools of holistic medicine. This is not so simple, for in a way everything can be a tool, and in another way there is only one tool: the physician or holistic therapist him or herself. From an abstract point of view healing comes from love. On a concrete level healing comes from thousand small things that together make a whole; thousand words said, small actions, holding the patients hand when the time is exactly right etc. We have already presented the five principles of holistic healing; they are very important, but we will not repeat them; instead we encourage the reader who forgot them to read the introduction to section one again. We have also mentioned the five derived formal errors of holistic therapy in the same section.

In this section we will look at holistic healing from a more concrete perspective: as something the holistic physician or holistic psychiatrist does. We look at the fundamental job of talking, touching and setting philosophical perspective. This is the well-known job of the practitioner of mind-body medicine. Then we look at the same, but from the angle of "Primum non nocere" – using the tools in a strategic way as to minimize the damage and inconvenience caused by the therapeutic interventions.

In a way this is highly practical, as it always will allow the holistic medical practitioner to pick a tool that is useful and not too big. In spite of the elegance of this approach it is not too helpful. Holistic medicine is not a science; healing and helping is not really a question of methods and skills as we would like it to be. It is really about "crazy wisdom" and without a huge measure of intuition and emotional intelligence the process of holistic healing cannot be done. So beware not to take the methods described in these chapters to literally. If you do you will fail miserably in order to help your patient.

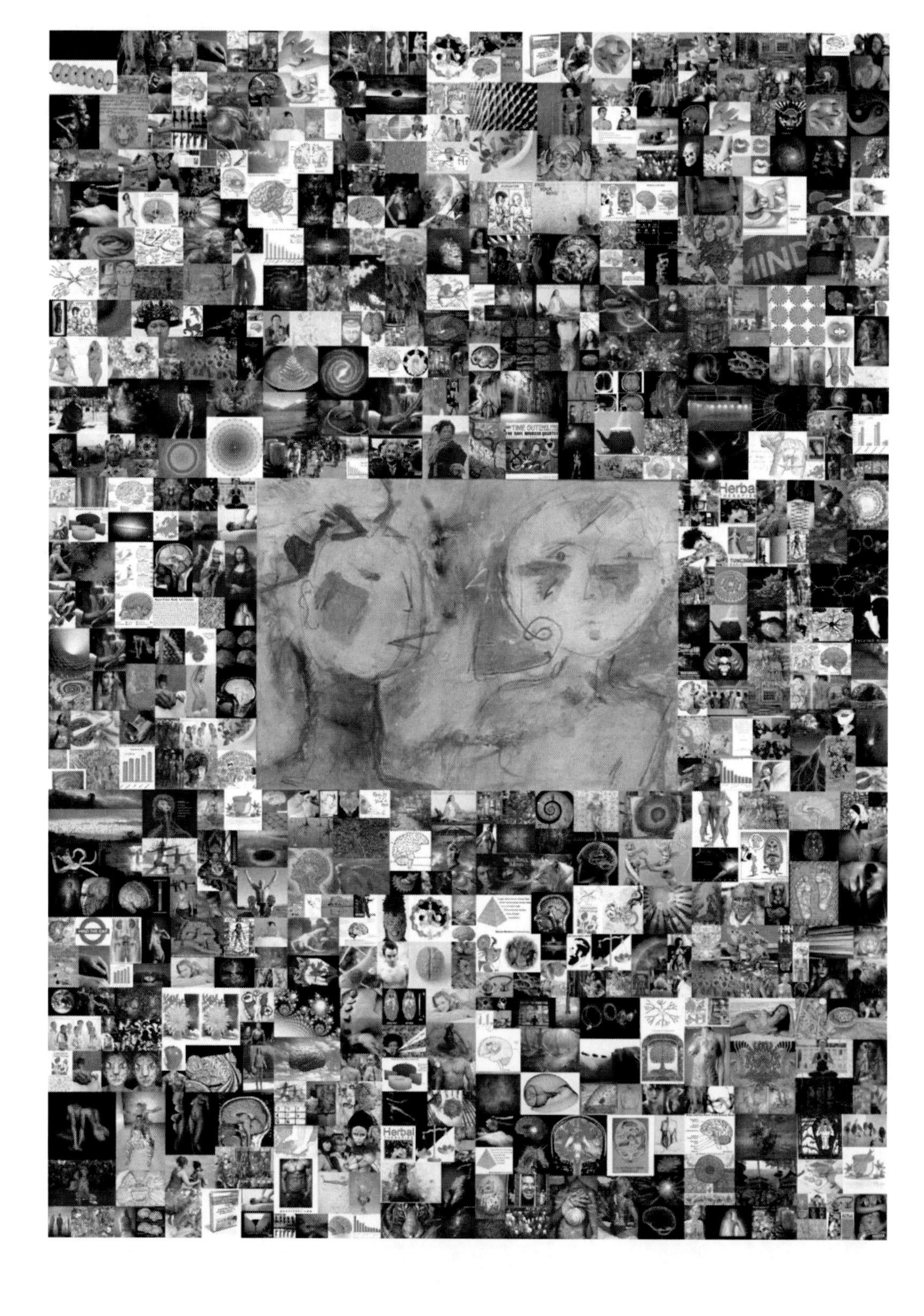

Chapter V

# Quality of life as the realization of life potential

Holistic medicine is also called "quality of life as medicine". The reason for this is simple. When the patients improve their quality of life they also improve their health, both their physical and mental health. So another approach to holistic healing is the improvement of the patient's quality of life in general. To help the patient improve his or her quality of life, it is necessary to know what quality of life is. A help is the quality-of-life theory. The chapters of this section all present some theoretical framework on the improvement of the patient's quality of life.

This chapter presents one of the eight theories of the quality of life (QOL) used for making the SEQOL (self-evaluation of quality of life) questionnaire or *the quality of life as realizing life potential.* This theory is strongly inspired by Maslow and the review furthermore serves as an example on how to fulfil the demand for an overall theory of life (or philosophy of life), which we believe is necessary for holistic medicine as well as for global and generic quality-of-life research.

Whereas traditional medical science has often been inspired by mechanical models in its attempts to understand human beings, this theory takes an explicitly biological starting-point. The purpose is to take a close view of life as a unique entity, which mechanical models are unable to do. This means that things considered to be beyond the individual's purely biological nature, notably the quality of life, meaning in life and aspirations in life, are included under this wider, biological treatise.

Our interpretation of the nature of all living matter is intended as an alternative to medical mechanism, which dates back to the beginning of the twentieth century. New ideas such as the notions of the human being as nestled in an evolutionary and ecological context, the spontaneous tendency of self-organizing systems for realization and concord and the central role of consciousness in interpreting, planning and expressing human reality are unavoidable today in attempts to scientifically understand all living matter, including human life.

## Introduction

This chapter presents one of the eight theories of the quality of life (QOL) used for making the SEQOL (self-evaluation of quality of life) questionnaire or the quality of life as realizing life potential. This theory is strongly inspired by Maslow (1,2) and has been presented in several publications (3,4). The present overview furthermore serves as an example on how to fulfil the demand for an overall theory of life (or philosophy of life), which we believe (5,6) is necessary for global and generic quality-of-life research.

Whereas traditional medical science has often been inspired by mechanical models in its attempts to understand human beings, this theory takes an explicitly biological starting-point. The purpose is to take a close view of life as a unique entity, which mechanical models are unable to do. This means that things considered to be beyond the individual's purely biological nature, notably the quality of life, meaning in life and aspirations in life, are included under this wider, biological treatise.

Trying to include such lofty qualities of life in a biological theory will probably raise the suspicion that these qualities are going to be reduced to something more primitive. We hope that this analysis will make it clear that this is not the case. The purpose is to show a respect for life rather than to reduce it to mere trivial mechanisms.

## The hierarchy of life

What is life from a modern biological viewpoint? If we look at how life is organized, we will immediately have a picture of a pyramid before our eyes: an organization of hierarchies with levels of biological systems nestled in one another, from the tiniest molecule, cell and organism, to ecosystems and the biosphere (3,7).

In recent decades the belief has arisen that the essence of this hierarchy of life is not any material substance but the information that organizes the hierarchy (8). What interest us are the self-reproducing patterns that contain these particles of matter. They are of interest, because they contain what is life in a unique sense and not just the few grams of hydrogen, carbon and other elements found in every living organism.

Recent surveys stress the ability of the physical, chemical and biological world to generate new patterns spontaneously, where hitherto there were none (9,10). This process is known as self-organization, and it has been an on-going process, since the “Big Bang”. This is how the planets and the galaxies came into existence, and life has developed in this manner over 4 billion years. During the evolutionary process, biological systems developed more and more complex hierarchies with organisms and ecosystems forming through mutual interaction with the physical-chemical environment.

Higher-level organisms, such as animals and human beings, are colonies of cells that have united to form ever more complex systems with more and more cells for the past billion years (11). To uphold the unity of the organism, the cells constantly exchange information to achieve maximum adaptation and coordination. This is because the subsystems of the organism have to carry out certain functions: they monitor the development and health of the organism as a whole. This life-maintaining communication between cells is called the biological information system.

The biological information system keeps the organism together and is found in all living beings – one-celled organisms, animals and plants. The system that monitors the regulation and communication, including the hormones, the nervous system and the immune system, is also responsible for the overall creation of form, known as ontogenesis: the creation of each individual, regeneration of damaged tissue, etc.

Through evolution, the biological data system in more complex animals has generated a nervous system that processes the sensory input from the environment, ensuring that the body reacts at maximum potential. An image of the external world is contained at the site where all sensory data is processed. In humans, this forum is the brain. Consciousness can be seen as an emergent quality of the organism. This quality emerges at a sufficiently high degree of complexity in the biological information system.

The human brain contains representations of external reality in the form of abstract maps of reality containing detailed descriptions of the external and internal world and the human self (the ego). Using these maps, we guide ourselves in our inner lives as well as in our external physical and social environment; as a consequence, these maps determine our ability to function in the world. All things being equal, poor maps will create poor lives and good maps good lives. This is because good maps of reality enable us to acknowledge, internally, our potential as well as the rich opportunities of our external lives, to identify these when they arise and to make constructive choices throughout life. The good map becomes the bridge to the world and ensures the optimal balance between the deep dreams and opportunities in life.

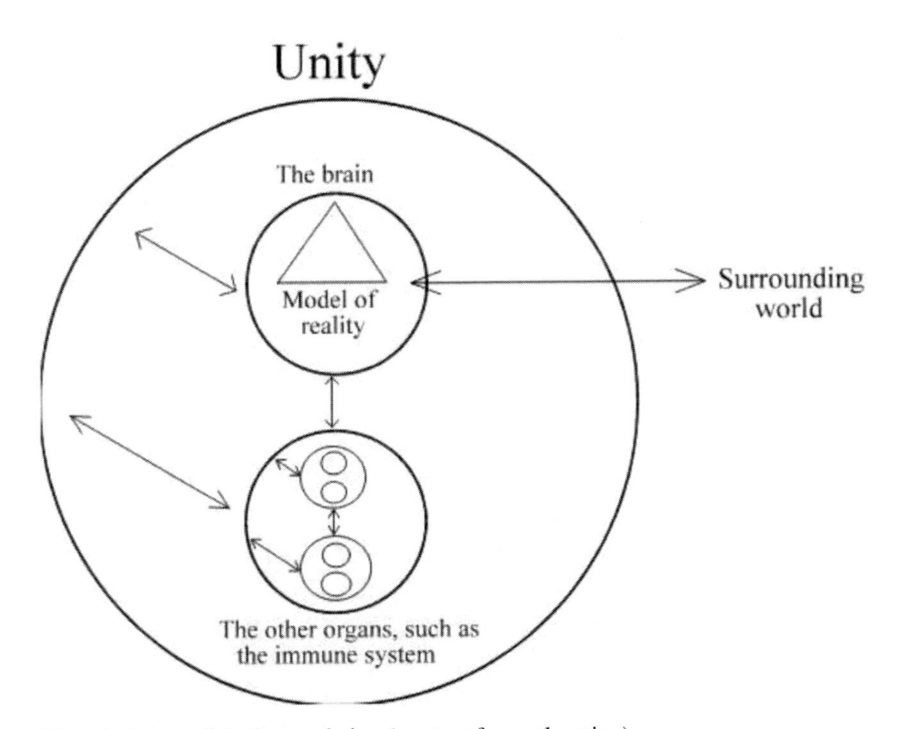


Figure 1. The wholeness of the human being (see text for explanation).

Figure 1 presents a holistic model of the human being. The brain contains the map of reality, which, in the figure, is symbolized by a triangle. The map may be in good or poor shape, reflecting the person's understanding of life, himself and the surrounding world. The brain is located within the unity and serves this unity through an image of the world (the map) by connecting it to the external world. The map stems from personal history and is thus related to reason – everything we have learned about reality. The unity is linked to our actual existence and our deep lives; it contains the history of life as it has developed from the very beginning of life on this planet - a history the human being only has access to intuitively.

The theory of realizing life potential tells us that, by nature, human beings are capable of living: able to love and to connect to the world. The key to the good life is to have activities that allow you to use all your talents and contribute with what is needed in this world. The real problem in life is to weed out the wrong and the outdated ideas such that the map is evolving internally in a proper balance with the inner being as well as the external reality.

The unity of the human being is created through a complex interaction between all parts of the organism, even at the cellular level, symbolized by the smaller levels in the bottom circle of figure 1 and all the arrows. Likewise, the unity of the world is created by integrating all living organisms into the global ecosystem. Thus, understanding ourselves does not entail discovering our own ego, but rather discovering the nature of our relationship to the world.

## The biological potential and life intentions

Each living organism contains a store of information that reflects the evolution of that particular species. In recent decades we have become accustomed to viewing this mass concentration of piled-up information as carried by the genes. However, it is now becoming increasingly clear that both the cell surrounding the DNA strands and the data attached to the organism play a significant role in the formation and further development of biological form.

Let us then move one step further and state that living organisms have biological potential as a result of evolution. If we combine this notion with the universal tendency towards self-organization, we can conclude that biological potential requires the realization of life potential.

This urge of the biological potential to realize itself is termed the will to live. All living organisms, from bacteria to humans, have a will to live: a self-organizing instinct, or urge, that realizes the biological potential. We do not wish to posit a metaphysical or parapsychological, let alone new (or old) life force beyond scientific description. Rather, we wish to give an intuitively plausible name to the tendency towards realization, a tendency that is no more mysterious than that tendency towards self-organization, spontaneous order and evolution that modern physics and biology have identified in numerous systems (12,13). In humans, the will to live is expressed by biological potential: in physical evolution from the fertilized ovum to the mature body as well as in all the psychological and social activities human life requires when lived to the full.

We seldom come across the will to live per se in our everyday lives. Rather we see its actual manifestations in life, which we will call life intentions or life purposes (14). Life intentions are the images of the present and the future that serve to give our lives the course we want them to take: the desire for a meaningful occupation, good social relations, family and children, stability or variety of life. As symbol-carrying images, often unconscious, life intentions form part of the values of life in the model of reality found in the brain. They are a part of our mental maps. As such they can further or inhibit the realization of life potential to varying degrees.

Life intentions are dormant seeds existing as dispositions of biological potential, dispositions that may shape the potential of a life. Nevertheless, our life intentions are really moulded in close encounters with culture, especially our parents or other caregivers.

Our life intentions determine our efforts to develop life in certain directions. They are frustrated when we do not succeed in realizing life in accordance with our intentions. When this happens and we cannot reshape our life intentions, we tend to give them up and adapt the realization of life potential to the reality we find – we dream less ambitious dreams.

We see the will to live, when we meet death. It is a powerful experience, because we are confronted with life, its intentions and the basic urge to live. When we meet death, one of the major crises in life, we have to discover whether we are sufficiently strong to re-evaluate our true intentions and way of life. We may even have to change our attitude to it entirely. This in itself may lead to new growth and a reassessment of our values.

## Ill health and meaning in life

In the search for causes of ill health, medical science tends to examine genetic reasons such as defective molecules that cause malfunction – or external stresses that cause traumas, such as traffic accidents, asbestos or smoking. Only certain disciplines, notably psychosomatic medicine, paediatrics and public health, are to a greater extent concerned with psychosocial factors.

Hence, medical science tends to believe that mechanical faults are the most important factors in the cause of ill health. Nevertheless, in the vast psychosocial field, the factors of the quality of life, may well be significantly more important than genetics and external stress factors. It could well be that the quality of life, and its many dimensions, is the major reason for ill health.

This is difficult to comprehend, because consciousness and our entire worldview contribute to creating the quality of life. Life is far greater and more spacious than our perception of being and reality. As evolution concerns everything, not just you and me, the biological information system is a collective system, which, like the hierarchy of life, encompasses all individuals, including the biosphere. This link with the world plays a major role in the realization of life potential of each organism.

If we view human beings as organisms with biological potential capable of realizing themselves mentally and socially, the purpose of life is the ability to let this potential blossom and develop in an individual and eco-social context. We may take this one step further so that the quality of life, a good life, means the ability to maximize life potential in a social and ecological context.

The acknowledgment of this and the ability to choose a good course in life (constantly adjusting one's life intentions in order to achieve the full realization of life potential) leading to a close connection to reality generate meaning in life. Meaning in life arises, when we experience a fruitful connection between the inner depths of our being and the external world. The given biological potential is then realized and a unified worldview is hereby developed. This unification or connection may be experienced as stages reached in the realization of life (that is, manifest results such as having a partner and children) or it may take shape as a feeling that things are happening, that development is taking place in which the different phases in life are explored and seized gradually.

The experience of meaning in life presupposes a high degree of contact with the depths of our being, the center of our existence, which we here call the biological information system. Meaning in life and hence the quality of life caused by our biological potential is how biology expresses itself subjectively in our lives. An objective expression of biological potential is found in our state of health.

A healthy body is proof that the biological potential is finding a healthy outlet. Likewise, illness means that the biological potential is hampered in realizing itself in a healthy body. The biological information system, which is responsible for the biological potential, is out of balance in the sick body. Hence, communication between the cells, which is crucial for the maintenance of the organism as a whole, is disturbed. A good example of this is cancer. Cancer is usually regarded as an illness in which the ability of the cells to fit into the organizational unity breaks down. This is the inevitable consequence of a breakdown in the mutual communication, regulation and coordination of the cells.

Likewise, many other illnesses can be seen as a communication failure at an elementary, cellular level or as problems in the biological information system. This is further complicated, when the immune system is affected.

Infection, allergy, eczema, insulin-dependent diabetes, arthritis, multiple sclerosis and other ailments can be explained, if we think of these illnesses as a result of malfunctioning of the immune system. This dysregulation is, according to our understanding, linked to disturbances in the global biological information-system of the organism (15,16). Unfortunately this global and integrative biological information system has yet no satisfying scientific description; we believe it to carry our consciousness.

The subjective meaning in life and objective state of health of the individual is then a common basis of the individual's inner being or the existential center. As the quality of life is closely linked with self-realization and the degree of meaning in life attained, the quality of life is closely linked with illness via the state of the biological feedback system. As our quality of life is enhanced or diminished by the way we live and our opportunities to realize our biological potential, changes in lifestyle and the realization of life potential will change the quality of life and state of health.

The relationship between the quality of life and illness is that both originate from the realization of life potential, that is, the ability to live out our life intentions. Figure 2 outlines the roles the quality of life and state of health play in life. Three types are shown:

- A good life with high quality of life and good health where the individual live to the full to the very end.
- An average life, where the life intentions, quality of life and the other subjective factors are neither quite right nor quite hopeless. This generates a poorer state of health and might end with thrombosis or cancer.
- A poor life, where life intentions, quality of life and maps of reality are bleak right from infancy. This leads to a life that is continuously downhill. Abandoning responsibility might lead to mental illness in which the individual no longer wishes to take part in collective reality.

We may choose to work with our fundamental notions of life and reality at any time. We can then adjust our course in life and thus achieve a better life (4,17-19). Usually we need to meet death before we accept that we are no experts in life.

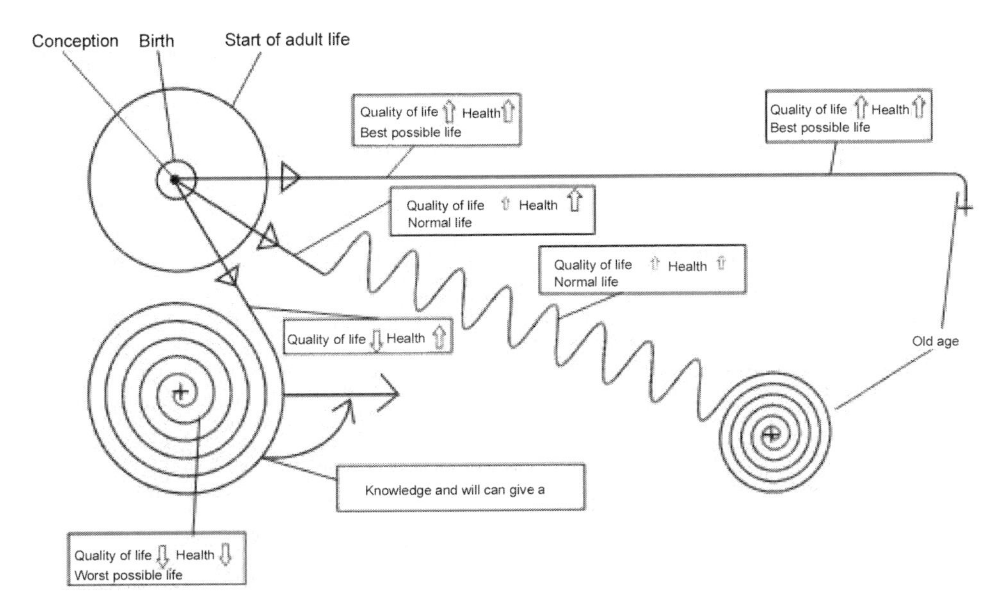


Figure 2. The three paths of life[4]: the good life with optimal QOL, health and ability of functioning, the average, normal, life with sub-optimal QOL, health and ability, and the poor life with low QOL, ill health and bad functioning, lived by a quartile of the Danish population.

**Table 1. The five central principles of healing in non-drug therapy (i.e. clinical medicine, holistic medicine, clinical holistic medicine, and CAM; see the major categories in table 2 from the curriculum of the EU-master in CAM**

1. The principle of salutogenesis: the whole person must be healed (existential healing), not only a part of the person. This is done by recovering the *sense of coherence*, character and purpose of life of the person.
2. The similarity principle: only by reminding the patient (or his body, mind or soul) of what made him ill, can the patient be cured. The reason for this is that the earlier wound/trauma(s) live in the subconscious (or body-mind).
3. The Hering's law of cure (Constantine Hering, 1800-1880): that you will get well in the opposite order of the way you got ill.
4. The principle of resources: only when you are getting the holding/care and support you did not get when you became ill, can you be healed from the old wound.
5. The principle of using as little force as possible (primum non nocere or first do no harm), because since Hippocrates (460-377 BCE) "declare the past, diagnose the present, foretell the future; practice these acts. As to diseases, make a habit of two things - to help, or at least to do no harm" has been paramount not to harm the patient or running a risk with the patient's life or health.

**Table 2. Classification of medicine according to the use of the healing principles of CAM into seven principal classes**

1. Chemical medicine (biomedicine, herbal medicine with bioactive molecules)
2. Body-medicine (massage, reflexology, physical therapy, physiotherapy, spa, sauna etc)
3. Mind-medicine (psychotherapy - psychodynamic, cognitive, gestalt etc.- psychoanalysis, meditation, no-touch sexology, couching, healing music)
4. Spirit-medicine (philosophical interventions, energy medicine, prayers, spiritual healing (i.e. Reichi), shamanism, spiritual CAM (i.e. crystal healing) etc.)
5. Mind-body medicine (acupuncture, acupressure, chiropractics, homeopathy, manual sexology, body-psychotherapy, Reichian bodywork, Rosen therapy, ergo therapy etc.)
6. Holistic (body-mind-spirit/existential) medicine (holistic medicine, clinical medicine, clinical holistic medicine, holistic body-psychotherapy, holistic bodywork, the sexological examination, holistic mind-body medicine, biodynamic bodypsychotherapy, tantric bodywork and massage, holistic sexology, Native American rituals).
7. Chemical-body-mind-spirit medicine (Shamanism with peyote, Ayahuasca, magic mushrooms, Grof's LSD-psychotherapy etc) (44-61)

**Table 3. Side effects/adverse effects caused by psychotherapy, bodywork, and psychotherapy combined with bodywork (80)**

**Psychotherapy**

1. Re-traumatization
2. Brief reactive psychosis
3. Depression (and hypomania)
4. Depersonalization and derealization
5. Implanted memories and implanted philosophy
6. Iatrogenic disturbances
7. Negative effects of hospitalization
8. Studies with no side effects, or side effects less than the side effects of drugs
9. Suicide and suicide attempts
10. Paradoxal findings: Psychotherapy diminished side effects

**Bodywork**

1. Brief reactive psychosis
2. High-energy manipulations of the body in chiropractics can cause damage to the spine of vulnerable patients.
3. Damage to the body if the therapist is unaware of illnesses or for example fractures.
4. Suicide and suicide attempts

**Psychotherapy and bodywork/ holistic medicine** (i.e. manual sexology like the sexological examination, clinical holistic medicine (CHM), and holotropic breath work)

1. Brief reactive psychosis
2. Implanted memories and implanted philosophy
3. (Developmental crises)
4. Suicide and suicide attempts

**Table 4. Side effects/adverse effects caused by Gerda Boyesen's body-psychotherapy on 13.500 patients**

| Side effects | N* | NNH** |
|---|---|---|
| 1. Re-traumatization | 0 | > 13,500 |
| 2. a) Brief reactive psychosis, with no history of previous psychotic, mental illness | 0 | > 13,500 |
| 3. b) Brief reactive psychosis, with a history of previous psychotic, mental illness | 0 | > 13,500 |
| 4. Depression | 0 | > 13,500 |
| 5. Depersonalization and derealization | 0 | > 13,500 |
| 6. Implanted memories and implanted philosophy | 0 | > 13,500 |
| 7. Iatrogenic disturbances | 0 | > 13,500 |
| 8. a) Side effects from manipulations of the body: Insignificant physical problems lasting less than one week (skin-abrasions, blue marks, and tenderness) | 0 | > 13,500 |
| b) Side effects from manipulations of the body: Problems lasting less than three months (fractures etc.) | 0 | > 13,500 |
| c) Side effects from manipulations of the body: Permanent physical problems | 0 | > 13,500 |
| 9. Damage to the body if the therapists are unaware of illnesses, fractures, etc | 0 | > 13,500 |

* Number of patients with side effects; ** number needed to harm

**Table 5. Adverse events during or three month after Gerda Boyesen's intervention with intensive, clinical holistic medicine on 13.500 patients**

| Adverse events | N* | NNH** |
|---|---|---|
| 1. Suicide attempt in relation to treatment on the training site/during treatment | 0 | > 13,500 |
| 2. Suicide attempt in relation to treatment up to 3 months after treatment | 0 | > 13,500 |
| 3. Committed suicide in relation to treatment on the training site/during treatment | 0 | > 13,500 |
| 4. Committed suicide in relation to treatment up to 3 months after treatment | 0 | > 13,500 |
| 5. Hospitalization for physical health problem, during or up to 14 days after treatment | 0 | > 13,500 |
| 6. Hospitalization for mental health problem during or up to 14 days after treatment | 0 | > 13,500 |

*Number of patients with side effects; ** number needed to harm

## Towards a new scientific understanding of humanity

This understanding of the realization of life potential has many traits of a popular understanding of life and may strike us as being self-evident. Unfortunately, this is not the case. Another widely accepted model for the life and health of the human being, the medical science model, states in its biomedical mechanism that the cause of illness is either genes or external trauma: accidents, infections, bacteria and other attacks on the body. The entire psychosocial field, including the mental maps of reality and life intentions, regarded in our model to be factors of affecting the quality of life, is not regarded as particularly meaningful in medical, molecular biology research. In fact, these factors are merely considered to be the background against which the factors causing the illness unfold and they are thus often ignored in scientific discussions of sickness and health.

The most important scientific hypothesis of our quality-of-life project is precisely that the quality of life, in the truest and deepest meaning of the concept, is the real cause of most illnesses, notably cancer, cardiovascular diseases and allergies, and that these illnesses can be prevented by improving the quality of life in time (19). If this hypothesis is confirmed and/or more explicitly formulated, it can lead to a new and far more comprehensive discipline of medicine than the one we know today.

Our interpretation of the nature of all living matter is intended as an alternative to medical mechanism, which dates back to the beginning of the twentieth century. New ideas such as the notions of the human being as nestled in an evolutionary and ecological context, the spontaneous tendency of self-organizing systems for realization and concord and the central role of consciousness in interpreting, planning and expressing human reality are unavoidable today in attempts to scientifically understand all living matter, including human life.

## References

[1] Maslow A. Toward a psychology of being. New York: Van Nostrand, 1962.
[2] Ventegodt S, Merrick J, Andersen NJ. QOL Theory III. Maslow revisited. ScientificWorld Journal 2003;3:1050-7.
[3] Ventegodt S. Review of quality of life with a biological theory on global quality of life. Agrippa 1991;13:58-79. [Danish].
[4] Ventegodt S. Measuring the quality of life. Copenhagen: Forskningscentrets Forlag, 1996. [Danish]
[5] Ventegodt S, Henneberg EW, Merrick J, Lindholt JS. Validation of two global and generic quality of life questionnaires for population screening: SCREENQOL and SEQOL. ScientificWorldJournal 2003;3:412-21.
[6] Ventegodt S, Hilden J, Merrick J. Measurement of quality of life I: A methodological framework. ScientificWorldJournal 2003;3:950-61.
[7] Køppe S. Levels of reality. The new science and its history. Copenhagen: Gyldendal, 1990. [Danish]
[8] Bateson G. Mind and nature: A necessary unity. New York: Ballantine, 1972.
[9] Yates FE, ed. Self-organizing systems (the introduction): the emergence of order. New York: Plenum, 1987.
[10] Davies P. The cosmic blueprint. London: Heineman, 1987.
[11] Margulis L, Sagan D. Microcosmos: Four billion years of evolution. New York: Simon Schuster, 1989.

[12] Yates FE, ed. Self-organizing systems: The emergence of order. New York: Plenum, 1987.
[13] Kaufman S. The origins of order: Self- organization and selection in evolution. Oxford: Oxford Univ Press, 1993.
[14] Ventegodt S. The life mission theory: A theory for a consciousness-based medicine. Int J Adolesc Med Health 2003;15(1):89-91.
[15] Ventegodt S. The connection between quality of life and disease.Stockholm: Federation Soc Insurance Officers, 1994.
[16] Ventegodt S, Ventegodt S. The connection between quality of life and health. Theory and practice. Copenhagen: Acad Appl Philosophy, 1994. [Danish]
[17] Ventegodt S, Poulsen DL. What advice to give on a better quality of life. Meet the person, where he/she is. Farmaci 1992;139-40. [Danish]
[18] Lindholt JS, Ventegodt S, Henneberg EW. Development and validation of QOL5 for clinical databases. A short, global and generic questionnaire based on an integrated theory of the quality of life. Eur J Surg 2002;168:107-13.
[19] Ventegodt S, Merrick J, Andersen NJ. Quality of life as medicine: A pilot study of patients with chronic illness and pain. ScientificWorldJournal 2003;3:520-32.

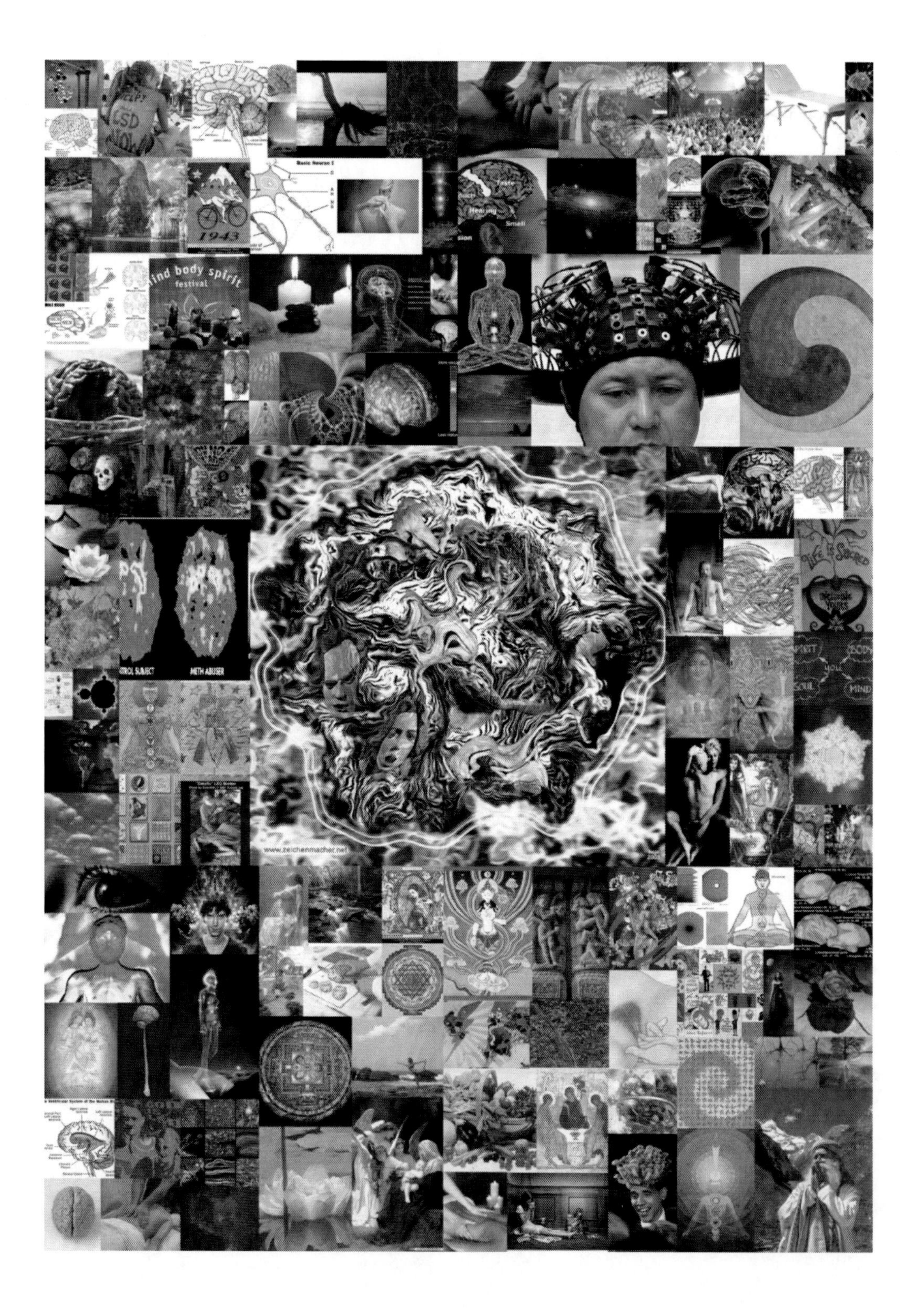
LSD NOW
mind body spirit festival
1943
Basic Neuron
Taste
Hearing
Smell
METH ABUSER
www.zeichenmacher.net
LIFE IS SACRED
SPIRIT
BODY
YOU
SOUL
MIND

*Chapter VI*

# Mental disorders form a holistic perspective

From a holistic perspective psychiatric diseases are caused by the patient's unwillingness to assume responsibility for his life, existence and personal relations. The loss of responsibility arises from the repression of the fundamental existential dimensions of the patients. Repression of love and purpose causes depersonalization (i.e. a lack of responsibility for being yourself and for the contact with others, loss of direction and purpose in life). Repression of strength in mind and emotions give de-realisation – the breakdown of the reality testing, often with mental delusions and hallucinations. The repression of joy and gender give devitalisation – emotional emptiness, loss of joy, personal energy, sexuality, and pleasure in life.

The losses of the existential dimensions are invariably connected to traumas with life-denying decisions. Healing the wounds of the soul by holding and processing will lead to the recovery of the person's character, purpose of life and existential responsibility. It can be very difficult to help a psychotic patient. The physician must first love his patient unconditionally and then fully understand the patient in order to meet and support the patient to initiate the holistic process of healing. It takes motivation and willingness to suffer on behalf of the patients in order to heal, as the existential and emotional pain of the traumas resulting in insanity is often overwhelming. We believe that most psychiatric diseases can be alleviated or cured by the loving and caring physician who masters the holistic toolbox. Further research is needed to document the effect of holistic medicine in psychiatry.

## Introduction

Genuine mental disorders are characterized by the condition medically referred to as "psychosis": a state of severe mental illness making normal function impossible for the patient. Psychosis is a difficult and much debated concept, and over the years various psychiatrists and schools of psychiatry have fought over the definition and delimitation of the term. Indeed, it is difficult to draw a clear line between psychosis and the normal, neurotic and disturbed mental state that characterizes a large fraction of people in the western world.

In for example the Danish society, often said to be one of the richest and most healthy communities in the world, one in every fourth person is severely mis-thriving (1,2). Only every second has close friends with whom they share everything, every second has some kind of sexual problems and only one in three are really satisfied with their job (1,2). From the high numbers of prevalence and incidence presented by the major textbooks (3) about one in five will be treated by a psychiatrist during their lifetime, and presumably many more will experience severe life crisis.

## A general holistic theory of mental illness

The interesting question is whether there is a smooth transition from the normal state of consciousness into what we label as the psychotic state, or whether an actual qualitative shift occurs, when people become mentally ill. Holistic medicine regards most dimensions of the mind as continuous, while conventional psychiatry insists that there is a discrete leap from the normal mental state to the psychotic state. Admittedly, one easily gets the impression that the mentally ill, hallucinatory patient has had a sharp break from reality. We have followed patients closely in and out of psychosis as we have done many times now; we have never observed such leaping in and out of the psychotic state. Instead we find gradual shifts from severe existential pain though degrees of escapes from the overwhelming emotions to sheer denial and total repression of the emotionally painful content and finally into the state of hallucination, as the ultimate escape from unbearable emotional pain. There seems to be a general agreement that psychosis is characterized by a combination of the following:

- De-realization – breakdown of the reality-testing, mental delusions and hallucinations
- Devitalisation – emotional emptiness, loss of joy, personal energy, sexuality and pleasure
- Depersonalization – lack of responsibility for being oneself and for the contact with others, loss of direction and purpose in life

Together the break down in these three vital areas of human existence (corresponding to the fundamental dimensions of existence in the theory of talent) (4) constitute a mental and existential state that prevents the patient from assuming responsibility for his or her own life and for normal functioning, which are the core characteristics of the psychotic state of being.

In our opinion, the most important single dimension of psychosis and "madness" in general is that the person disclaims responsibility for his or her own life. Accordingly, we consider psychosis a defense against the emotional and existential suffering associated with assuming responsibility. It might seem rather surprising that assuming responsibility can cause such emotional problems. In the therapy the extreme and intolerable pain of the psychotic patient reveals itself as raising from being yourself fully as a child (so vulnerable and open as you enter life) and failing completely in giving what you have to offer to the people you trusted fully and loved so unconditionally. As most children do not receive the holding they need (4,5), it is not so surprising that most people carry deep wounds in their soul. These wounds can burst open when life becomes rough. The real mystery is why some people choose to dig into this old, painful material voluntarily seemingly with the intention to integrate what was left of being and thus heal their existence, while other people keep the mind extrovert and the machinery of the facade intact through life, thus avoiding the turmoil connected with confronting the most serious of our human traumas.

As psychosis comes in a gradual spectrum, its most common manifestation is "silent" and indistinguishable to lay people, such as the quiet young girl who confess to her physician that her home has been equipped with surveillance cameras, only she cannot find them. It may also have very dramatic manifestations as when the patient poses a danger to himself and to others, as in classic madness. In this situation a conflict is often building over time and the patient often chooses to be evil in order to avoid emotional pain (6).

When encountering a psychotic patient in the holistic clinic, we have to examine the following conditions to assess the nature and severity of the psychosis. For the patient's own safety, in particular, it is important to assess whether the severity of the psychosis prevents surviving in a normal everyday life. The degree of reduced functioning and the severity of the psychosis call for special precautions:

- Cognitive disturbances – is the patient's perception impaired or distorted, for example by hallucinations?
- Emotional disturbances – is the basic mood lowered as in the case of depression or elevated as in the case of mania? Is the sex life affected?
- Disturbances in meaning, content and direction of life – is the patient realistic in respect to his or her project in life? Is the patient assuming responsibility for own existence and the relations to other? Is the patient consciously choosing to be evil?

Healthy individuals are in control of their fantasy world and do not mix it with the perception of the external world, while psychotic patients tend to hallucinate, create their own perceptions, like an internal picture partially overlapping the perception of the external world. When studied extremely carefully, it can be demonstrated that everybody projects something on other people from their own subconscious mind - like the inner man or woman when fallen in love. Everybody is slightly hallucinatory, what really matters is the degree.

In some psychotic patients the perception of reality includes a few, perceptional elements created unconsciously. The classic example of such acute psychosis is delirium tremens in alcoholics, where spiders and snakes crawl out of the walls. As a medical student, one of the authors (SV) once helped a patient with acute delirium get the spiders out of the window. That really calmed him down, but the nurse reprimanded afterwards for doing this act. The cause of delirium in alcoholics is the brain compensating for the sedative effect of alcohol by increasing activity, including the neurotransmitter system that use a substance called GABA. When the alcoholic suddenly drinks less than usual, brain activity becomes so high and productive that the symbols and images otherwise belonging to the dream world and the subconscious mind cannot be contained within the imagination, but are projected onto the walls and doors of the physical world.

The examination will often reveal that any patient is to some extent living in his or her own world, which is one way of disclaiming responsibility. A total lack of reality testing – where the patient lacks the ability to respond appropriately to the external environment and has withdrawn completely into his or her own reality – is rare. Even in the most hallucinatory state of being, most aspects of reality still are interpreted normally (there might be non-existent spiders in the state of delirium but they still climb the real wall and table).

The spontaneous hallucinations observed in most mentally ill patients are difficult to understand. Urgent matters in the subconscious mind, while at the same time the patient is unwilling to take responsibility for the pain from the traumatic moments in the past, probably cause them.

The problem manifests itself symbolically in the present: old poisonous comments become poisonous gas flowing into the house, old condemnation becomes hazardous irradiation, childhood traumas from excessive control become a sense of camera surveillance at home, the parents' unbearable criticism turns into constantly audible voices.

Another strategy for disclaiming responsibility is to depreciate the existence, value, power and possession of yourself, of life and the world, obviating all requirements for achievement and performance. When the person is so insignificant and has so little value or knowledge and the world is so impossible – the perception observed in many depressive patients – the person no longer has any particular responsibility for his or her life. No one is committed beyond one's power.

Conventional psychiatry distinguishes between two main types of mental illness: schizophreniform disorders, which primarily occur in schizophrenic patients and borderline patients and affective mood disorders, which occur in depressive patients, manic patients and patients with manic-depressive disorders. The former type is generally associated with increased brain activity and can be treated with psychotropic drugs, which reduce the brain activity appropriately. By contrast, a depressive patient's brain activity is too low. This can be treated with drugs that stimulate brain activity. Anxiety is related to specific neurotransmitter systems and can be treated with drugs that suppress the activity of these systems.

Psychotropic drugs have come into wide use in our culture and at least one in five people in Denmark will at some point in life receive such drugs. There is consensus that psychotropic drugs affect the symptoms, but not the actual disorder. To heal the disease the patients must heal his or her existence and human character (7) and in this process recover the clearness of mind, the spaciousness of feelings, the strength of being present in the body, the acceptance of gender and sexuality and the acknowledgment of the essence of his wholeness and being (the soul) and in the core of this: the purpose of life (8).

Before we address the question of how the psychiatric patient can be helped by the holistic physician we take a closer look at the holistic process of healing. It is important to notice that the holistic theory of mental illnesses presented here is derived from a general theory of loss of health, quality of life and ability (4-10). From a holistic perspective psychiatric diseases are caused by the patient's unwillingness to assume responsibility for their own life, existence and personal relations.

This loss of responsibility is caused by the repression of the patient's fundamental existential dimensions, which we normally call love and purpose, strength and power, joy, gender and sexuality (4). Repression of love and purpose gives depersonalization or the lack of responsibility for being oneself and for the contact with others, as well as loss of direction and purpose in life.

Repression of power and strength in mind, feelings and body gives de-realization or the breakdown of the reality testing, often with mental delusions and hallucinations. The repression of joy, gender and sexuality gives devitalisation or emotional emptiness, loss of joy, personal energy, sexuality and ability to feel pleasure and happiness in life. The loss of the physical, mental and spiritual character seems to be the price the patient has to pay for this multidimensional repression of his or her true self.

## Clinical holistic medicine

Please allow us to repeat below what we think is at the core of scientific holistic medicine. The life mission theory (4-10) states that everybody has a purpose of life, or huge talent. Happiness comes from living this purpose and succeeding in expressing the core talent in your life. To do this, it is important to develop as a person into what is known as the natural condition, a condition where the person knows himself and uses all his efforts to achieve what is most important for him. The holistic process theory of healing (11-14) and the related quality of life theories (15-17) state that the return to the natural state of being is possible, whenever the person gets the resources needed for the existential healing. The resources needed are holding in the dimensions: awareness, respect, care, acknowledgment and acceptance with support and processing in the dimensions: feeling, understanding and letting go of negative attitudes and beliefs. The preconditions for the holistic healing to take place are trust and the intention for the healing to take place. Existential healing is not a local healing of any tissue, but a healing of the wholeness of the person, making him much more resourceful, loving and knowledgeable of himself and his own needs and wishes. In letting go of negative attitudes and beliefs the person returns to a more responsible existential position and an improved quality of life. The philosophical change of the person healing is often a change towards preferring difficult problems and challenges, instead of avoiding difficulties in life (18-25). The person who becomes happier and more resourceful is often also becoming more healthy, more talented and able of functioning (26-28).

## Dimensions of the mental disorders

A skilled psychiatrist will immediately "scan" his patient for a dozen or so different symptoms, more or less well defined. Some of them are so well defined that they can be rated on various psychometric scales, which will indicate the severity of the patient's condition: depression, mania, anxiety, psychosis (e.g. hallucinations), neuroticism or introversion. Other dimensions can be sensed, but are difficult to quantify: the degree of delusion, somatisation, grief, hypochondria, arousal level (e.g. panic), liveliness, untruthfulness, hysteria, and quality of attention or alertness.

Based on these observations, the psychiatrist can form an impression on the degree of the patient's suffering, functional capacity, the degree to which the patient assumes responsibility for his or her own life and relations, the patient's level of consciousness, insight and finally the severity of the disorder. The complexity of human consciousness makes it difficult to become a good holistic psychiatrist, because of the numerous paths that one has to know and be able to follow, as the patient enters them.

Conventional psychiatric treatment typically involves psychotropic drugs or electro-convulsive therapy (ECT). In the short run the drugs and ECT are efficient in about half the patients, generally there is insufficient evidence on the long-time effect of the drugs, and little scientific knowledge about any lasting effect of ECT's often serious temporary side effects like discomforts and memory impairment (29). It seems from a search in MedLine (www.pubmed.gov) that the long term side effects has not been well examined but it seems fair to expect from this extremely violent treatment that at least some side effects will last. Conventional psychiatric treatment seeks to alleviate the symptoms that prevent the patient from functioning and coping with life. It is generally agreed that while medication can be effective in many cases, it hardly ever leads to recovery. Many health professionals would therefore prefer a new psychiatric approach that deals more with the causes of the disorders. In order to adopt such an approach we have to understand the causes of psychiatric disorders.

> *Female, aged 27 years, where the psychiatrist only prescribes medication.*
> Patient is dissatisfied because her psychiatrist only prescribes medication. Physiotherapy has had little effect on her headache. Patient has had physiotherapy ten times, and there is no reason to continue. I recommend her to read books about people who have had the same experience and have solved their problems. Perhaps the librarian can help her. She has to be honest with her psychiatrist and verbalize her discontent.

As physicians, we must to be careful not to destroy each other's work. When the psychiatrist has put the patient on medication, in principle, we should not interfere with his field of work, but since she is dissatisfied with the psychiatrist and seeks help from a holistic physician, she obviously feels a need to get help and support to confront the biomedical paradigm (30,31). We believe that reading books is important, as they can provide words with which to think. They will also make it easier for the patient to communicate with the psychiatrist. In this case the helper is therefore the librarian.

## Biomedical versus holistic perspectives of the mental disorders

In a conventional (biomedical) psychiatric perspective, mental disorders are caused by certain disturbances in brain activity, considered to be genetically controlled. Depression and schizophrenia are assumed to be hereditary, although there is insufficient evidence of any genetic causes. Twin studies with identical twins, who grew up away from each other showed that in 25-50% of the twin pairs, both twins were schizophrenic (the concordance) (32-36). This is generally considered to support the hypothesis that schizophrenia has a genetic cause, but in our opinion it confirms the belief that factors other than genetics determine, whether the disorder develops. There are of course some genetically determine vulnerability which might differ from individual to individual, but the genetic patterns has never been identified with any certainty, so this is still speculative. When we take mentally ill or disturbed patients into deep regressive therapy, many patients reveal traumatic episodes going all the way back into the womb. It is very likely that identical twins being genetically identical are in closer mental contact in the womb than non-identical twins, making them to a higher extent share the content of their early consciousness, also the traumatic content. Such considerations seem to favour the hypothesis of early psychosocial factors causing schizophrenia, and weaken the evidence for the genetic hypothesis.

From our holistic perspective, mental disorders are generally not caused by genetics. People may be genetically predisposed, but rather by traumas, emotionally difficult situations often occurring early in the individual's life that lead to negative decisions denying life, self and reality. The decisions lie as deep structures in the conscious and subconscious mind and compromise the patient's relations with himself, his inner life and the outside world. The inner conflicts are manifested as suffering and reduced capacity in relation to mental and social functioning, love, sex or work.

The traumas in the mentally ill patient often involve severe emotional pain, leading to dramatic and destructive statements such as: "I am outside", "Nobody likes me", "I am nothing but trouble", "I am crazy", "I am dead", "You are dead", "It is unreal", "It is not now". Often, these statements include a directly social hereditary element, for instance if the patient's mother has had a mental disorder and experiences with her lead to conclusions such as: "She is mentally ill," and if one attempts to excuse the mother's illness: "I am mentally ill," etc.

## Holistic healing induces recovery of character, purpose and responsibility

Recovery is known to happen in one out of four even in the most severe psychiatric cases. The recovery literature shows several kinds of recovery from schizophrenia (32), the most interesting being full recovery happening in one study in 13,7% of the patients after 5 years (33) and in about 25% of the patients long term (34,35) in the western countries and, quite surprisingly, much more often in the third world (36), Since third world countries are mostly without a developed biomedical psychiatry, this may indicate that many of the therapeutic procedures which seem beneficial in the short run (month) might actually be contra-therapeutic with a perspective of years. It is important to cooperate with this spontaneous recovery process and to enhance it, if and when possible. This is the mission of the holistic approach to the psychiatric illness.

According to the holistic medicine perspective, the major mental disorders are caused by traumas with painful emotional content and life-denying decisions. Therefore, the causal cure consists in helping the patient to heal his or her existence by the integration of the old traumas. The existential healing is induced by applying the obligatory steps of holistic process of healing on the mental diseases (13):

- Make the patients become aware of what lies behind the symptoms they display.
- Let them sink into the feeling until they understand what it is about.
- Help them apply words to the feelings and support them in letting go of all decisions that make themselves or their lives less good and real.

In practice, the process is complicated. The greater the old emotional pain, the stronger the patient's mental defense against entering the old now and more support and holding – attention, respect, care, acceptance and acknowledgment – are required to get the patient through the trauma. In principle, holistic medicine can help any psychiatric patient, who is willing to assume responsibility for his or her own life, provided that there is sufficient support and that the holistic physician fully understands the patient, his/her situation, and his/her state of being. The latter is absolutely crucial. A patient who does not experience being seen and met will not be able to show any trust. Without trust the patient will not allow the physician to give him/her holding and support.

To understand mentally ill people in sufficient depth, the therapist must possess great personal insight and acknowledge the corresponding problems in his own life, naturally on a smaller scale. In our opinion, we are all tarred with the same brush regardless of the nature and severity of the particular human problem. The purpose of conventional, biomedical, psychiatric treatment of psychosis is to make the symptoms of the psychosis disappear, while the purpose of holistic treatment of mental disorders is to eliminate their cause and in that way help the patient return fully to life, health and ability. The essence of holistic treatment of mental disorders is to help the patient recommence and take full responsibility for his or her life. As they disclaimed their responsibility under extreme pressure patients frequently, in order to recover, have to relive difficult events and temporarily experience increased aggravation and suffering during the sessions, in order to recover. This constitutes a distinct difference between biomedical and holistic psychiatry. The former approach does not allow the patient to suffer, because suffering is unnecessary, while the latter approach allows suffering, if it helps the patient to move on. In addition, existential pain is actually an important element of life of which the patient should not be deprived without the most careful of thoughts. In the holistic clinic, it is to some extent rational to apply the conventional (biomedical) psychiatric diagnoses. This allows for consensus among professionals, when cooperating in helping the patient and when doing research. However, the holistic physician has to supplement the traditional diagnosis with a description of the dimensions that are relevant for the holistic therapy. For example: What resources, internal and external, does the patient possess? What is the patient's reality? Is the patient, for example, an institutionalized, experienced user of psychiatry, with little motivation for a major change, or is it a new patient with no experience with the established psychiatric system? Is there an insatiable appetite for learning and a will to recover?

The latter questions are very important, because patients can survive in the psychiatric system with a much lower level of responsibility, than is required to survive in the real world. Patients who have become accustomed to being hospitalized know that it is acceptable for them to disclaim responsibility, unlike patients who lack that experience. In a way, the biomedical, psychiatric system of today inadvertently rewards patients who disclaim responsibility, which is most unfortunate.

In the field of holistic psychiatry the physician's kindness, his human generosity and emotional capacity are the primary tools for helping the patient. The physician's love of his patient is the patient's primary resource and the ethical standard of the holistic physician is also an important prognostic factor. The physician's good intention restores confidence and provides an opening. If a therapist has a patient that he cannot accommodate, it is absolutely essential to say so immediately and refer the patient to someone, who can. Incidentally, kindness is neither sympathy nor empathy, but rather the willingness to give something to the patient without receiving anything in return, a generous quality closely related to the love we share with our relatives.

# Suicidal thoughts

Naturally, suicidal thoughts are a central issue, since a patient with very low self-esteem may have a spontaneous death wish in order not to be in the way or cause trouble for other people. The way we see it, a death wish is actually social. We all, deep down, need to feel useful and if we are not of value to anybody we will not live as a burden.

Specific plans to commit suicide mean that the patient has to be treated in cooperation with an experienced psychiatrist. If the situation is clearly life threatening there is no alternative to admission for treatment, by force if necessary. As force will almost invariably inflict new traumas on the patient and therefore cause a setback in the patient's development, force should only be applied in extreme cases. If the physician succeeds in making the patient let go of the decisions that are the cause of low self-esteem and the death wish, a crisis can sometimes be avoided, but it is important to ensure that the patient's condition subsequently remains stable. With this said, it really is a difficult ethical (and classical philosophical) question. Are we allowed to compromise the patient's autonomy to save his life? What is more important: the life or the survival of the patient? If we have to choose most people will say that surviving with no living is pointless. Of course living is not possible without survival either. With this said, we have found that holistic medicine is known to prevent suicide. A recent review has documented that about hundred patients who had decided to take their own life actually survived by the help and intervention of holistic medicine (37).

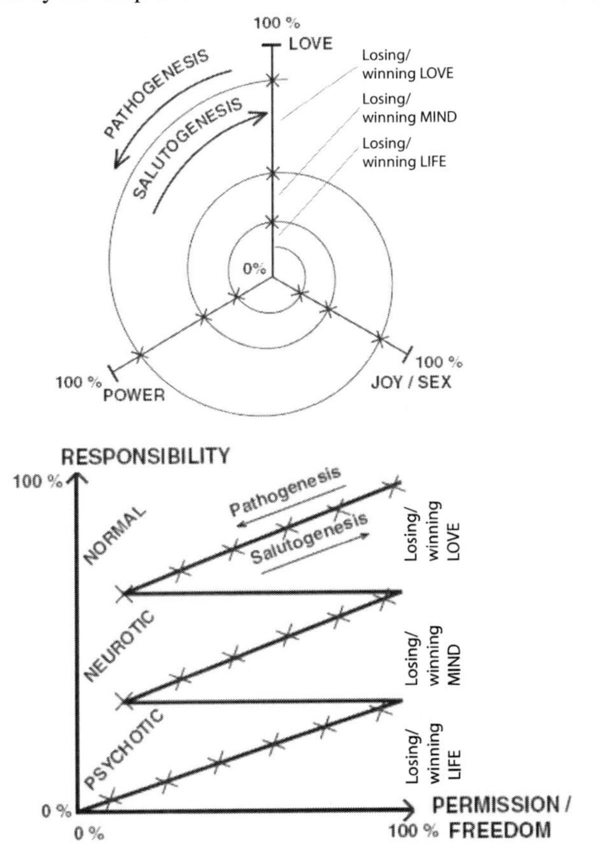


Figure 1.5. (Continued).

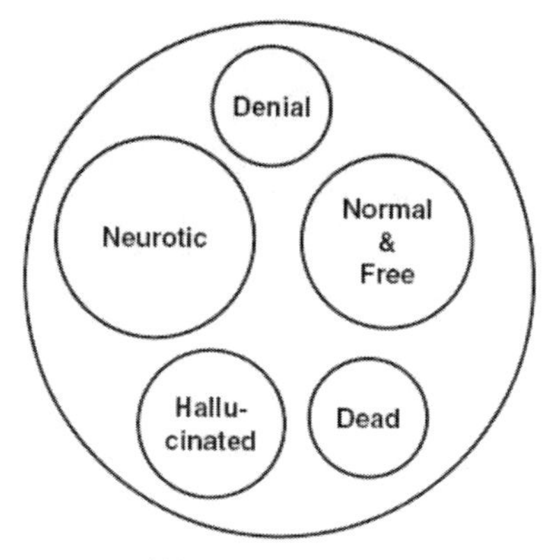


Whole Person

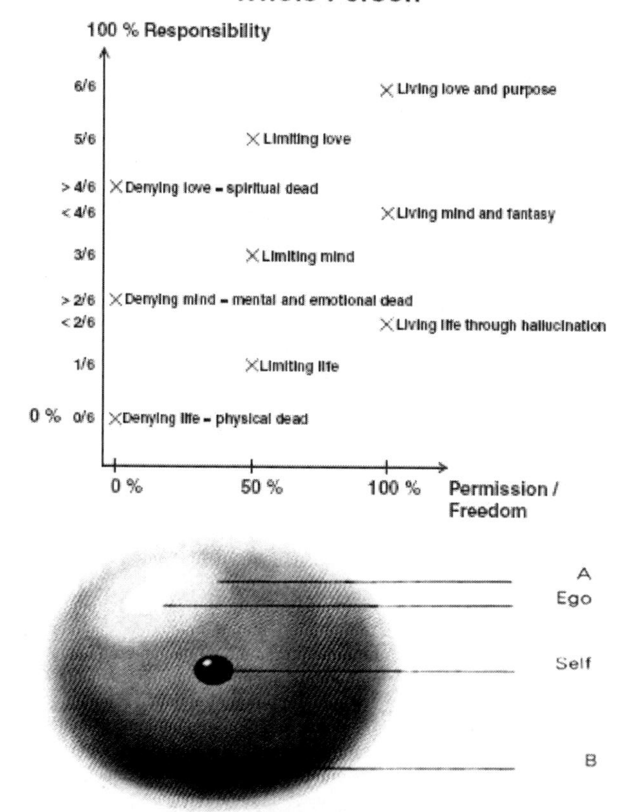


The psyche can be compared to a sphere with a bright field (A) on its surface, representing consciousness. The *ego* is the field's center (only if "I" know a thing is it conscious). The *Self* is at once the nucleus and the whole sphere (B); its internal regulating processes produce dreams.

Figure 1.5. Theories of human existence.

## Discussion

Patients with acute psychosis, who do not pose any danger to themselves or others, are highly susceptible to contact and care founded on profound empathy and endless patience. Acute psychosis is a common condition in connection with severe traumas and may also be provoked by recreational substances, such as LSD, ecstasy or cannabis. Follow-up should include a brief series of conversations. If the patient remains in a psychotic state, a psychiatric specialist can provide help by means of appropriate, small doses of antipsychotic medication.

Unipolar depression, including major depression and minor depression can often be treated with holistic medicine. A therapeutic course lasting six months should be expected in major depression. Antidepressants can often remove the symptoms in a couple of months, but the tendency towards depression will usually persist for the rest of the patient's life. Once the holistic treatment has been completed successfully and the patient has learned from the experience there is justified hope that the depression is gone forever.

In our experience, the bipolar disorder is difficult to treat, because this type of patient tends to shift rapidly from one mental state to the next to avoid contact with the underlying existential pain. In young people who have not been admitted for psychiatric treatment, but have a tendency to become psychotic, holistically oriented conversational therapy appears to be effective in preventing mental illness, but more research is required to confirm this. Schizophreniform psychosis: schizophrenia, borderline psychosis and similar disorders can be treated, if the therapist understands and feels great kindness towards the patient. A long therapeutic course should be anticipated, because psychosis usually reveals a hidden flaw in the patient's character in respect of responsibility.

In elderly psychotic patients or patients with a history of repeated hospitalization in a psychiatric ward, treatment may be extremely difficult and require substantial resources. For example, in the case of the patient's resources – for example because of the patient adapting to a life as mentally ill with all the privileges of not being responsible – and in that case holistic treatment without psychotropic medication is deemed impracticable. A mentally ill patient often undergoes thorough assessment and a detailed treatment and development plan prior to receiving holistic therapy, which is frequently provided in close cooperation with a psycho-dynamically oriented psychiatrist. Now and again, we let the specialist do the initial work with the patient, particularly in patients who require many resources, then we step in as a coach for personal development, when the patient has been stabilized and gained access to his own resources. People with development perspective are generally more susceptible to holistic treatment than people, who are ignorant of the notion of personal development.

From a holistic perspective most psychiatric diseases are caused by the patient's unwillingness to assume responsibility for his life, existence and personal relations. The loss of responsibility arises according to the holistic theory of mental illnesses from the patient's repression of the fundamental existential dimensions (called love, strength and joy in the theory of talent). Repression of love and purpose gives depersonalization – lack of responsibility for being oneself and for the contact with others and loss of direction and purpose in life. Repression of strength in mind and emotions give de-realization – the breakdown of the reality testing, often with mental delusions and hallucinations. The repression of joy and gender give devitalisation – emotional emptiness and loss of joy, personal energy, sexuality, and pleasure in life.

The loss of the existential dimensions is invariably connected to traumas with life-denying decisions. Healing the wounds of the soul by holding and processing in accordance with the holistic process theory of healing will lead to the recovery of the persons character, purpose of life, and existential responsibility. It can be very difficult to help a psychotic patient. The physician must first love his patient unconditionally and then fully understand the patient and his/her state of being. Only then can he meet and support the patient and initiate the holistic process of healing. It takes a lot of motivation and willingness to suffer on behalf of the patient, so that he can heal, as the existential and emotional pain of the traumas giving insanity is often overwhelming. We believe that most psychiatric diseases can be alleviated or cured by the loving and caring physician, who masters the holistic toolbox.

A recent metaanalysis has documented that holistic medicine actually prevented suicide making holistic medicine a treatment also when the patient is suicidal (37). If it is necessary to use force to prevent suicide we recommend this, but we acknowledge that it is a fundamental ethical problem, if suicidal thoughts should make the physician neglect the patient's fundamental human right of autonomy.

# References


[1] Ventegodt S. [Livskvalitet i Danmark.] Quality of life in Denmark. Results from a population survey. Copenhagen: Forskningscentrets Forlag, 1995. [Danish]

[2] Ventegodt S. [Livskvalitet hos 4500 31-33 årige.] The Quality of Life of 4500 31-33 year-olds. Result from a study of the Prospective Pediatric Cohort of persons born at the University Hospital in Copenhagen. Copenhagen: Forskningscentrets Forlag, 1996. [Danish]

[3] Fauci AS, Braunwald E, Isselbacher KJ, Wilson JD, Martin JB, Kasper, DL, et al, eds. Harrison's principles of internal medicine, 14th ed. New York: McGraw-Hill, 1998.

[4] Ventegodt S, Andersen NJ, Merrick J. The life mission theory III: Theory of talent. ScientificWorldJournal 2003;3:1286-93.

[5] Ventegodt S, Merrick J. The life mission theory IV. A theory of child development. ScientificWorldJournal 2003;3:1294-1301.

[6] Ventegodt S, Andersen NJ, Merrick J. The life mission theory V. A theory of the anti-self and explaining the evil side of man. ScientificWorldJournal 2003;3:1302-13.

[7] Ventegodt S, Kromann M, Andersen NJ, Merrick J. The life mission theory VI: A theory for the human character. Healing with holistic medicine through recovery of character and purpose of life. ScientificWorldJournal 2004;4:859-80.

[8] Ventegodt S. The life mission theory: A theory for a consciousness-based medicine. Int J Adolesc Med Health 2003;15(1):89-91.

[9] Ventegodt S, Andersen NJ, Merrick J. Editorial: Five theories of human existence. ScientificWorldJournal 2003;3:1272-6.

[10] Ventegodt S, Andersen NJ, Merrick J. The life mission theory II: The structure of the life purpose and the ego. ScientificWorldJournal 2003;3:1277-85.

[11] Ventegodt S, Andersen NJ, Merrick J. Holistic medicine: Scientific challenges. ScientificWorldJournal 2003;3:1108-16.

[12] Ventegodt S, Andersen NJ, Merrick J. Holistic Medicine II: The square-curve paradigm for research in alternative, complementary and holistic medicine: A cost-effective, easy and scientifically valid design for evidence based medicine. ScientificWorldJournal 2003;3: 1117-27.

[13] Ventegodt S, Andersen NJ, Merrick J. Holistic Medicine III: The holistic process theory of healing. ScientificWorldJournal 2003;3: 1138-46.

[14] Ventegodt S, Andersen NJ, Merrick J. Holistic Medicine IV: The principles of the holistic process of healing in a group setting. ScientificWorldJournal 2003;3:1294-1301.

[15] Ventegodt S, Merrick J, Andersen NJ. Quality of life theory I. The IQOL theory: An integrative theory of the global quality of life concept. ScientificWorldJournal 2003;3:1030-40.
[16] Ventegodt S, Merrick J, Andersen NJ. Quality of life theory II. Quality of life as the realization of life potential: A biological theory of human being. ScientificWorldJournal 2003;3:1041-9.
[17] Ventegodt S, Merrick J, Andersen NJ. Quality of life theory III. Maslow revisited. ScientificWorldJournal 2003;3:1050-7.
[18] Ventegodt S, Andersen NJ, Merrick J. Quality of life philosophy: when life sparkles or can we make wisdom a science? ScientificWorldJournal 2003;3:1160-3.
[19] Ventegodt S, Andersen NJ, Merrick J. QOL philosophy I: Quality of life, happiness, and meaning of life. ScientificWorldJournal 2003;3:1164-75.
[20] Ventegodt S, Andersen NJ, Kromann M, Merrick J. QOL philosophy II: What is a human being? ScientificWorldJournal 2003;3:1176-85.
[21] Ventegodt S, Merrick J, Andersen NJ. QOL philosophy III: Towards a new biology. ScientificWorldJournal 2003;3:1186-98.
[22] Ventegodt S, Andersen NJ, Merrick J. QOL philosophy IV: The brain and consciousness. ScientificWorldJournal 2003;3:1199-1209.
[23] Ventegodt S, Andersen NJ, Merrick J. QOL philosophy V: Seizing the meaning of life and getting well again. ScientificWorldJournal 2003;3:1210-29.
[24] Ventegodt S, Andersen NJ, Merrick J. QOL philosophy VI: The concepts. ScientificWorldJournal 2003;3:1230-40.
[25] Merrick J, Ventegodt S. What is a good death? To use death as a mirror and find the quality in life. BMJ. Rapid Response 2003 Oct 31.
[26] Ventegodt S, Merrick J, Andersen NJ. Quality of life as medicine. A pilot study of patients with chronic illness and pain. ScientificWorld Journal 2003;3:520-32.
[27] Ventegodt S, Merrick J, Andersen NJ. Quality of life as medicine II. A pilot study of a five day "Quality of Life and Health" cure for patients with alcoholism. ScientificWorld Journal 2003;3: 842-52.
[28] Ventegodt S, Clausen B, Langhorn M, Kromann M, Andersen NJ, Merrick J. Quality of Life as Medicine III. A qualitative analysis of the effect of a five days intervention with existential holistic group therapy: a quality of life course as a modern rite of passage. ScientificWorld Journal 2004;4:124-33.
[29] Stromgren LS. Therapeutic results in brief-interval unilateral ECT. Acta Psychiatr Scand 1975;52(4):246-55.
[30] Ventegodt S, Morad M, Merrick J. Clinical holistic medicine: The "new medicine", the multi-paradigmatic physician and the medical record. ScientificWorldJournal 2004;4:273-85.
[31] Ventegodt S, Morad M, Andersen NJ, Merrick J. Clinical holistic medicine Tools for a medical science based on consciousness. ScientificWorldJournal 2004;4:347-61.
[32] Jorgensen P. Recovery and insight in schizophrenia. Acta Psychiatr. Scand 1995;92(6):436-40.
[33] Robinson DG, Woerner MG, McMeniman M, Mendelowitz A, Bilder RM. Symptomatic and functional recovery from a first episode of schizophrenia or schizoaffective disorder. Am J Psychiatry 2004;161(3):473-9.
[34] Torgalsboen AK. Full recovery from schizophrenia: the prognostic role of premorbid adjustment, symptoms at first admission, precipitating events and gender. Psychiatry Res 1999;88(2):143-52.
[35] Torgalsboen AK, Rund BR. "Full recovery" from schizophrenia in the long term: a ten-year follow-up of eight former schizophrenic patients. Psychiatry 1998;61(1):20-34.
[36] Warner R. Recovery from schizophrenia in the Third World. Psychiatry 1983;46(3):197-212.
[37] Ventegodt S, Andersen NJ, Kandel I, Merrick J. Effect, side effects and adverse events of non-pharmaceutical medicine. A review. Int J Disabil Hum Dev 2009;8(3):227-35.

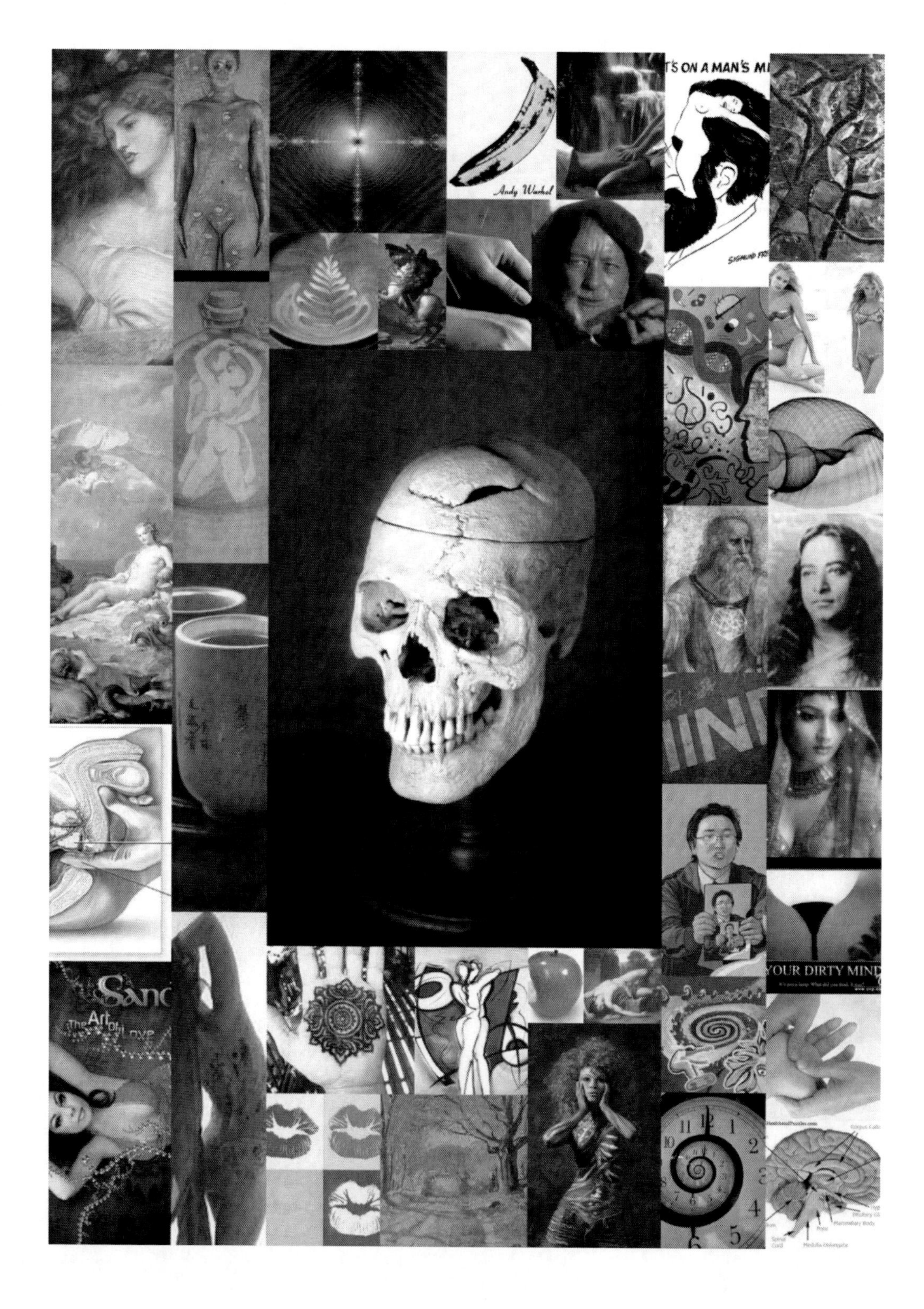
Andy Warhol
YOUR DIRTY MIND

*Chapter VII*

# Consciousness

Consciousness is the source of our being and the way we deal with our own consciousness often become our destiny, also concerned with our physical and mental health. Every physician should be willing to go beyond his/her own limits and to upgrade attitudes and personal belief systems for the sake of his or her patients. This is what creates the real, full and rich life. And this is also what creates health and prevents diseases. How can medical students be taught this? Well, it is not too complicated and in some of our publications we have dealt explicitly with the philosophy of life needed for being able to handle these difficult aspects of medicine. Philosophy can be read and understood, and it can be taught at medical school. Allow us to recommend that all medical students get such training.

## Introduction

You could ask how much our moral values influence clinical decisions (1). Seen from a holistic perspective, the human being is much more than his body. Mind has psychic dimensions difficult to measure and turn into science, especially the soul, the spiritual level of man, that is normally acknowledged to be a wordless domain of our existence. Unfortunately, consciousness is a soul-thing. The place within our self, where we take the final judgment of our life values and major decisions in life, is hidden, unpredictable, and un-material (2).

Consciousness is the source of our being and the way we deal with our own consciousness often become our destiny, also concerned with our physical and mental health. The Danish existential philosopher Søren Kierkegaard (3) recommended to always make the most arduous and difficult choice, when confronted with a choice of something easy or something challenging.

The physician (usually the family physician) will often be the person discussing these life-forming decisions with the patient. Unfortunately, the modern physician is so absorbed in his own profession that it can be very difficult to understand how it is to be a truck driver, a cleaner, or a shopkeeper. Often the physician is not really taking the hardest of alternatives himself in his own personal life.

So the person that the patient is most likely to entrust his or her life to might be the person least able to give the inspiriting advice of seeking the challenge and running the risk.

In life the real emotional risk is too lose yourself. To put you own existence to the test. To go beyond your own limits. To upgrade your attitudes and personal belief system. This is the game of consciousness in which every physician should be involved for the sake of his or her patients. This is what creates the real, full and rich life. And this is also what creates health and prevents diseases according to our research from the Copenhagen Prospective Birth Cohort (4).

How can medical students be taught this? Well, it is not too complicated. In the recently published first and second volumes of our new book series "Principles of Holistic Medicine" (5,6), we have dealt explicitly with the philosophy of life needed for being able to handle these difficult aspects of medicine.

Philosophy can be read and understood, and it can be taught at medical school. Allow us to recommend that all medical students get such training.

# References


[1] Godlee F. Learning for life. BMJ 2006;332:0-f.

[2] Ventegodt S, Flensborg-Madsen T, Andersen NJ, Merrick J. The life mission theory VII. Theory of existential (Antonovsky) coherence: A theory of quality of life, health and ability for use in holistic medicine. ScientificWorldJournal 2005;5:377-89.

[3] Eremita V, ed. Enten-Eller. Et Livs-Fragment [Either-Or: A fragment of life]. Copenhagen: CA Reitzel, 1843. [Danish]

[4] Ventegodt S, Flensborg-Madsen T, Andersen NJ, Nielsen M, Morad M, Merrick J. Global quality of life (QOL), health and ability are primarily determined by our consciousness. Research findings from Denmark 1991-2004. Soc Indicator Res 2005;71:87-122.

[5] Ventegodt S, Kandel I, Merrick J. Principles of holistic medicine. Philosophy behind quality of life. Victoria, BC: Trafford, 2005.

[6] Ventegodt S, Kandel I, Merrick J. Principles of holistic medicine. Quality of life and health. New York: Hippocrates Sci Publ, 2005.

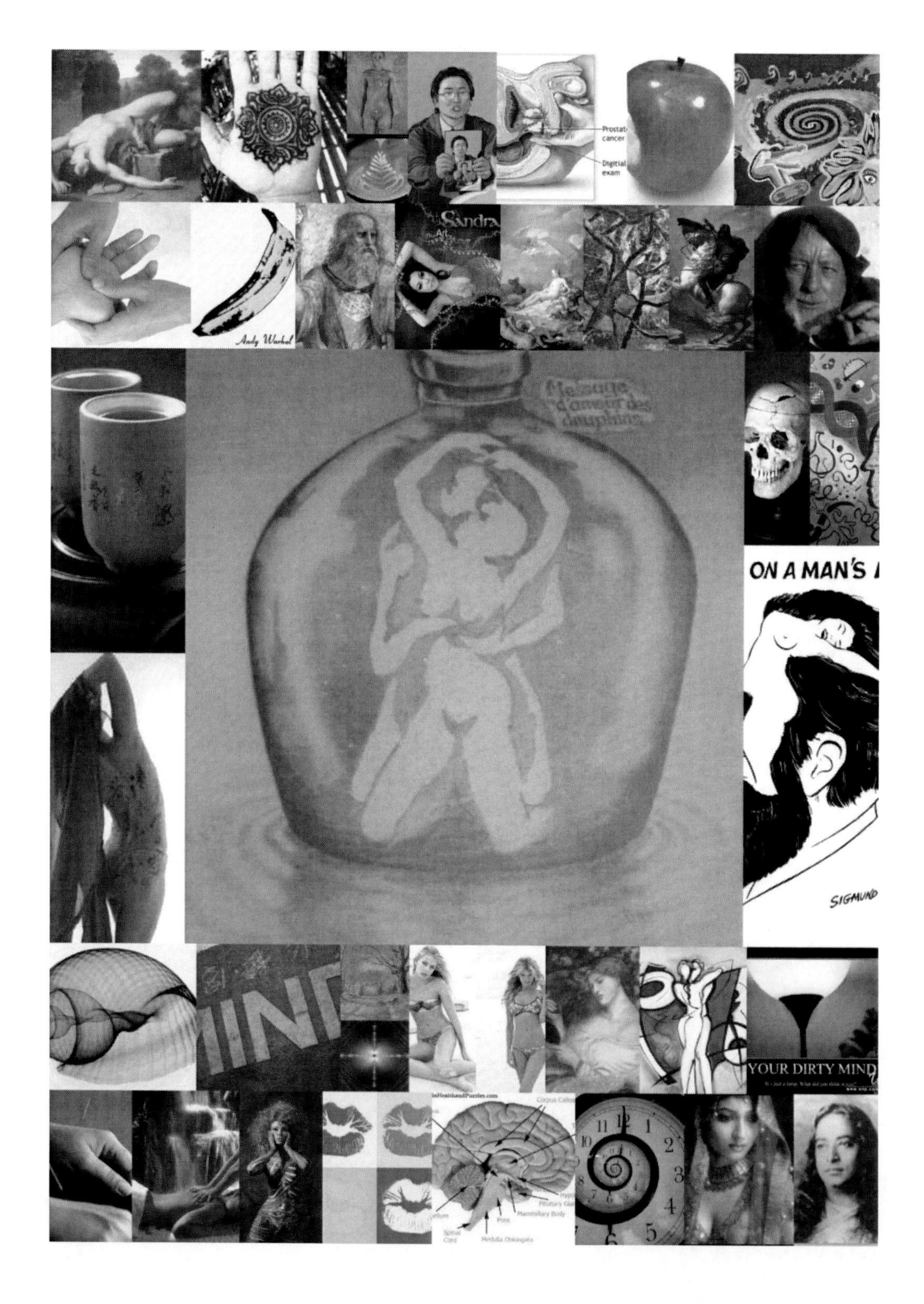
Prostate cancer
Digitial exam
Sandra
Andy Warhol
ON A MAN'S
SIGMUND
YOUR DIRTY MIND
Corpus Callo
Pituitary Gla
Mammillary Body
Pons
Spinal Cord
Medulla Oblongata

*Chapter VIII*

# Holistic treatment of mental disorders

We have analysed how responsibility, perception and behaviour decays in the pathogenesis of mental disease, the hypothesis being that mental illness is primarily caused by low existential responsibility. We have mapped the subsequent loss of responsibility into an eight-step responsibility-for-life scale: 1) Full responsibility and free perception, 2) Overwhelming emotional pain, 3) Denial of life purpose (psychic death/ego death), 4) Escaping into low responsibility perspectives, 5) Denial of reality, 6) Destruction of own perception,7) Freedom of hallucination, 8) Suicide, unconsciousness, coma, and dead. The scale seems to be a valuable tool for understanding both pathogenesis and salutogenesis: the states of consciousness a mentally sick patient must go through to recover.

The scale can help the holistic physician to guide the patient through the process of assuming responsibility and recovering; in the process of salutogenesis the patient enters into an altered state of consciousness, which we call "being in holistic healing". This happens when the patient receives unconditional love - sufficient intense care – by a physician or therapist; being fully at the patient's service the physician wins the trust of the patient and gets allowance to give the sufficient support and holding. In the holistic existential therapy old childhood traumas are re-experienced and integrated. Repressed painful emotions reappear to the surface of the patient's consciousness and a new more constructive understanding of life emerges; in this process the patient gradually lets go of negative beliefs and assumes responsibility for own life.

To recover responsibility for life the patient must rehabilitate the three fundamental dimensions of existence from "theory of talent": 1) love including purpose of life (the life mission), 2) power of mind, feelings and body, and 3) gender including character and sexuality. It seems that even severely mentally ill patients can recover fully if they let go of all the negative attitudes and beliefs rising from the sufferings and causing the disease.

Interestingly, just a few hours of existential holistic therapy where the patient enters the state of holistic healing and confronts the core existential problems seems to be of significant help, especially to the young patient with the emerging disease, who has not yet been given psychotropic drugs or institutionalized. This gives great hope for prevention and early intervention. Many somatically severely ill patients like cancer patients can also benefit from assuming responsibility as most diseases have a psychosomatic element.

## Introduction

In this chapter we will demonstrate how to heal some mental disorders through love, trust, holding and processing (1-9) using the general holistic theory of mental diseases. Many physicians and psychiatrists from the biomedical paradigm seems to believe that mental diseases cannot be healed, but the biomedical approach can alleviate the symptoms and give many patients the possibility to lead a normal or almost normal life. The recovery-literature on the spontaneous healing of mental disease, with the recovery of schizophrenia as the most radical example, shows that about one in four of even the very sick mental patients will eventually be well again without the intervention of a physician.

The recovery literature shows several kinds of recovery from schizophrenia (10), the most interesting being full recovery happening in one study in 13,7% of the patients after five years (11) and in about 25% long term (12,13) in the western countries and quite surprisingly much more in the third world (14). Coming from the holistic paradigm we believe strongly that everybody has huge hidden resources and the organism contains strong self-healing powers, which can be mobilized by the intervention in the holistic medical clinic. Before we give a series of examples of this induction of spontaneous recovery and holistic healing, we would like to introduce the reader to our previous work in this field. The chapter will explain through a number of case stories why holistic healing can work on the patient with mental illness.

## What is insanity?

In our way of looking at holistic medicine we define insanity as the degeneration of our state of consciousness and the subsequent degeneration of our behaviour. From a theoretical perspective it is caused by the repression of our purpose of life (5). Spiritual, mental, physical and sexual character (15) is also repressed, and so are the mental, emotional and physical strength (7) together with gender and sexuality (16).

We aim to integrate all these dimensions in the much simpler perspective that insanity is simply caused by the loss of responsibility for our own existence; recovery from mental illness is therefore a question of re-assuming responsibility for life.

In theory, there are three dimensions of existence to be responsible for: Love, power and joy (7). Love is about purpose of life, or out personal mission. Power is the personal power of mind, feelings and body.

Joy is the dimension of gender, character and sexuality. If the three dimensions collapsed randomly, or if they collapse in parallel, we would pretty much have the pattern of a spiral or whorl, going from full responsibility for the three key areas to zero (see figure 1).

From our clinical findings this is not the pattern we normally observe; it seems that first love is lost, then the feelings and the rational mind, and finally sexuality and life itself. Another interesting finding is that the dimension is normally not lost in one traumatic, but the persons own freedom or permission to use the dimensions are withdrawn before the dimensions are completely lost in a qualitative shift of the patients existence, changing both state of consciousness, perception and behaviour (figure 2). It therefore seems possible to create a one-dimensional scale of existential responsibility (see table 1).

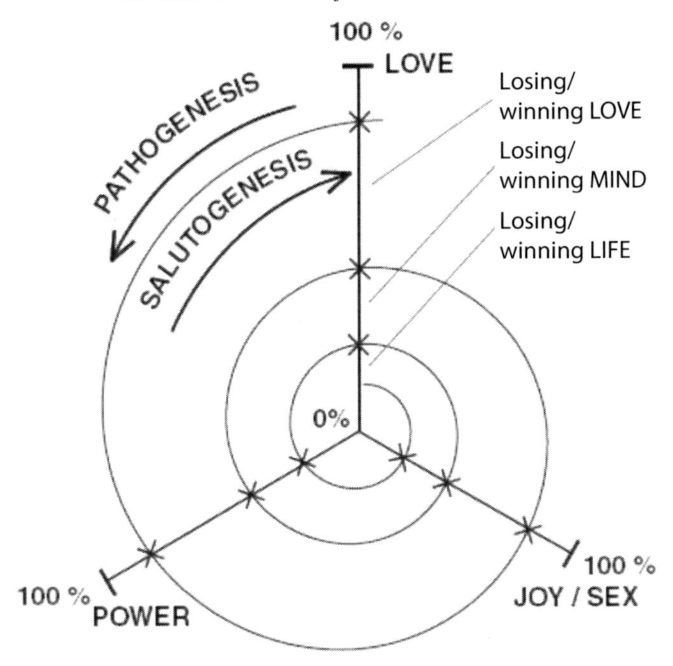


Figure 1. How the loss of existential responsibility causes insanity – theoretical model. If the three dimensions of love, power and joy (from theory of talent[7]) are collapsed randomly, or if they collapse in parallel, we would pretty much have the pattern of a spiral or whorl, going from full responsibility for the three key dimensions down to zero. Responsibility can be defined as responsiveness to all experienced gabs, the gabs being between self and others, in self or in others, or even on the group level (in "the space"). ("X" represents a traumatic life event).

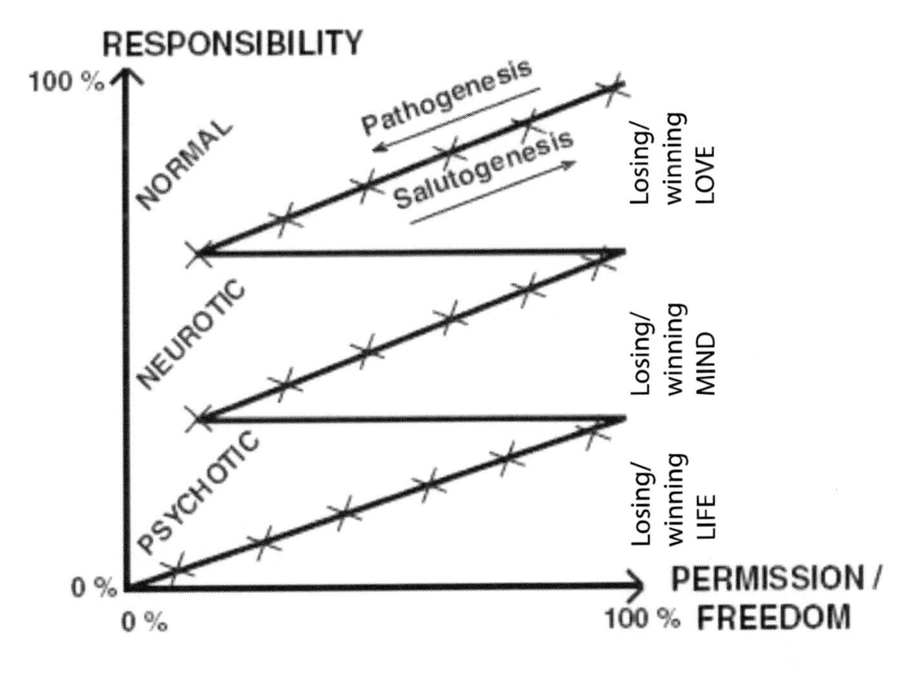


Figure 2. How the loss of existential responsibility causes insanity – clinical findings.

Clinical findings where patients are regressing back to their childhood traumas in holistic existential therapy demonstrate that love is lost first, then power, and finally "sexuality" in its most primitive sense. Every dimension of love, power and joy/sex is lost gradually, until it goes under in a qualitative shift, changing state of consciousness, perception and behaviour at the same time. ("X" represents a traumatic life event).

The different qualities of perceptions related to mental diseases can be understood as the gradual loss or recovery of responsibility and permission, gradually de/reconnecting the patient with reality and urge. As a general rule, first love is lost, then mind and feelings, and at last the fundamental coherence in life itself. Permission can be defined to the level of giving in to the experienced urges (the urge of love, the urge of mind and feelings, the urge of sex and biological life).

**Table 1. Pathogenesis of mental diseases seen as an 8-step responsibility for life scale**

| | |
|---|---|
| 1. | Free perception (fully conscious and happy) |
| 2. | Painful perception (perceiving something unwanted) |
| 3. | Psychic death (overwhelmed by emotional pain) |
| 4. | Escape (changing perspective) |
| 5. | Denial (lying) |
| 6. | Destruction of own perception ("blacking out") |
| 7. | Hallucination (seeing what is wanted instead of reality) |
| 8. | Suicide, unconsciousness, coma, physical death |

When a person meets resistance and bad luck, life turns painful; when it turns to painful, we escape; when we cannot escape, we lie; when we cannot lie, we black out; when we cannot black out because the roof is falling down on our head, we hallucinate; and when this is impossible, we die (i.e., commit suicide). The theory of pathogenesis is also, when read bottom up, the path of salutogenesis and, thus, helpful when we work with low-responsibility patients, which are normally almost impossible to cure and help, i.e., suicidal patients. Some cancer patients and other somatically ill patients who are actually dying seem to be awfully low on this scale too, and might be helped in the same way, as there is a psychosomatic element in most disease.

In table 1 the pathogenesis of mental diseases is seen as an 8-step responsibility for life scale. When a person meet resistance and bad luck, life turns painful; when it turns to painful we escape; when we cannot escape we lie, when we cannot lie we black out; when we cannot black out because the roof is falling down on our head we hallucinate, and when this is impossible we die (i.e. commit suicide). The theory of pathogenesis is also when read bottom up the path of salutogenesis, and thus helpful when we work with low-responsibility patients, which are normally almost impossible to cure and help, i.e. suicidal patients. Some cancer patients and other somatically ill patients who are actually dying seem to be awfully low on this scale too, and might be helped in the same way, as there is a psychosomatic element in most disease.

This scale can be further elaborated into a highly structured and logical scale of responsibility (see table 2) which can be further elaborated into a detailed scale of the parallel decay of existential responsibility, perception, and behaviour (see table 3). This scale has proven clinically useful, when we as holistic physicians want to help patients to assume responsibility; as the scale illustrate the normal pathogenesis of mental diseases, we have tested the hypothesis that we can induce healing – salutogenesis with the famous expression of Aaron Antonovsky – using the scale as a staircase upwards to full health for our patients. The responsibility-scale is thus guiding the holistic physician's induction of the mentally ill patient's recovery (2). As we shall illustrate with clinical examples below, this seems to work surprisingly well, supporting the hypothesis, that the fundamental causal element in mental disease, which of cause co-exist with genetic vulnerability, are the traumatic life events which makes the human escape existential responsibility as it becomes overwhelmed by painful feelings and emotions. The patient then first enters a states of no-love, then it goes to ego-death; it reappears in the head as a reasonable although neurotic being, when overwhelmed again it starts to produce lies, and ends completely blacked out and in reality psychotic, before going further into an blossoming hallucinatory state, and further down to "negative symptoms" – not even hallucinating any more - helplessness, shock, unconsciousness, suicide, coma, and death.

Theoretically the scale is easy to understand, as it is a product of the gradual loss of first love, then mind, and finally life itself. As the patient goes "down under", he or she loses the ability to love, feel, think, be, enjoy, do, and live as a sexual being. At a first glance into the mentally ill patients personality, mind and sub-consciousness, the deterioration of existence including quality of life health, ability, character, gender, meaning, and coherence with the world happens rather chaotically as the negative and self-destructive decisions are taken; interestingly there seems to be yet another pattern, the famous pattern of multiple personalities, a famous pattern obvious in from some types of schizophrenia, and much less obvious in most other patients until looked for. This pattern is illustrated on figure 3. As the different parts are returning to normal during the therapy, they are integrated and merging into the wholeness of the person.

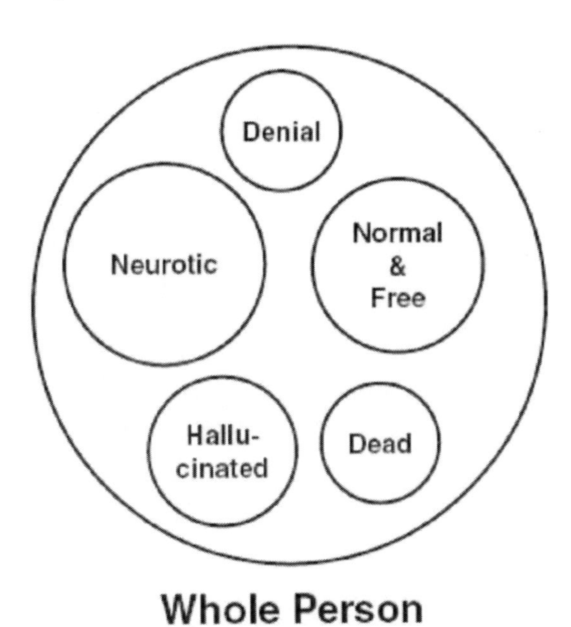


Figure 3. In practice the patient is almost always containing multiple personalities as the wholeness early in life is participated, and the parts are living their own life to a large extend. This means that different parts of the person co-exist on different states. This is the analysis from holistic existential therapy of a 26-year old female breast-cancer patient, made during the session to educate her to confront and assume responsibilities for all her "inner parts". One part of her is romanticizing and not meeting the real world (called hallucinated), another part of her is completely dead, while the largest part of her is neurotic.

The loss of sanity during a traumatizing personal history and the recovery during holistic existential therapy of love, mind and life itself is excellently illustrated with the case of the patient Anna (17), who took literally hundreds of negative life-denying decisions as she was abused during her childhood, and recovered from a borderline state as she confronted her different inner parts and the repressed emotions and decisions connected to them and let go of these decisions. To help the most severely ill patients, the advanced toolbox of holistic medicine must be taking into use (18); be warned that this takes some years of training in clinical holistic medicine to be able to use the most powerful tools. What is important is to take care of the patients safety; as one repressed inner part might with to commit suicide, this part must be confronted with extreme attention; we call this "to push the patient down", and it is a necessary part of deep existential therapy, as the repressed parts cannot be healed into the patient without this confrontation, but the existential crises reappearing to the surface of the patients consciousness must be taken well care of.

The transformations of perception in this scale can be understood if we look at a two-dimensional presentation, with permission and responsibility as the two axes (see figure 1), we see the theoretical background for the Responsibility scale, namely the repression of the three existential dimensions of man (cf. the theory for talent: love, power, and joy (7).

**Responsibility × Permission Diagram**

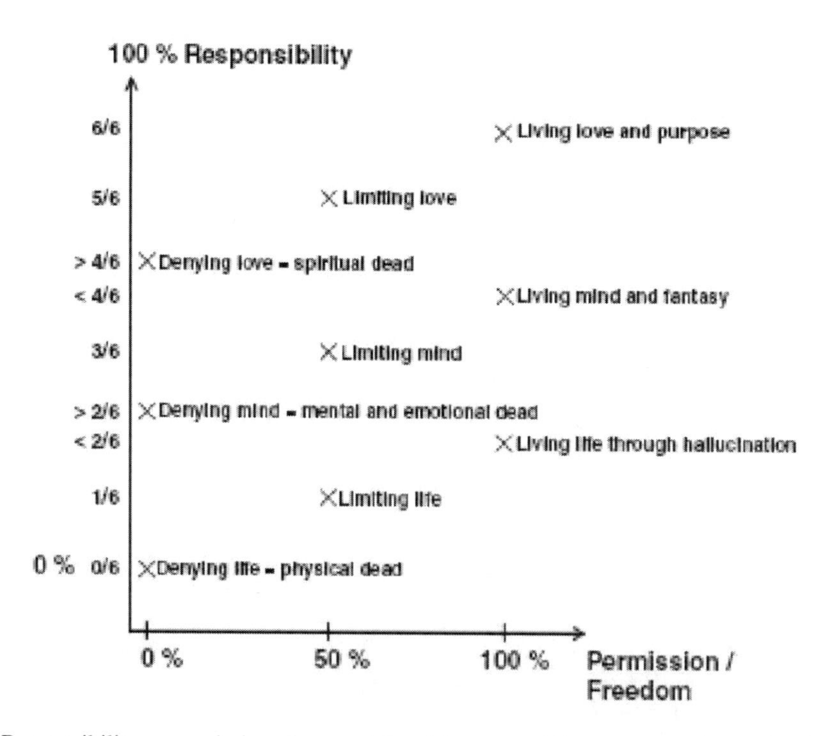


Figure 4. Responsibility x permission diagram. The different qualities of perceptions related to mental diseases can be understood as the gradual loss or recovery of responsibility and permission, gradually de/reconnecting the patient with reality and urge. First love is lost; then mind, and at last the fundamental coherence with life itself.

**Table 2. Responsibility-for-life scale**

**Responsibility-for-Life Scale**

| Degree of Responsibility for Your Own Existence (Estimated Percentage) | State of Consciousness (Many Substates Exist) | Behavior (Other Patterns Might Exist) |
|---|---|---|
| 100% responsibility **Mentally healthy** | Present, fully aware, interpreting the world according to your purpose of life | Succeeding, playing |
| 90–80% | Emotional pain (denying and repressing the feelings) | Fighting, attacking |
| 66% **Neurotic** | Emotionally overwhelmed, psychic death (denying the purpose of life) | Fighting, defending |
| 50% | Escaping from here and now | Flight, running |
| 40% | Cannot escape, denying here and now | Freezing, helplessness |
| 33% **Psychotic** | Destruction of the perception (wiping out, "blackness", "closing eyes", denying the mind) | Shocked, numb, lame |
| 20–10% **Hallucinating** (substituting perception) | Dreaming (perception and behavior not related to the outer world) | Dream state |
| 0% responsibility **Dead** | Unconscious, in coma (denying the body) | Physically dying, suicidal, evil and destructive |

The scale describes how existential responsibility - seen from inside (the state of consciousness) and outside (the behaviour) – is first lost and then found as the patient climb the ladder of hallucination, blacking out, denial, escape, psychic death, unbearable emotional pain, to freedom of perception. To rehabilitate a psychotic patient in a hallucinatory state of consciousness, you need to help him/her confront the chocking trauma that originally motivated the escape into hallucination; in doing this you must carefully avoid to push them deeper down into suicide (see text).

# Healing the mentally ill patient

The general principle in healing the mentally ill patient and inducing recovery is to process the repressed emotional pain and negative decisions (4-44). When this is done, the patients will gradually assume more responsibility for life and existence. To follow the patient step-by-step up the scale demands that the holistic physician masters the compassionate meeting of the patient in a series of specific states of consciousness (see table 1).

It is also important that the physician follows the patients as he or she moves spontaneously along the timeline, and the physicians must also follow the internal shifts from one inner part ("multiple personality") to another; often the mentally ill patient will shift mood, perception and behaviour fast and it takes a great deal of training to process the most ill patients. The more competent assistants the physician has giving holding to the patient in the session, the smoother the therapy will run. Below we present a strategy for meeting the patient on the different levels of existential responsibility.

### Step 8: No responsibility, evil, suicidal

This patient is the most difficult to handle. It can be the anorectic patient starving herself to death, it can be the insane serial killer or simply the patient determined to end life by his own hand. The fundamental problem is to love this person, who has so little love for him/herself or others. Can you love a person who wants to kill you? This is the art of the physician dealing with the evil patient, the patient who has chosen to be evil (9). Can you love a patient who destructs him- or herself?

This is the problem of the many anorectic girls and psychotic incest victims often with borderline diagnosis. Can you love a person who intent to end his own meaningless life? Well, the answer to all the questions: you can if you can see and acknowledge their beautiful souls, their talents and their gifts. So the state of unconditional love is needed to deal with the most difficult patients.

### Step 7: Hallucinating

This patient needs to be met in his or her own world. This takes a lot of training and will to let go of one own ego and preconceptions of the world. But it is not impossible to visit the psychotic patient in his or her own psychotic universe and if you can do that you can take the patients by the hand and "walk him or her out of there". This is all it takes to help an acute psychotic patient out of the psychosis.

On entering into the world of the emotional pain that caused the psychosis it will reappear to be processed. The difficult part is to make an alliance with the patient in the psychotic state that is so strong that he or she will not let go of your hand, while taking him/her through the "terrifying walls of black smoke and burning fire". That is the art of holding, when it becomes most intense.

### Step 6: Blacking out, destroying the perception

Helping the patient to integrate his destruction of perception, which is what makes the blank screen to project hallucinations on; this state if often experienced by the patient as blackness and the processing is often difficult, because of the lack of responsibility for perception in such events.

Making the patient perceive the blackness i.e. as "a strange shadow", and just by talking about this experience of blackness in precise words, the patient will find another perspective and soften up. The holistic medical tools of touch (36,41) are often much more efficient that anything else in this phase. Shame is often an important part of these traumas, making acceptance through touch (16) a useful tool, if the patient can accept this. Basic care is often very helpful. Sometimes advanced tools must be used (18).

### Step 5: Denying

Timeline therapy and even better spontaneous regression is excellent with these patients, who now assume so much responsibility that holding and processing often is quite easy.

### Step 4: Escaping

This patient is almost back into reality. During the therapy it can almost always be understood what the escape was about; most often the reason for the escape is not present anymore. Just by realizing this, much of the emotional pain is integrated.

### Step 3: Overwhelmed

This is the phase of emotional recovery, where the patient returns to normal life and functioning. It is the recovery of character.

### Step 2: Emotional pain

Holistic existential standard therapy runs smoothly. It is the stage of recovery of purpose of life.

### Step 1: Full responsibility

The patient is back; fully alive, aware of his or her purpose of life and able to use all his/her talents. This is the stage of optimal QOL, health and ability. To the frustration of some therapist, the patient will often start a new round presenting another of the inner parts needing the therapist attention, when one part (one of the "multiple personalities") is healed. This seemingly repetitive procedure, which slowly is processing many years of intense childhood suffering, often makes the therapy go on for years. Patience and deep devotion making every moment with the patient joyful and interesting is a must for working with the most traumatized patients. Now, let us see how this fits in with working on the different categories of the mental illnesses.

## Depression and mania – Affective disorders

We become depressive, when we run away from the responsibility for our own lives by describing the world, life and ourselves as impossible. Similarly, we can escape from the world by describing ourselves as unrealistically well (the world as fantastic), which is the manic strategy. The most advanced strategy is to have both descriptions and then alternate between them at your own convenience. This is characteristic of the bipolar disorder.

Systematic and categorical denial of the value of the life inside us and in our external world leads to a life in a bleak, dark and disconsolate world – the depressive universe. In this case, the nature of reality is the problem, including our own unbearable, but unfortunately un-improvable personality. Thus, the problem is not that we, as responsible souls, have made some existential choices with unfortunate consequences, which we now have to learn from and revise. That would be the responsible, existential perspective. Classic depression has a cognitive, an emotional and a physical dimension. The cognitive dimension is the negative description of self, life and reality. The emotional dimension concerns the low emotional basic mood. Depression is also associated with a number of bodily symptoms, such as reduced speed of speech and movement, waking in the early hours of the day, loss of appetite and sexual desire (libido). It is also common for depressive patients to experience chronic pain that is resistant to medication.

The depressive patient needs help to cope with being depressive and control when the depression occurs. Instead of being "full-time depressed", controlled by the dark side, the patient can learn to become "part-time depressed", so that the patient controls when the depression should come and go, and how long it should last. By being willing to enter the depression and feel all aspects of it, and then being willing to leave it again with the knowledge from that experience, the patient can overcome his depression and no longer be enslaved by his pattern of survival. The healing process has commenced and as the patient confronts and deals with the existential pain, he recovers.

Treatment of a depressive and psychotic patient must have due regard for the patient's safety. The therapist should handle both the structure of the patient's defense and the underlying pain. The dark side of a psychotic or depressive patient may appear as a "helping agent", which can be very shrewd and cunning and require great skill on the part of the holistic therapist. Some patients can be very self-destructive and the "agent" inside – the dark side – is virtually authorized to kill the patient, before the existential pain is uncovered completely. This aspect demands the utmost professional expertise, which in our clinic means a referral to a psychiatrist at the slightest suspicion of specific plans for suicide, in order to ensure that the patient survives.

*Female, aged 48 years with bipolar affective disorder and obsessive thoughts.*

Manic-depressive with fixed pattern: Manic for two and a half months, depressive for two and a half months. She has been manic for nearly three months now. She describes her depressive state as follows: "My head is severed," "I only have gloomy thoughts," "I only think about how to get away from here with my daughter". Major problems with ex-husband, who will not talk to her. They have had a dependency relationship, her being his obedient little dog. She still is and she feels that he is "pissing on her and that she still accepts being pissed on by him". The authorities have granted them 12 months to become good parents; otherwise their 10-year-old son will be removed. All in all, the patient is in a miserable state, but not beyond therapeutic reach. EXERCISE 1 – in relation to ex-husband and other people: Say no, do not put up with being messed about, express your anger when you feel it, do not submit. EXERCISE 2 – win the case about your son – take responsibility for his entire parenthood and make sure that he gets what he needs. Or bring him here perhaps, so we can look at the interaction between the two of you. EXERCISE 3 – be depressed for 15 min. a day. Sit on a chair and be depressed. Find statements such as: "Everything is hopeless." "There's nothing good awaiting me," and let go of them. PLAN: Rosen session once a month, with physician (SV) once a month.

This patient is in a miserable state. When you spend half the time wishing to get away from here – and take your child with you – the situation is really serious. Since she has not killed herself and has suffered from her illness for half her life, the risk of suicide is not great. She will not be redeemed, until she confronts the underlying pain, which led to the negative decisions that now control her life.

> *Male, aged 55 years with manic-depressive disorder.*
>
> QOL conversation: The patient has responded to body therapy with mania. Has a history of manic-depressive disorder going back many years. Treated by his own psychiatrist with lithium. Treated by anthroposophical doctor for 13 years with Cikorium [chicory root] and gold D 6 against mania, Terraxikum (dandelion), gold D 30 and other substances. Muscle pain throughout the body, tension headache and fatigue. On examination: Appears somewhat bleary-eyed, all trigger points tender /fibromyalgia/. Instructed to "feel, understand, and let go." PLAN: Wishes to go into psychotherapy and can start here with one of our psychiatric consultants. The topic would be to take responsibility for his own feelings: Six gestalt therapy sessions, then appointment again. Then, he should be encouraged to choose the doctor he wants in future. EXERCISE: Read three good books on personal development – find a new life philosophy, ideally one that concerns responsibility.

Here the patient is merely supported in helping himself by getting a grip on the concept of responsibility in theory and in practice. We guide him, as gently as possible, into acknowledgement. A patient, who has received treatment for 13 years without any progress is likely to begin to wonder whether the treatment is working. Many alternative therapists tell their patients that the beneficial effect sets in slowly and imperceptibly, so they have to be patient. A surprisingly large number of patients undergo all sorts of peculiar courses of treatment, before painfully acknowledging that they are not being helped. We believe that patients should experience being helped from the very first appointment at our clinic, including when we provide holistic treatment. If they do not, they should find another therapist. It is a general rule that if everything is exactly the same as before you had the treatment, you should not expect it to be effective in the long run either. Good therapy is effective and leads to immediate improvement, but naturally it may take long to resolve the problem completely. If we are initially unable to help the patient just a little bit, we doubt that we will be able to help the patient at all. Our advice to a patient asking whether acupuncture, for instance, is effective, is therefore as follows: feel for yourself whether it is effective.

## The class of schizophreniform psychosis

We can also run away from existential pain by escaping from the world in general, prompted by decisions that deny the existence of ourselves, life and/or the world around us. This causes the classic psychosis characterized by depersonalization (I am not real), de-realization (the outside world is not real) and devitalisation (life is not real, but merely something mechanical and inanimate).

The primary characteristic of psychosis is the lack of reality-testing (that is, poor contact with reality) and emotional blunting. Denial goes here all the way through blackness to hallucination. Occasionally, but not always, we see the split personality that led to the disease being named schizophrenia.

The split implies that two different sides cannot be united in the person's character, one side being for instance vibrant and driven by instinct, and the other side being conscious, inhibited and conscientious. According to a holistic interpretation, the split personality stems from the negative decisions.

> *Female, aged 29 years with acute psychosis.*
> The patient has spontaneously entered something old and very painful. She is contactable, not in the present. She becomes agitated and tries to hit me (the physician) with the furniture. She then smashes up the furniture systematically in a classic catharsis /acute psychosis/. Guarded so that she does not hurt herself and kept under observation to determine appropriate treatment.

In rare cases we come across the classic picture of "madness" where the patient is furious, evil, and very destructive. Psychosis is often a quite subtle diagnosis and fairly inconspicuous to lay people. This particularly applies to patients with borderline personality, where we sense that the patient "has a screw loose".

> *Male, aged 29 years with borderline condition?*
> QOL conversation: Very pensive as a child. Assaulted by bikers at the age of 18 years, anxiety since then. Has seen a psychologist. Degree in engineering. At the age of 20 years he was furiously angry with the system, smoked a lot of cannabis. Smashed up his room, had a psychotic episode with 5 days in closed psychiatric unit. Admitted to closed psychiatric unit again with cannabis psychosis for three weeks at the age of 21. The patient is writing his autobiography. The patient believes that he is harbouring so much pain that he is at risk of dying from it. According to his records he has suffered from depression and paranoid psychosis with delusions. He has therefore received: Zoloft [sertraline] and Zyprexa [olanzapine] for the past couple of years. Prescribe Zoloft 50 mg bid /suspected borderline/. Analysis: The patient is a truth-seeking person, who early in his life encountered the injustices of the world and raged about them. Anger and aggression are major problems here, because in my opinion the patient harbours a great deal of suppressed anger. PLAN: This patient has to restore his balance without taking a wrong turn. The patient's intelligence must be mobilized. He must stop being a destructive and maladapted element. Does a lot of reading already, but should pick relevant books that can help the patient. Perhaps books about philosophy. EXERCISE: Write down the facts of the events: what happened, how did you feel. Come back in two weeks with your autobiography, then we shall look at the way you work, so that you can obtain maximum benefit from it.

Like any other patient, the psychotic patient has certain defense against facing and integrating the problematic gestalts. The holistic therapist has to "meet and understand" the patient and handle the patient's defense in an intelligent manner. Basically, they are defense against feeling the pain, but a psychiatric patient often finds it particularly difficult to begin to work with himself, since recognition of the disorder is particularly difficult together with the stigmatization of mental illness in modern society. If modern society adopted a more relaxed attitude towards mental illness and possessed greater faith in the patients' ability to solve their problems through personal development, it would become much easier to be mentally ill and the illness would probably last much shorter than the case today, when mental illness is often for life.

The fear of mental illness is understandable as we experience that schizophrenics, for example, are a great burden on themselves and the people near them throughout their lives. Some experience has shown, that 20 to 30 per cent of schizophrenic persons recover spontaneously. In our view, they attain recovery, when they succeed in finding a genuine and intimate relationship that provides them with sufficient support to spontaneously heal the old wounds to their soul. Treatment of depressive or psychotic patients can be difficult and protracted, but may also be simple, fast and surprisingly painless, if the patient manages to obtain a clear and precise understanding of his situation. When the patient realizes the real nature of his "opponent", he will often experience fast, effective and lasting recovery. Complete recovery often requires years of treatment.

## Delusions

According to the "feel, acknowledge, let go" hypothesis, it is possible to help patients who can confront the pain behind their illness. Making an exact diagnosis is therefore not important. The important thing is to obtain an accurate understanding of the patient's existential dilemmas. The next patient is suffering from delusions. If the physician understands the problem, it is often possible to make the patient understand it as well in a short time. The patient is often hallucinated in a smart and well-hidden way.

> *Male, aged 49 years with obsessive thoughts.*
>
> Obsessive thoughts about having to take off his shoes, before stepping on to the carpet, about killing – children and adults, etc. Wants to die. His family physician has put him on antidepressive medication, apparently with no effect. A few years ago, he ran into a 45-year-old man with his car and killed him, has felt very bad since then. We talk about the death of his father, when the patient was 12 years old, which made him think that everybody around him would die and that he, too, would soon die. Cries. EXERCISE: Write your autobiography and come to terms with your difficult relationship with death, one hour a day. Can return in a month.

The feeling of guilt is hard, difficult and we tend to repress it. If such a feeling is repressed early in life, an event occurring later in life can create an opening that will make all the old skeletons jump out of the cupboard. The patient killed a man by accident and he already has the death of his father on his conscience (children assume responsibility for everything the adults do not). So now he is falling apart, and he needs to sort things out. If the patient succeeds in discovering the key problem he will soon make progress and recover. The next patient suffers from paranoia, a very unpleasant condition with basic distrust of everything and everybody.

> *Female, aged 64 years with paranoia.*
>
> QOL conversation: Appears somewhat paranoid, her neighbours steal her mail and do other wicked things. I think that if the patient focuses on what she is good at and the useful things she can do, then the problem with her neighbours will diminish. The patient would like to change her personality, to become more extrovert and social. We talk about

the patient being able to improve. EXERCISE 1: Call more on your friends and acquaintances – the patient's own suggestion. EXERCISE 2: Ignore the wicked neighbours. EXERCISE 3: Her son, whom the patient has rejected, deserves a postcard.

In this case, we choose a behavioural approach: practical exercises. The actual treatment is in exercise 3. According to our analysis, the patient becomes frightened by the wickedness, which she herself is still practicing in relation to her son, who deep down psychologically is herself. A classic example of mental disorder is querulous paranoia. Such a patient is running away from his or her life and is engaged in constant battle with society and the authorities; soon the patient spends all his or her time writing letters of complaint. It is a very agonizing condition and the patients are often completely unaware of their illness. In the following case report, the driving force behind the complaints is the loss of a child.

*Female, aged 41 years with possible querulous paranoia.*

QOL conversation: Alone with her 14-year-old son. Husband left her three years ago. Three months into the last relationship she became pregnant, but gave birth to a stillborn daughter. It seems as though the patient is living in the past instead of living here and now. Will not let go of her past, which means so much to her. She is very involved in a complaint concerning compulsory treatment at a psychiatric hospital. We talk about letting go of the past /suspected querulous paranoia/. EXERCISE 1: If you want to, you can turn your back on the past and face the present and the future by asking yourself: What do I need? How can I achieve that? Do not concern yourself with the past, with writing letters to the authorities, with thinking about things that happened in the past. But you need to cry and mourn the death of your daughter, so do that. EXERCISE 2: Read "The Power of Now" by Eckhart Tolle, and other good books about living in the present. EXERCISE 3: Make a complete list of all your problems in the present, write half a page about each of them – about 20 major problems. PLAN: Next appointment in one month.

## Anxiety

Anxiety afflicts about one in ten people in Denmark. A suitable amount of anxiety is a natural element of life, but when it grows into an uncontrollable fear of death and overshadows one's entire existence, it becomes a psychiatric disorder.

*Female, aged 44 years with anxiety and grief.*

First visit: Having difficulties with feelings in the form of fear of death and grief that overwhelm her. We talk about how to cope better with her strong feelings – by regarding them as an acceptable part of her. The feelings are strong, but not dangerous, and they are a part of her, which she needs. On examination: not suicidal or psychotic-depressive. She can return in two weeks if problems persist.

Second visit: Abdominal pain, attacks reported to last one hour a day for a month. No fever, affective pattern apparently normal, but poorly observed. On examination: Abdomen soft with no palpable tumours, no significant tenderness except minute McBurney tenderness and diffusely around navel. Rectal exploration shows no blood, normal faeces. Pelvic examination: Vulva, vagina natural, no cervical motion tenderness of the uterus, no tenderness corresponding to adnexa. No tumours, mucous membrane smooth, sphincter tone slightly above average. Other gynaecological findings: no

> complaints, in particular no vaginal discharge. PLAN: To be observed to see what induces the pain – e.g. related to meals? Movement? Waking? Agitation? etc. Also faeces to be observed, plus urine dipsticks. Blood tests. Prescribe Voltaren [diclophenac] suppositories 100 mg as required.
>
> Third visit: She is doing much better. Barely any problems for two weeks, although anxiety is still lurking beneath the surface. She recalls that it began after a serious accident at work eight years ago. Now she can handle the anxiety when it occurs, but is still scared of dwelling on it. We shall look at that next time. Once she becomes able to enter her anxiety, she will also be able to enter other feelings, also positive ones such as love and sex, which she finds difficult at present because she feels "reserved" in relation to her boyfriend. On examination: Marked improvement. Appears happy today.

By allowing the patient to harbour her feelings and assuring her that they are in no way dangerous – on the contrary – although they may be difficult, we open the waste bin, which virtually explode, having built up an enormous pressure for years in the form of denial and repression of feelings. We perceive her abdominal pain as being psychosomatic, but since the health service is founded on biomedicine, such a diagnosis is an exclusion diagnosis, which can only be made following a thorough physical assessment. We have to rule out several somatic possibilities. But everything turns out well, and the patient reaches the other side, happy and free, both of abdominal complaints and of her fear of death. As an unexpected bonus, the process lead to an improved love life.

> *Male, aged 28 years with anxiety and headache.*
>
> Frequent anxiety, suffers from fear of death – thinks of when his heart will stop beating, does not sleep. Has started seeing a psychiatrist, who prescribed Seroxat [paroxetine] for panic disorder. Also very severe headache daily. On examination: Appears very tormented and afraid, his back is tense as a rock from Os Sacrum to atlas /tension headache/ /fear of death/. Cannot suppress anxiety with Alopam [oxazepam] 15 mg 3 times daily. Prescribe physiotherapy. EXERCISE: Sit down and feel the anxiety, when it emerges. Do not run away from it – otherwise it will pursue you for the rest of your life. Come back next week for conversation.

Suppressed anxiety will lead to tension, typically manifested as headache as in this patient. He is a young man full of energy and inclined not to repress, but to integrate things. That is the reason why his fear of death surface in the first place. So a better solution would be for him to name the monster and invite it in, make friends with it and then release it.

> *Female, aged 24 years with anxiety.*
>
> Conversation: Acute counseling during the weekend following anxiety attack. Now composed, but worried. Watched her father stab her mother with a bread knife, when she was five years old. That incident is coming back to her now. At that time she used to think: "If only they would hold onto him, because he is sick in his head". EXERCISE: Describe every detail of the incident – everything that happened, everything you felt. When you become afraid, feel yourself as the little girl again, and look at the world from her perspective. Next appointment in two weeks, when she will bring what she has written with her. Is able to work.

When the father and mother are in a life-and-death struggle, the children suffer terrible wounds to their soul. Mercifully almost all such wounds can be healed over time.

## Discussion

The concept of loss of existential responsibility and subsequent degeneration of human perception is highly complex and the 8-step Responsibility-for-Life Scale we have presented in this chapter is clearly too simple. Every mental patient contains many "inner parts" living their own life, and needing individual processing along the scale. A lot of gestalts are working in the patient's mind at the same time and all the decisions that modify perception and consciousness are there at the same time, making the patient's perception spread out all over the scale, instead of being at one single point of it. This means that a patient that can be seemingly completely normal in his/her behaviour can be 30% hallucinated and only while dealing with special persons or in specific situations will this show. Interestingly, when sitting with a patient you can easily feel the "insane" quality of the patient and as you work your way downwards the time line using the holistic medical techniques of holding and processing, inducing the spontaneous regression to the patients' traumas, you will suddenly see the patient entering a psychotic state that was there all the time. It seems fair to talk about the web of consciousness, because our mind is woven of so many perceptual gestalts, memories, decisions and philosophical attitudes.

The question is, if a scale like the presented is meaningful at all. We think it is, as a general scheme for the degeneration of our consciousness. In the holistic clinical practice it serves very well as a map of states and transformations. It is very interesting that you cannot hallucinate, before you have cleaned your tabular and you do this by repressing the content of your mind so efficiently that the perception turns black. Now, on the blackness, you can add anything you want. The psychotic patient has many aspects of his/her perception repressed in the same time, but still there often is a basic orientation. You can talk to the insane person, because he or she sees you in some form, maybe severely disturbed, but you are still there and you can discuss reality. The psychotic patient will perceive reality very different from you, but if you are into symbolic language, even the discrepancies will make fine meaning to you and using this ability to understand you can actually help the patient to heal.

What we are doing in these examples are not very difficult; all it takes is really the intention to be of service to the patient and to come with love or intense care, win trust, give holding and lead the processing. Interestingly, a similar idea of levels or scales of responsibility seems to be the foundation of many systems of therapy and healing, from gestalt therapy[45] to energy healing[46] using the healer as a saviour and channel of divine energy, to the new-religious movements, where a scale of responsibility sometimes is used together with peculiar star war-like axioms of reincarnation. The use of the scale of responsibility for spontaneous regression and existential healing following love, trust, and full holding (the combination of care, respect, awareness, acceptance through touch and acknowledgement) are normally not used in neither gestalt therapy, healing or religious ceremonies and seems thus to be a characteristic of holistic medicine.

In contrast to the normal belief, it is possible to help the mentally ill patients to heal, if you can love them, win their trust and get allowance to give them support and holding. Even the most psychotic schizophrenic patient can heal if you can make him or her feel the existential pain in its full depth, understand what the message of the suffering is and let go of all the negative attitude and beliefs connected with the disease. While healing the most severe schizophrenic patients, especially those with a long carrier in mental institutions, might take many years to heal and even be out of reach, because of limited resources and lack of motivation for participate in their own healing, most mentally ill young people will benefit from existential holistic processing and many might even get healed completely. This would make it possible for them to get a good life and thus be saved from the long carrier as mental patients, so painful for anybody involved and close to the person, and so expensive for society.

The "trick" of helping the mentally ill patient seems to understand the level of responsibility the patient take and help him or her process the trauma and decisions that made him escape responsibility for his or her own life and destiny. A scale from free perception over emotional pain to psychic death (denial of life purpose making love impossible) further down to escape and denial to destruction of own perception and hallucination seems to be a valuable tool to understand the state of consciousness of the patient and the nature of the process of healing the patient must go through.

In the holistic existential therapy old childhood traumas are re-experienced and integrated. Repressed painful emotions reappear to the surface of the patient's consciousness and a new more constructive understanding of life emerges; in this process the patient gradually lets go of negative beliefs and assumes responsibility for own life.

To recover responsibility for life the patient must rehabilitate the three fundamental dimensions of existence from "theory of talent": 1) love including purpose of life (the life mission), 2) power of mind, feelings and body, and 3) gender including character and sexuality. It seems that even severely mentally ill patients can recover fully if they let go of all the negative attitudes and beliefs rising from the sufferings and causing the disease. The use of the Responsibility-for-Life Scale can be used on patients who need a path to assume responsibility for life, both mentally and somatically ill patients including cancer patients.

Interestingly, just a few hours of existential holistic therapy where the patient enters the state of holistic healing and confronts the core existential problems seems to be of significant help, especially to the young patient with the emerging disease, who has not yet been given anti-psychotic drugs or been institutionalized. This gives great hope for prevention and early intervention.

# References

[1] Ventegodt S, Andersen NJ, Neikrug S, Kandel I, Merrick J. Clinical holistic medicine: Mental disorders in a holistic perspective. ScientificWorldJournal 2005;5:313-23.

[2] Ventegodt S, Andersen NJ, Merrick J. Holistic Medicine III: The holistic process theory of healing. ScientificWorldJournal 2003;3:1138-46.

[3] Ventegodt S, Andersen NJ, Merrick J. Holistic Medicine IV: The principles of the holistic process of healing in a group setting. ScientificWorldJournal 2003;3:1294-1301.

[4] Ventegodt S, Andersen NJ, Merrick J. Editorial: Five theories of human existence. ScientificWorldJournal 2003;3:1272-6.

[5] Ventegodt S. The life mission theory: A theory for a consciousness-based medicine. Int J Adolesc Med Health 2003;15(1):89-91.

[6] Ventegodt S, Andersen NJ, Merrick J. The life mission theory II: The structure of the life purpose and the ego. ScientificWorldJournal 2003;3:1277-85.

[7] Ventegodt S, Andersen NJ, Merrick J. The life mission theory III: Theory of talent. ScientificWorldJournal 2003;3:1286-93.

[8] Ventegodt S, Merrick J. The life mission theory IV. A theory of child development. ScientificWorldJournal 2003;3:1294-1301.
[9] Ventegodt S, Andersen NJ, Merrick J. The life mission theory V. A theory of the anti-self and explaining the evil side of man. ScientificWorldJournal 2003;3:1302-13.
[10] Jørgensen P. Recovery and insight in schizophrenia. Acta Psychiatr Scand 1995;92(6):436-40.
[11] Robinson DG, Woerner MG, McMeniman M, Mendelowitz A, Bilder RM. Symptomatic and functional recovery from a first episode of schizophrenia or schizoaffective disorder. Am J Psychiatry 2004;161(3):473-9.
[12] Torgalsboen AK. Full recovery from schizophrenia: the prognostic role of premorbid adjustment, symptoms at first admission, precipitating events and gender. Psychiatry Res 1999;88(2):143-52.
[13] Torgalsboen AK, Rund BR. "Full recovery" from schizophrenia in the long term: a ten-year follow-up of eight former schizophrenic patients. Psychiatry 1998;61(1):20-34.
[14] Warner R. Recovery from schizophrenia in the Third World. Psychiatry 1983;46(3):197-212.
[15] Ventegodt S, Kromann M, Andersen NJ, Merrick J. The life mission theory VI: A theory for the human character. Healing with holistic medicine through recovery of character and purpose of life. ScientificWorldJournal 2004;4:859-80.
[16] Ventegodt S, Morad M, Hyam E, Merrick J. Clinical holistic medicine: Holistic sexology and treatment of vulvodynia through existential therapy and acceptance through touch. ScientificWorldJournal 2004;4:571-80.
[17] Ventegodt S, Clausen B, Merrick J. Clinical holistic medicine: The case story of Anna. I. Long term effect of physical maltreatment, incest and multiple rapes in early childhood. ScientificWorldJournal
[18] 2006;6:1965-76.
[19] Ventegodt S, Clausen B, Nielsen ML, Merrick J. Clinical holistic medicine: Advanced tools for holistic medicine. ScientificWorldJournal 2006;6:2048-65.
[20] Ventegodt S, Andersen NJ, Merrick J. Holistic medicine: Scientific challenges. ScientificWorldJournal 2003;3:1108-16.
[21] Ventegodt S, Andersen NJ, Merrick J. Holistic Medicine II: The square-curve paradigm for research in alternative, complementary and holistic medicine: A cost-effective, easy and scientifically valid design for evidence based medicine. ScientificWorldJournal 2003;3:1117-27.
[22] Ventegodt S, Merrick J, Andersen NJ. Quality of life theory I. The IQOL theory:An integrative theory of the global quality of life concept. ScientificWorldJournal 2003;3:1030-40.
[23] Ventegodt S, Merrick J, Andersen NJ. Quality of life theory II. Quality of life as the realization of life potential: A biological theory of human being. ScientificWorldJournal 2003;3:1041-9.
[24] Ventegodt S, Merrick J, Andersen NJ. Quality of life theory III. Maslow revisited. ScientificWorldJournal 2003;3:1050-7.
[25] Ventegodt S, Andersen NJ, Merrick J. Quality of life philosophy: when life sparkles or can we make wisdom a science? ScientificWorldJournal 2003;3:1160-3.
[26] Ventegodt S, Andersen NJ, Merrick J. QOL philosophy I: Quality of life, happiness, and meaning of life. ScientificWorldJournal 2003;3: 1164-75.
[27] Ventegodt S, Andersen NJ, Kromann M, Merrick J. QOL philosophy II: What is a human being? ScientificWorldJournal 2003;3:1176-85.
[28] Ventegodt S, Merrick J, Andersen NJ. QOL philosophy III: Towards a new biology. ScientificWorldJournal 2003;3:1186-98.
[29] Ventegodt S, Andersen NJ, Merrick J. QOL philosophy IV: The brain and consciousness. ScientificWorldJournal 2003;3:1199-1209.
[30] Ventegodt S, Andersen NJ, Merrick J. QOL philosophy V: Seizing the meaning of life and getting well again. ScientificWorldJournal 2003;3:1210-29.
[31] Ventegodt S, Andersen NJ, Merrick J. QOL philosophy VI: The concepts. ScientificWorldJournal 2003;3:1230-40.
[32] Merrick J, Ventegodt S. What is a good death? To use death as a mirror and find the quality in life. BMJ. Rapid Response 2002 Oct 31.
[33] Ventegodt S, Merrick J, Andersen NJ. Quality of life as medicine. A pilot study of patients with chronic illness and pain. ScientificWorld Journal 2003;3:520-32.

[34] Ventegodt S, Merrick J, Andersen NJ. Quality of life as medicine II. A pilot study of a five day "Quality of Life and Health" cure for patients with alcoholism. ScientificWorld Journal 2003;3: 842-52.

[35] Ventegodt S, Clausen B, Langhorn M, Kromann M, Andersen NJ, Merrick J. Quality of life as medicine III. A qualitative analysis of the effect of a five days intervention with existential holistic group therapy: a quality of life course as a modern rite of passage. ScientificWorld Journal 2004;4:124-33.

[36] Ventegodt S, Merrick J. Clinical holistic medicine: Applied consciousness-based medicine. ScientificWorldJournal2004;4:96-9.

[37] Ventegodt S, Morad M, Merrick J. Clinical holistic medicine: Classic art of healing or the therapeutic touch. ScientificWorldJournal2004;4:134-47.

[38] Ventegodt S, Morad M, Merrick J. Clinical holistic medicine: The "new medicine", the multi-paradigmatic physician and the medical record. ScientificWorldJournal2004;4:273-85.

[39] Ventegodt S, Morad M, Merrick J. Clinical holistic medicine: Holistic pelvic examination and holistic treatment of infertility. ScientificWorldJournal2004;4:148-58.

[40] Ventegodt S, Morad M, Hyam E, Merrick J. Clinical holistic medicine: Use and limitations of the biomedical paradigm ScientificWorldJournal2004;4:295-306.

[41] Ventegodt S, Morad M, Kandel I, Merrick J. Clinical holistic medicine: Social problems disguised as illness. ScientificWorldJournal 2004;4:286-94.

[42] Ventegodt S, Morad M, Andersen NJ, Merrick J. Clinical holistic medicine Tools for a medical science based on consciousness. ScientificWorldJournal 2004;4:347-61.

[43] Ventegodt S, Morad M, Hyam E, Merrick J. Clinical holistic medicine: When biomedicine is inadequate. ScientificWorldJournal2004;4:333-46.

[44] Ventegodt S, Flensborg-Madsen T, Andersen NJ, Morad M, Merrick J. Clinical holistic medicine: A Pilot on HIV and quality of life and a suggested treatment of HIV and AIDS. ScientificWorldJournal 2004;4:264-72.

[45] Ventegodt S, Morad M, Merrick J. Clinical holistic medicine: Induction of spontaneous remission of cancer by recovery of the human character and the purpose of life (the life mission). ScientificWorldJournal 2004;4:362-77.

[46] Perls F, Hefferline R, Goodman P. Gestalt therapy. New York: Julian Press, 1951.

[47] Brofman M. Anything can be healed. Findhorn: Findhorn Press, 2003.

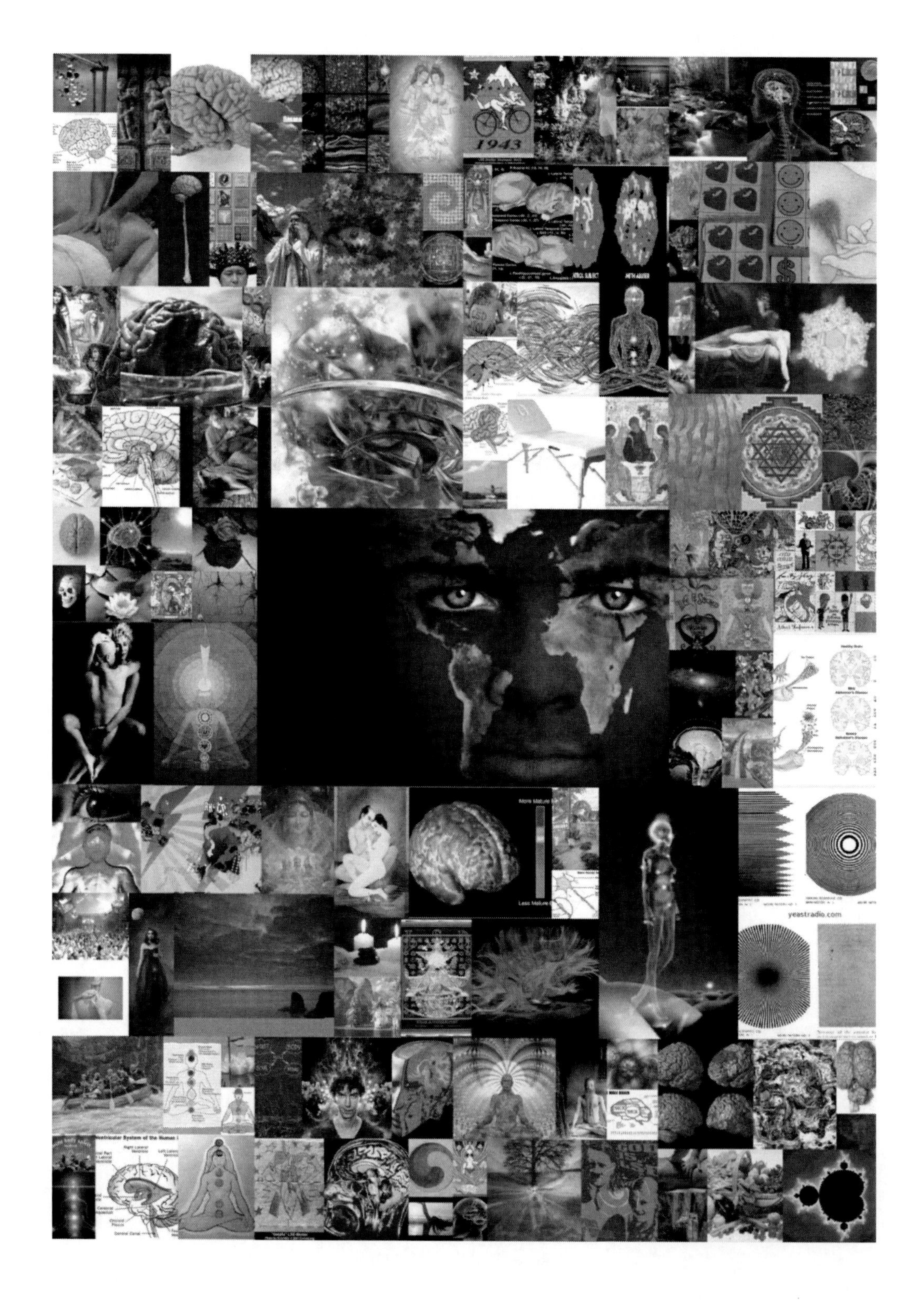
1943
More Mature
Less Mature
yeastradio.com

*Chapter IX*

# Self harm and death

Suicide is one of the most problematic issues in psychiatry; fortunately holistic medicine has recently been found to prevent suicide (1). A metaanalysis found that about 100 patients that entered therapy after taking the decision of committing suicide all survived. In the therapy the patient found resources to let go of the decision of killing themselves. In general holistic therapy therefore seems to be the preferred treatment for patients in danger of committing suicide.

But things are not that simple. Many countries have special laws installed to protect the life of patients wanting to commit suicide. Often force is used to save the patients, in spite of the use of force obviously violating the sacred principle of patient autonomy. The holistic physician or therapist must obey the laws in spite of these not being rational according to the latest scientific knowledge (1).

Death can be good or bad. In this section we also discuss what a good and a bad death is. Understanding this has by existential thinkers been seen as crucial for the whole understanding of life itself. We have included this chapter, which is of little practical value, to give the reader an example of contemporary holistic philosophy of life.

## Reference

[1] Ventegodt S, Andersen NJ, Kandel I, Merrick J. Effect, side effects and adverse events of non-pharmaceutical medicine. A review. Int J Disabil Hum Dev 2009;8(3):227-35.

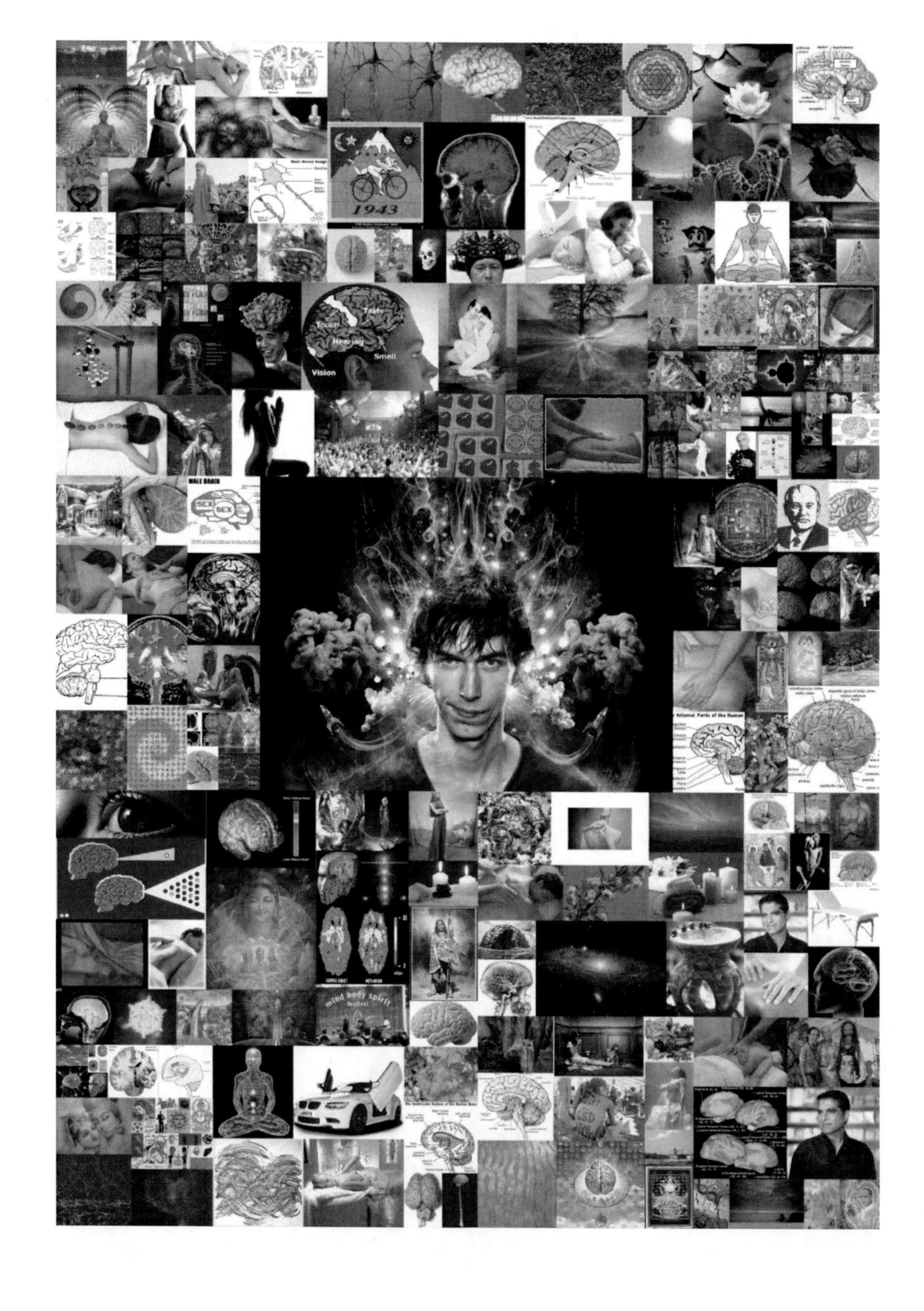

1943
Touch
Taste
Hearing
Smell
Vision
MALE BRAIN
SEX
SEX
mind body spirit
festival

*Chapter X*

# Personality disorders

Scientific holistic medicine has as mentioned several times its roots in the medicine and tradition of Hippocrates. Modern epidemiological research in quality of life, the emerging science of complementary and alternative medicine (CAM), the tradition of psychodynamic therapy, and the tradition of bodywork are merging into a new scientific way of treating patients. This approach seems able to help every second patient with personality disorders and mental illness in 20 sessions over one year. To treat personality disorders with holistic medicine the patients are first diagnosed in five dimensions based on the classical Hippocratic description of man: 1) body and sexuality, 2) consciousness and psyche, 3) feelings and emotions, 4) spirituality and ability to love, and 5) an integrative function of the I often called "the heart".

The patient can be normal, mentally ill or have a disturbed personality. The later goes from the mildest degree of low self-esteem, low self-confidence and nymphomania over mild personality disorders (the dependent, nervous/evasive, compulsive) to the borderline patients (the labile, narcissistic, hysteric/histrionic, dyssocial/antisocial, and paranoid), to the schizoid almost schizophrenic patient. The therapy address the level of psychosexual development; it facilitates development from infantile autoerotic over the immature (oral/anal/clitoral) to the mature, genital state where the patient can engage in mutually satisfactory coitus. The patient's affective and emotional state is developed from blocked over flat to vita. The patients mind are stimulated and developed from an immature to a mature level (on the scale: mature, immature, instable, deluded, deluded-instable, disintegrated).

The patient's spiritual state are also analysed and old defense like split and flattening are reversed often during intensive existential crisis where the patient regress to early childhood to heal his or her whole existence (the existential healing Antonovsky called "salutogenesis"). Finally when body, mind and spirit are ready, the heart or "I-Strength" can be recovered. The five-dimensional diagnostic system makes diagnosis and planning of the psychodynamic or holistic therapy easy and open op for a constructive dialog about the goal of therapy with the patient.

## Introduction

Hippocrates (460-377BCE) (1) and his students worked to help their patients to step into character, get direction in life, and use their human talents for the benefit of their surrounding world. For all that we know this approach was extremely efficient medicine that helped the patients to recover health, quality of life and ability. On other continents similar medical systems were developed. The medicine wheel of the native Americans, the African Sangoma culture, the Samic Shamans of northern Europe, the healers of the Australian Aboriginals, the Ayurvedic doctors of India, the acupuncturists of China, and the herbal doctors of Tibet all seems to be fundamentally character medicine (2-8). All the theories and the medical understanding from these pre-modern cultures are now being integrated in what is called integrative or transcultural medicine. Many of the old medical systems are reappearing in modern time as alternative, complementary and psychosocial medicine. This huge body of theory is now being offered as a European Union Master of Science degree (2-8).

## What is happening today?

If you recall our chapter on the history of scientific holistic medicine you can jump over this section. If not, you can keep on reading. We repeat this as we believe it to be important that the practitioner of holistic medicine thoroughly understands its historical roots.

Interestingly, two huge movements of the last century have put this old knowledge into use: psychoanalysis (9) and psychodynamic therapy (10,11) (most importantly STPP) (12,13) going through the mind on one hand, and bodywork (most importantly Reich) (14), Lowen (15) and Rosen (16)) and sexual therapy (especially the tantric tradition)(17) going through the body on the other. A third road, but much less common path has been directly though the spiritual reconnection with the world (18,19).

Our international research collaboration got interested in existential healing from the data coming from epidemiological research at the University Hospital of Copenhagen (Rigshospitalet) starting in 1958-61 at the Research Unit for Prospective Pediatrics and the Copenhagen Perinatal Birth Cohort 1959-61. Almost 20 years ago we were conducting epidemiological research on quality of life, closely examining the connection between global quality of life and health for more than 11,000 people in a series of huge surveys (20) using large and extensive questionnaires, some of them with over 3,000 questions. We found (quite surprisingly) from this huge data base that quality of life, mental and physical health, and ability of social, sexual and working ability seemed to be caused primarily by the consciousness and philosophy of life of the person in question, and only to a small extent by objective factors, like being adopted, coming from a family with only one breadwinner, mother being mentally ill, or one self being financially poor or poorly educated (which are obviously very much socially inherited) (20).

This scientific finding was not expected and so contra-intuitive for us that we were forced to investigate the subject going to the roots of western medicine, or the Hippocratic character of medicine. This meant that we had to look at transcultural and integrative medicine, the emerging science of alternative medicine (scientific CAM theory) and to the very much forgotten traditions of psychosomatic, psychodynamic, and bodily oriented therapies. Around

1994 we received substantial funding for our research project trying to embrace this huge heritage of medical wisdom

Philosophically (21-28), theoretically (29-49), epidemiologically/statistically (50-71). We have since 1997 with a great effort tried to take this knowledge into clinical practice (72-113) and with quite extraordinary results. Clinical holistic medicine has in our Research Clinic for Holistic medicine in Copenhagen helped every second patient with physical, mental, existential or sexual health issues or diseases over one year (114-119). Finally we have been looking at what seems to be the common denominator for all existential healing work in all cultures at all times: the sense of coherence, most clearly expressed by Aaron Antonovsky (1923-1994), a sociologist from the Faculty of Health Sciences at the Ben Gurion University of the Negev in Israel (18,19,120-125). We have also been debating many difficult issues related to modern day medical science, especially in the British Medical Journal (126-139) and finally we are now collecting most of what we consider essential knowledge for the holistic physician in a series of books on the “Principles of holistic medicine” (140-142). What we have learned from this long journey through the grand medical heritage from the different cultures on this planet is that we need to work on body, mind and spirit at the same time (medicine men has always combined talking, touching, and praying), and that being human and truly kind is what really heals the other person. This is what Hippocrates called “the Art” (1), not “the art of medicine” or “the art of right living”, but simply “the art” – the way of the human heart, cultivating existence into sheer compassionate behaviour and joyful being, which has always been the ultimate goal of all the great healers in our history.

We are more than happy to see our research project in scientific holistic medicine (clinical holistic medicine, CHM) developing. The most paradoxal aspect of this is that while we like to think we are taking medicine forward, we are actually just taking medicine back to its roots. The most important thing is that research and development in this field is made in a dialectic process between qualitative and quantitative research.

## What is a personality disorder?

The personality disorders are traditionally placed between the completely mentally healthy state and the most psychotic mentally ill schizophrenic state; historically the personally disorders are collectively characterized by causing unproductive conflicts in the persons inner and outer life. When only the patient himself is tormented by the mental disorder we often use the work “neurosis”, i.e. “anxiety neurosis”, but almost always anxiety will give the patient an evasive trait - paradoxically creating lots of conflicts around the patient as all the patient’s fears one by one materialize - turning the neurosis into a personality disorder. The concept of ”neurosis” is therefore well substituted with the concept of personality disorders. All mental illnesses are rooted in psychological defense and therefore also based in personality disorders. The distinction between personality disorders and mental illnesses are therefore also totally artificial. Theoretically there is no reason not to integrate the mental illnesses and the personality disorders, as we have done in our suggested 5-dimensional model of personality disorders (see table 1).

In the psychodynamic literature there seems to be an agreement that the outer conflicts is a materialization of the persons inner conflicts, which are understood as internalized early external conflicts, often going all the way back to the earliest childhood and even the womb. The reason for the internalization is adaptation to the environment and parents to increase the holding and love and thereby optimizing the basic conditions for personal development and survival. Traditionally the personality disorders have been categorized as mild, borderline, and psychotic.

We have developed a five-dimensional model, which we have tested in clinical practice and found that it allows successful healing work with both patients with personality disorders and with mental illnesses (118).

## Holistic medicine and biomedicine in treatment of personality disorders

Historically the treatment of personality disorders like hysteria goes all the way back to Hippocrates and the Greek physicians, who used massage of the uterus combined with conversational therapy to heal the sexual disturbances believed to be the primary cause of personality disturbances (1). Holistic medicine that combined conversational therapy with bodywork was the European medicine for more than 2000 years, and Freud started himself as holistic physician giving massage to the hysterical patient's legs (144). Freud left bodywork and initiated the tradition of psychodynamic psychotherapy; he struggled with the problem that contemporary culture was extremely negative towards physical touch and bodily intimacy and he gained great fame from developing a style of therapy that left bodywork behind to focus on the talking. This in spite of the fact that the psychosexual developmental problems were still seen as the primary cause of personality disorders.

During the 20th century psychiatry developed the neurobiological hypothesis for personality disorders and this resulted in mental problems becoming less treated with conversational therapy and more and more often treated with psychopharmacological drugs, often combined with ECT.

It is difficult to compare the results from the three different ways to treat personality disorders, but it seems that Philippe Pinel (1745-1826) could cure 70% of his patients – presumably a mixture of schizophrenics and borderline patients - with his version of holistic medicine, the "Traitement moral" that had a strong focus on philosophical and somatic aspects of the patient around the 1800 (145); psychodynamic psychotherapy with conversational therapy alone could cure around 33% of the patients with personality disorders and schizophrenia from 1900 to 1970 [146-9], while psychopharmacological treatment only have helped a few per cent of the patients with personality disorders since 1970 (150) and cured even less.

The reason for the use of psychopharmacological drugs in the treatment of the personality disorders in spite of lack of Cochrane or other studies documenting clinically significant effect is simple: First the belief that mental disorders are caused by chemical disturbances in the brain makes this natural; and secondly an extremely large number of patient can be treated with minimal physician time. The sad fact is that the urbanization, modernization and the shift to a strong focus on natural science and biochemistry in medicine seems to take the healing power out of medicine.

**Table 1. In clinical holistic medicine the personality are analysed and diagnosed according to five central dimensions: sexuality, emotion, mind, spirit and heart (see text)**

| | | I-Strength (integrative ability, "heart") | Sexual development | Affective (emotional) state | Mental state | Spiritual state |
|---|---|---|---|---|---|---|
| Normal, healthy person | - | Strong | Genital, free | Vital | Mature | Whole |
| | Low self-esteem * | Fair | Genital, free | Flat or blocked | Mature | Whole |
| | Low self-confidence * | Fair | Genital, free | Vital | Immature | Whole |
| | Nympho-mania * | Fair | Sexualised, often genital | Vital | Mature | Whole |
| Mild (neurotic) | Dependant | Fair | Often immature, free | Vital | Often immature | Whole |
| | Nervous/ Evasive | Fair | Often immature, free | Vital | Often immature | Whole |
| | Compulsive | Fair | Often immature, often blocked | Often flat | Often immature | Whole |
| Borderline | Emotionally labile | Moderate or weak | Immature, free | Vital | Often immature | Whole |
| | - | Moderate or weak | Infantile autoerotism, free | Vital | Often immature | Whole |
| | Histrionic (Hysteric) | Often weak | Sexualised, often genital | Vital | Often immature, instable | Whole |
| | Dyssocial | Weak | Immature, sexualised or blocked | Often flat | Often immature | Flat |
| Psychotic | Paranoid | Weak | Immature, blocked | Often flat or blocked | Immature, deluded | Flat |
| | Schizoid | Weak | Immature or infantile autoerotism, blocked | Blocked | Immature | Split |
| | (Autistic) | Weak | Infantile autoerotism,blocked | Blocked | Immature, deluded | Split |
| Schizophrenia * | Schizophrenia * | Weak | Infantile Autoerotism, blocked | Blocked | Immature, deluded, dis-integrated | Split |

*Not considered a personality disorder.

After a decade of treatment experimentation and research into the process of holistic healing we have come up with a theoretical framework that can be used to explain and map all major personality disorders (see table 1) together with the mental diseases (33). We have learned that we are indeed capable of understanding and also curing most of the patients with these disorders and illnesses using the simple tools of clinical holistic medicine (28). Of course one can disagree with the holistic description of man as consisting of body, mind, spirit and heart, and with the idea of the sexual energy as the fundamental life energy of man. Without this perspective the presented theory of personality disorders and the holistic cures will be of little value. On the other hand one can argue that the fine results of the methods derived from this understanding can be taken as an empirical confirmation of the holistic theory of man.

## The definition of personality

In holistic medicine the personality is different from the being (34). The entity, or real person, is behind every appearance always intact and can be revitalized just by letting go of all the many layers of existential learning and adaptation that we call personality. The personality is in this sense *neurotic and created for survival and adaptation,* and very different from the person's character (35) and life mission (33,35-40), that is the person's real talents given already at conception intended for *living and growing*. So in this sense a completely healthy person does not have a personality, but is striving to create it for self-realization in order to be able to create value in this world. A mentally healthy person can create conflicts, but these conflicts will always be about maximizing value and taking down hindrances for what is considers good by the individual.

On the other hand will personality disorders always lead to neurotic conflicts that will consume a lot of time and energy and only lead to modest results if any. More often the conflicts will be destructive to the individual in spite of the experience of the conflicts being necessary and for the good of all. A person with severe personality disturbances will always blame the surrounding world for the problems and conflicts, while a mentally healthy person will assume full responsibility for all conflicts. Conflicts can be made actively and passively; the psychodynamic concept of "passive aggression" is often very well used in relation to personality disorders. Autism can be seen as the pure crystallization of passive aggression towards the parents; it can also be seen as a product of arrested psychosexual development around the foetal or infantile state called "infantile autoerotism" by Freud (41).

## Holistic theory of personality disorders

Man is seen holistically as body, mind, spirit and heart with sexuality as a penetrating ubiquitous energy, which circulates in the energetic system and connects all parts of it. The mild personality disorders (the dependent, the nervous, the narcissistic and the labile) are characterized by in open heart, and whole and functionally intact spirit, often a normal emotional life, but a somewhat immature mind and sexuality.

The borderline, or intermediate, personality disorders (the compulsive, the hysteric (histrionic), the anti-social (psychopathic), the depressive, the manic, and the schizotypical) are characterized by a blocked heart making connections to people very difficult; often a "flat" spirit, flat or labile emotions, a somewhat immature mind, and often a blocked sexuality.

The psychotic personality disorders (the autistic, the bi-polar, the paranoid, and the schizoid) are characterized by a blocked heart making connections to people very difficult; a split spirit, flat, an immature and deluded mind, and most often a completely blocked or little developed sexuality. The schizophrenic patient is at the extreme end of the spectrum with infantile auto-erotic and no objects-related sexuality, split spirit, often highly underdeveloped, strongly deluded mind, and most often complete, emotional flatness. In principle, body and sexuality must be rehabilitated first, then emotions and mind, and finally spirit and heart. In practice the course of therapy is always strongly dependent on the patient; the therapist needs to invent a new cure for every new patient.

Table 1, which we have already met in the previous section, shows the system of personality disorders and the underlying sexual, mental, spiritual and integrative (I/heart) problems that must be addressed in therapy to cure the patient.

# The five dimensions of mental health

## 1. Sexuality

Sexuality has been known to play a central role in personality disorders all the way back to Hippocrates and the Greek physicians and this perspective has been kept in today's psychoanalysis, psychodynamic psychotherapy, and holistic medicine from Hippocrates to Freud, Jung, Reich, Searles and many other great therapists. Sexuality lies at the core of human existence and the level of psychosexual development and the free or blocked flow of sexual energy is easily observed in clinical practice from the level of libido, sexual aggression, will to live, level of life energy etc. The development goes from object-less, infantile autoerotism through immature sexuality to the mature, genital sexuality needed for mutually satisfying, sexual intercourse. Freud described the immature sexuality as oral or anal. It has in the literature of erotic tantra been suggested that immature female sexuality can be seen as "clitoral" opposed to mature, vaginal sexuality. Sexuality (the sexual energy) can be free, blocked or sexualized. Sexualized energy is neurotically boosted; compare this with the classical diagnosis of "nymphomania", which is neurotically boosted sexuality in an otherwise normal patient (nymphomania is therefore included in table 1 as a normal condition and not a disorder).

Many hysteric patients are strongly sexualized and have an obvious nymphomaniac trait. Promiscuous behaviour is sometimes the behavioural derivate of sexualisation also in normal people, but this is not a mental disorder as we see it. This problem and many other related sexual problems like vulvodynia belongs to the field of sexology in spite of obvious presence of personality disorders in these patients; eating disorders are often more strongly related to sexual than to mental problems and should therefore also be treated with under the specialty of sexology. In the future psychiatry and sexology might also be integrated into a more holistic model; as physical health are also strongly related to mental and sexual problems we must always remember that body and mind cannot truly be separated in medicine. A few minutes talk about sexuality will reveal the patient's level of psychosexual developmental status; often just the way the patient dresses and contact you will let you know.

## 2. Affect/emotions

The emotional state of a human being goes from vital and healthy to flat and further to completely blocked. A person can contain a whole palette or rainbow of emotions, every moment being like a colourful painting; or emotional life can be flat and simplistic, one single emotion at the time, and no symphony of tones, no profoundness and mystery; or emotional life can be completely blocked. The palette can be dominated by dark colours in depression, or light colours in mania, and the whole palette can be changing unpredictably as in cyclothymia and emotional lability. The emotional status of the patient is easily experiences in personal contact.

## 3. Mind

The mind can be immature or maturely developed; it can contain complex concepts and fine language for describing the world, and intelligent and creative processes to model the surrounding world and meet the multiple challenges from inside and outside. It can be sharp, precise, stable, and useful tool, a reliable source of information and true resource for problem solving. When mind is immature, its description of the world can be instable, deluded, an unreliable source of information, or even a severe burden insisting compulsively on the patient doing or thinking specific thoughts or actions, and in the psychotic patient deluded thoughts and ideas can lead to highly destructive acts. In the most undeveloped and disturbed form the conception is confused and disintegrated. An hour of conversation will allow the therapist to estimate the level of development of patient's mind.

## 4. Spirit

In this important, but abstract dimension of man lies our ability to love and give unconditionally; if wholeness or the concept of soul is denied in the patient's personal philosophy, the ability to love unconditionally is often destroyed. The spiritual dimension also holds our mission of life, i.e. our core talents, which we need for being of true value in our social relationships. The spiritual dimension can be whole and vital, flat and reduced, or split in two or more parts, giving the most severe personality disorders. The split spirit is a well-known defense mechanism. Splitting is our normal reaction to traumas early in life when mind is still too immature to cope; in holistic therapy we often find these traumas under deep regression to the womb, where they can be healed.

The clinical assessment of this is quite difficult. A split spirit should not be mistaken for the phenomenon of multiple personalities that we all, sound as sick, contains as a condition for normal mental functioning; normally our multitude of "personalities" are not visible due to a high level of integration. But split spirit often materializes though the phenomenon of inner conflicts between the inner personalities, and this is the extreme examples of this that have given name to the illness schizophrenia, meaning "split spirit" in Greek. Other manifestations of the split defense is ambivalence; in marriage seen as a strong tendency to adultery; in work seen as a strong tendency to change work places, in friendship seen as a high rhythm of meeting and sacking friends.

Diagnosing the patient's spirit is the most difficult part of the diagnosing process; to master diagnoses and holistic therapy with patients with split-spirit problems the therapist needs to go through deep and regressive therapy himself, allowing for deep self-exploration into the spiritual domain. But even the inexperienced student will soon learn to identify ambivalence and strong inner conflicts in the patient coming from the obvious split defense.

### 5. Heart

The experience of an integrated I is a function of a complex integrative function developed though childhood and adolescence; we often call this function the "human heart". The heart integrates body, mind and spirit, or more accurately the patient's Id, Ego and Self/soul. The function of the heart makes it possible for us to meet another person as a subject (Though) and not an object ("it") (151). If a person becomes emotionally wounded the heart can be temporarily "broken" or more permanently blocked (a "closed heart"), and relating becomes difficult. This influences the whole experience and appearance of the person. Psychiatry has often understood the concept of I-Strength as a mental quality, while holistic medicine traditionally has seen is as an existential quality. Holistic medicine is aligned with the more common understanding of the heath; people who "have a heart" or "an open heart" are able to meet the world and other people in an open-minded, assertive, empathic, accepting, involved, respectful, interested, and loving way. The status of the heath is thus easily observed in clinical practice.

## How to diagnose with the 5-dimensional system

The power of the 5-dimensional system lies in its practicality in daily work. To use the system we always start with an interview about the patient's status in the five dimensions; the therapist's global impression grows organically out of this dynamic interaction. After rating this general global impression and also the five dimensions (on the 6 scales), the diagnosis is easily found using table 1. It is strongly recommended also to use a patient-rated questionnaire like QOL1, QOL 5 or QOL10 (60), and compare the two ratings to secure a reasonable concordance between the two sets of ratings. If the ratings differ much, the reason for the discrepancy must be thoroughly analyzed. In general, holistic therapy will not run smothery without a fundamental agreement between the therapist and the patient about what the patient's problem is, and what the solution and goal of therapy is. Therapist rated questionnaire for diagnosing the personality disorders and mental illnesses (The holistic 5-dimensional system suggested for ICD-11 and DSM-V):

**Q1: Therapist's global impression:**
Normal (no significant personality disorder or mental illness)
Normal, low self-esteem
Normal, low self-confidence

Normal, nymphomaniac
Dependant
Nervous/evasive (including anxiety)
Compulsive
Labile
Narcissistic
Hysteric (Histrionic)
Dyssocial/Antisocial
Paranoid
Schizoid
Mentally ill

**Q2: How I-strong is the patient (heart open/closed)?**
Strong ("open heart")
Fair
Moderate ("broken heart")
Weak ("closed heart")

**Q3: How developed is the patient's sexuality?**
Genital (mature)
Autoerotism (immature clitoral/oral/anal)
Infantile autoerotism (no object)

**Q4: How blocked or sexualized is patient's sexual energy?**
Free
Sexualized
Blocked

**Q5: How vital are the patient's emotions?**
Vital
Flat
Blocked

**Q6: How developed is the patient's mind?**
Mature
Immature
Immature, instable
Deluded
Deluded, instable
Deluded, disintegrated

**Q7: How whole is the patient's spirit?**
Whole
Flat (remote)
Split

## Principles of treatment

There were four core principles for the treatment:

- Induce healing of the whole existence of the patient and not only his/her body or mind (18,19). The healing often included goals like recovering purpose and meaning of life by improving existential coherence and ability to love, understand and function sexually.
- Adding as many resources to the patient as possible, as the primary reason for originally repressing the emotionally charged material was lack of resources - love, understanding, empathy, respect, care, acceptance and acknowledgement - to mention a few of the many needs of the little child. The principle was also to use the minimal intervention necessary by first using conversational therapy, then in addition philosophical exercises if needed, then adding bodywork or if needed adding role plays, group therapy and finally when necessary in a few cases, referring to a psychiatrist for psychotropic intervention. If the patient was in somatic or psychiatric treatment already at the beginning of the therapy, this treatment was continued with support from the holistic therapist.
- Using the similarity principle that seems to be a fundamental principle for all holistic healing. The similarity principle is based on the belief that what made the person sick originally will make the patient well again, when given in the right, therapeutic dose. This principle leads to often dramatic events in the therapy and to efficient and fast healing, but seems to send the patient into a number of crises that must be handled professionally. The scientific background for a radical and fast healing using the similarity principle is analyzed in.
- Using Hering's Law of Cure (Constantine Hering, MD, 1800-1880) supporting the patient in going once again through all the disturbances and diseases – in reverse order - that brought the patient to where he or she is now. Other important axioms of Hering's Law of Cure is that the disease goes from more to less important organs, goes from the inside out, and goes from upside down. The scientific rationale for the last three axioms is less clear than for the first: the patient must go back his time-line to integrate all the states and experiences s/he has met on her/his way to disease. Going back in time is normally done though spontaneous regression in holistic existential therapy.

## Discussion

Psychodynamic psychotherapy has a long tradition of doing it (41-44) and in our experience is not at all difficult to cure the personality disorder in therapy. A therapist that understands the basic principle of healing can cure mental illnesses; a skilled therapist like Searles cured 33% of even the most severely ill schizophrenic patients even after years of hospitalization with 900 hours of psychoanalysis (148); in our study we found that 57% of the mentally ill patients experienced to be cured with clinical holistic medicine (118). In our experience it is important to work with a broad variety of patients, also including the most ill patients, for the therapist to fully understand the basic constitution of the personality and the problems connected to it. Only in the most severely ill patients the whole structure of man becomes transparent and visible. When you can deal with schizophrenia, everything else becomes easy.

Working with the patient's sexuality is normally the biggest problem for a modern physician, because of the strong sexual taboo of society; we must stress that this is an absolutely necessary step in helping most patients with severe personality disorders, and not only a thing that should be cared about when rehabilitating patient with explicit sexual traumas. It is also important to remember that one girl in seven are still being sexually abused and these girls very often become the adult patients that seek therapy for personality disorders and mental problems. The therapist needs to be without prejudice, generous, caring and containing, to help patients re-integrate their ability to feel sexual interest, desire and arousal. Often the patents need to verbalize many sexual issues that normal people would never care about verbalize, i.e. their experience of the bodily reactions or orgasm. Most therapist feel quite awkward and embarrassed in the beginning working explicitly with patent's sexuality, but it is really worth getting past this point because it give the patient motivation and energy to raise a mind.

The use of therapeutic touch is paradoxically reducing the need of verbalizing and is also dramatically reducing the intensity of sexual transferences, but they will never completely disappear, making supervision and Balint Group work mandatory for holistic therapists. Written consent is always a good idea, and the medical record must contain detailed record of all procedures and emotionally charged wordings.

If patient-physician "chemistry" is bad, with little love and affection, it is wise to allow the patient to change therapist. If the relation is healing up, this is a sign of patients sexuality heeling; in this case it is wise not to abrupt therapy as it can set the patient seriously back; of cause the therapist is responsible for keeping the sexual boundaries and respecting the ethical rules of holistic therapy. We recommend the rules of International Society for Holistic Health (www.internationalsocietyforholistichealth.org).

# References


[1] Jones WHS. Hippocrates. Vol. I–IV. London: William Heinemann, 1923-1931.

[2] Antonella R.Introduction of regulatory methods, systematics, description and current research. Graz: Interuniversity College, 2004.

[3] Blättner B. Fundamentals of salutogenesis. Health promotion and individual promotion of health: Guided by resources. Graz: Interuniversity College, 2004.

[4] Endler PC. Master program for complementary, psychosocial and integrated health sciences Graz, Austria: Interuniversity College, 2004.

[5] Endler PC. Working and writing scientifically in complementary medicine and integrated health sciences. Graz, Austria: Interuniversity College, 2004.

[6] Kratky KW. Complementary medical systems. Comparison and integration. New York: Nova Sci, 2008.

[7] Pass PF. Fundamentals of depth psychology. Therapeutic relationship formation between self-awareness and casework Graz, Austria: Interuniversity College, 2004.

[8] Spranger HH. Fundamentals of regulatory biology. Paradigms and scientific backgrounds of regulatory methods. Graz: Interuniversity College, 2004.

[9] Jones E. The life and works of Sigmund Freud. New York: Basic Books, 1961.

[10] Jung CG. Man and his symbols. New York: Anchor Press, 1964.

[11] Jung CG. Psychology and alchemy. Collected works of CG Jung, vol 12. Princeton, NJ: Princeton Univ Press, 1968.
[12] Leichsenring F, Rabung S, Leibing E. The efficacy of short-term psychodynamic psychotherapy in specific psychiatric disorders: a meta-analysis. Arch Gen Psychiatry 2004;61(12):1208-16.
[13] Leichsenring F. Are psychodynamic and psychoanalytic therapies effective?: A review of empirical data. Int J Psychoanal 2005;86(Pt 3):841-68.
[14] Reich W. [Die Function des Orgasmus]. Köln: Kiepenheuer Witsch, 1969. [German]
[15] Lowen A. Honoring the body. Alachua, FL: Bioenergetics Press, 2004.
[16] Rosen M, Brenner S. Rosen method bodywork. Accessing the unconscious through touch. Berkeley, CA: North Atlantic Books, 2003.
[17] Anand M. The art of sexual ecstasy. The path of sacred sexuality for Western lovers. New York: Jerymy P Tarcher/Putnam, 1989.
[18] Antonovsky A. Health, stress and coping. London: Jossey-Bass, 1985.
[19] Antonovsky A. Unravelling the mystery of health. How people manage stress and stay well. San Franscisco: Jossey-Bass, 1987.
[20] Ventegodt S, Flensborg-Madsen T, Andersen NJ, Nielsen M, Morad M, Merrick J. Global quality of life (QOL), health and ability are primarily determined by our consciousness. Research findings from Denmark 1991-2004. Soc Indicator Res 2005;71:87-122.
[21] Ventegodt S, Andersen NJ, Merrick J. Quality of life philosophy: When life sparkles or can we make wisdom a science? ScientificWorldJournal 2003;3:1160-3.
[22] Ventegodt S, Andersen NJ, Merrick J. Quality of life philosophy I. Quality of life, happiness and meaning in life. ScientificWorldJournal 2003;3:1164-75.
[23] Ventegodt S, Andersen NJ, Merrick J. Quality of life philosophy II. What is a human being? ScientificWorldJournal 2003;3:1176-85.
[24] Ventegodt S, Andersen NJ, Merrick J. Quality of life philosophy III. Towards a new biology: Understanding the biological connection between quality of life, disease and healing. ScientificWorldJournal 2003;3:1186-98.
[25] Ventegodt S, Andersen NJ, Merrick J. Quality of life philosophy IV. The brain and consciousness. ScientificWorldJournal 2003;3:1199-1209.
[26] Ventegodt S, Andersen NJ, Merrick J. Quality of life philosophy V. Seizing the meaning of life and becoming well again. ScientificWorldJournal 2003;3:1210-29.
[27] Ventegodt S, Andersen NJ, Merrick J. Quality of life philosophy VI. The concepts. ScientificWorldJournal 2003;3:1230-40.
[28] Ventegodt S, Merrick J. Philosophy of science: How to identify the potential research for the day after tomorrow? ScientificWorldJournal 2004;4:483-9.
[29] Ventegodt S, Merrick J, Andersen NJ. Quality of life theory I. The IQOL theory:An integrative theory of the global quality of life concept. ScientificWorldJournal 2003;3:1030-40.
[30] Ventegodt S, Merrick J, Andersen NJ. Quality of life theory II. Quality of life as the realization of life potential: A biological theory of human being. ScientificWorldJournal 2003;3:1041-9.
[31] Ventegodt S, Merrick J, Andersen NJ. Quality of life theory III. Maslow revisited. ScientificWorldJournal 2003;3:1050-7.
[32] Ventegodt S, Andersen NJ, Merrick J. Editorial: Five theories of human existence. ScientificWorldJournal 2003;3:1272-6.
[33] Ventegodt S. The life mission theory: A theory for a consciousness-based medicine. Int J Adolesc Med Health 2003;15(1): 89-91.
[34] Ventegodt S, Andersen NJ, Merrick J. The life mission theory II. The structure of the life purpose and the ego.ScientificWorldJournal 2003;3:1277-85.
[35] Ventegodt S, Andersen NJ, Merrick J. The life mission theory III. Theory of talent. ScientificWorldJournal 2003;3:1286-93.
[36] Ventegodt S, Andersen NJ, Merrick J. The life mission theory IV. Theory on child development. ScientificWorldJournal 2003;3:1294-1301.
[37] Ventegodt S, Andersen NJ, Merrick J. The life mission theory V. Theory of the anti-self (the shadow) or the evil side of man. ScientificWorldJournal 2003;3:1302-13.

[38] Ventegodt S, Kromann M, Andersen NJ, Merrick J. The life mission theory VI. A theory for the human character: Healing with holistic medicine through recovery of character and purpose of life. ScientificWorldJournal 2004;4:859-80.

[39] Ventegodt S, Flensborg-Madsen T, Andersen NJ, Merrick J. The life mission theory VII. Theory of existential (Antonovsky) coherence: A theory of quality of life, health and ability for use in holistic medicine. ScientificWorldJournal 2005;5:377-89.

[40] Ventegodt S, Merrick J. Life mission theory VIII: A theory for pain. J Pain Management 2008;1(1): 5-10.

[41] Hermansen TD, Ventegodt S, Rald E, Clausen B, Nielsen ML, Merrick J. Human development I. Twenty fundamental problems of biology, medicine and neuropsychology related to biological information. ScientificWorldJournal 2006;6:747-59.

[42] Ventegodt S, Hermansen TD, Nielsen ML, Clausen B, Merrick J.Human development II. We need an integrated theory for matter, life and consciousness to understand life and healing. ScientificWorldJournal 2006;6:760-6.

[43] Ventegodt S, Hermansen TD, Rald E, Flensborg-Madsen T, Nielsen ML, Clausen B, Merrick J. Human development III. Bridging brain-mind and body-mind. Introduction to "deep" (fractal, poly-ray) cosmology. ScientificWorldJournal 2006;6:767-76.

[44] Ventegodt S, Hermansen TD, Rald E, Flensborg-Madsen T, Nielsen ML, Clausen B, Merrick J. Human development IV. The living cell has information-directed self-organization. ScientificWorldJournal 2006;6:1132-8.

[45] Ventegodt S, Hermansen TD, Flensborg-Madsen T, Nielsen ML, Clausen B, Merrick J. Human development V: Biochemistry unable to explain the emergence of biological form (morphogenesis) and therefore a new principle as source of biological information is needed. ScientificWorldJournal 2006;6:1359-67.

[46] Ventegodt S, Hermansen TD, Flensborg-Madsen T, Nielsen M, Merrick J. Human development VI: Supracellular morphogenesis. The origin of biological and cellular order. ScientificWorldJournal 2006;6:1424-33.

[47] Ventegodt S, Hermansen TD, Flensborg-Madsen T, Rald E, Nielsen ML, Merrick J. Human development VII: A spiral fractal model of fine structure of physical energy could explain central aspects of biological information, biological organization and biological creativity. ScientificWorldJournal 2006;6:1434-40.

[48] Ventegodt S, Hermansen TD, Flensborg-Madsen T, Nielsen ML, Merrick J. Human development VIII: A theory of "deep" quantum chemistry and cell consciousness: Quantum chemistry controls genes and biochemistry to give cells and higher organisms consciousness and complex behavior. ScientificWorldJournal 2006;6:1441-53.

[49] Ventegodt S, Hermansen TD, Flensborg-Madsen T, Rald E, Nielsen ML, Merrick J. Human development IX: A model of the wholeness of man, his consciousness and collective consciousness. ScientificWorldJournal 2006;6:1454-9.

[50] Hermansen TD, Ventegodt S, Merrick J. Human development X: Explanation of macroevolution — top-down evolution materializes consciousness. The origin of metamorphosis. ScientificWorldJournal 2006;6:1656-66.

[51] Ventegodt S, Merrick J, Andersen NJ. Editorial-A new method for generic measuring of the global quality of life. ScientificWorldJournal 2003;3:946-9.

[52] Ventegodt S, Hilden J, Merrick J. Measurement of quality of life I: A methodological framework. ScientificWorldJournal 2003;3:950-61.

[53] Ventegodt S, Merrick J, Andersen NJ. Measurement of quality of life II: From the philosophy of life to science. ScientificWorldJournal 2003;3:962-71.

[54] Ventegodt S, Merrick J, Andersen NJ. Measurement of quality of life III: From the IQOL theory to the global, generic SEQOL questionnaire. ScientificWorldJournal 2003;3:972-91.

[55] Ventegodt S, Merrick J, Andersen NJ. Measurement of quality of life IV: Use of the SEQOL, QOL5, QOL1 and other global and generic questionnaires. ScientificWorldJournal 2003;3:992-1001.

[56] Ventegodt S, Merrick J, Andersen NJ. Measurement of quality of life V: How to use the SEQOL, QOL5, QOL1 and other and generic questionnaires for research. ScientificWorldJournal 2003;3: 1002-14.
[57] Ventegodt S, Merrick J, Andersen NJ. Measurement of quality of life VI: "Quality-adjusted life years" (QALY) is an unfortunate use of quality of life concept. ScientificWorldJournal 2003;3:1015-9.
[58] Ventegodt S, Merrick J. Measurement of quality of life VII: Statistical covariation and global quality of life data. The method of weight-modified linear regression. ScientificWorldJournal 2003;3:1020-29.
[59] Ventegodt S, Henneberg EW, Merrick J, Lindholt JS. Validation of two global and generic quality of life questionnaires for population screening: SCREENQOL and SEQOL. ScientificWorldJournal 2003;3:412-21.
[60] Lindholt JS, Ventegodt S, Henneberg EW. Development and validation of QOL5 for clinical databases. A short, global and generic questionnaire based on an integrated theory of the quality of life. Eur J Surg 2002;168:103-7.
[61] Ventegodt S. Sex and the quality of life in Denmark. Arch Sex Behav 1998;27(3):295-307.
[62] Ventegodt S. A prospective study on quality of life and traumatic events in early life – 30 year follow-up. Child Care Health Dev 1998;25(3):213-21.
[63] Ventegodt S, Merrick J. Long-term effects of maternal smoking on quality of life. Results from the Copenhagen Perinatal Birth Cohort 1959-61. ScientificWorldJournal 2003;3:714-20.
[64] Ventegodt S, Merrick J. Long-term effects of maternal medication on global quality of life measured with SEQOL. Results from the Copenhagen Perinatal Birth Cohort 1959-61. ScientificWorldJournal 2003;3:707-13.
[65] Ventegodt S, Merrick J. Psychoactive drugs and quality of life. ScientificWorldJournal 2003;3: 694-706.
[66] Ventegodt S, Merrick J. Lifestyle, quality of life and health. ScientificWorldJournal 2003;3: 811-25.
[67] Ventegodt S, Flensborg-Madsen T, Andersen NJ, Merrick J. The health and social situation of the mother during pregnancy and global quality of life of the child as an adult. Results from the prospective Copenhagen Perinatal Cohort 1959-1961. ScientificWorldJournal 2005;5:950-8.
[68] Ventegodt S, Flensborg-Madsen T, Andersen NJ, Merrick J. Factors during pregnancy, delivery and birth affecting global quality of life of the adult child at long-term follow-up. Results from the prospective Copenhagen Perinatal Birth Cohort 1959-61. ScientificWorldJournal 2005;5:933-41.
[69] Ventegodt S, Flensborg-Madsen T, Andersen NJ, Merrick J. Events in pregnancy, delivery, and infancy and long-term effects on global quality of life: results from the Copenhagen Perinatal Birth Cohort 1959-61. ScientificWorldJournal 2007;7:1622-30.
[70] Ventegodt S, Flensborg-Madsen T, Andersen NJ, Morad M, Merrick J. Quality of life and events in the first year of life. Results from the prospective Copenhagen Birth Cohort 1959-61. ScientificWorldJournal 2006;6:106-15.
[71] Ventegodt S, Flensborg-Madsen T, Andersen NJ, Merrick J. What influence do major events in life have on our later quality of life? A retrospective study on life events and associated emotions Med Sci Monit 2006;12(2):SR9-15.
[72] Ventegodt S. Every contact with the patient must be therapeutic. J Pediatr Adolesc Gynecol 2007;20(6):323-4.
[73] Ventegodt S, Merrick J. Psychosomatic reasons for chronic pains. South Med J 2005;98(11): 1063.
[74] Ventegodt S, Andersen NJ, Merrick J. Holistic medicine: Scientific challenges. ScientificWorldJournal 2003;3:1108-16.
[75] Ventegodt S, Andersen NJ, Merrick J. Holistic Medicine II: The square-curve paradigm for research in alternative, complementary and holistic medicine: A cost-effective, easy and scientifically valid design for evidence based medicine. ScientificWorldJournal 2003;3:1117-27.
[76] Ventegodt S, Andersen NJ, Merrick J. Holistic medicine III: The holistic process theory of healing. ScientificWorldJournal 2003;3:1138-46.
[77] Ventegodt S, Andersen NJ, Merrick J. Holistic Medicine IV: Principles of the holistic process of healing in a group setting. ScientificWorldJournal 2003;3:1294-1301.
[78] Ventegodt S, Merrick J. Clinical holistic medicine: Applied consciousness-based medicine. ScientificWorldJournal 2004;4:96-9.

[79] Ventegodt S, Morad M, Merrick J. Clinical holistic medicine: Classic art of healing or the therapeutic touch. ScientificWorldJournal 2004;4:134-47.
[80] Ventegodt S, Morad M, Merrick J. Clinical holistic medicine: The “new medicine”, the multiparadigmatic physician and the medical record. ScientificWorldJournal 2004;4:273-85.
[81] Ventegodt S, Morad M, Merrick J. Clinical holistic medicine: Holistic pelvic examination and holistic treatment of infertility. ScientificWorldJournal 2004;4:148-58.
[82] Ventegodt S, Morad M, Hyam E, Merrick J. Clinical holistic medicine: Use and limitations of the biomedical paradigm. ScientificWorldJournal 2004;4:295-306.
[83] Ventegodt S, Morad M, Kandel I, Merrick J. Clinical holistic medicine: Social problems disguised as illness. ScientificWorldJournal 2004;4:286-94.
[84] Ventegodt S, Morad M, Andersen NJ, Merrick J. Clinical holistic medicine Tools for a medical science based on consciousness. ScientificWorldJournal 2004;4:347-61.
[85] Ventegodt S, Morad M, and Merrick J. Clinical holistic medicine: Prevention through healthy lifestyle and quality of life. Oral Health Prev Dent 2004;1:239-45.
[86] Ventegodt S, Morad M, Hyam E, Merrick J. Clinical holistic medicine: When biomedicine is inadequate. TheScientificWorldJOURNAL 4, 333-346.
[87] Ventegodt S, Morad M, Merrick J. Clinical holistic medicine: Holistic treatment of children. ScientificWorldJournal 2004;4:581-8.
[88] Ventegodt S, Morad M, Merrick J. Clinical holistic medicine: Problems in sex and living together. ScientificWorldJournal 2004;4:562-70.
[89] Ventegodt S, Morad M, Hyam E, Merrick J. Clinical holistic medicine: Holistic sexology and treatment of vulvodynia through existential therapy and acceptance through touch. ScientificWorldJournal 2004;4:571-80.
[90] Ventegodt S, Flensborg-Madsen T, Andersen NJ, Morad M, Merrick J. Clinical holistic medicine: A pilot on HIV and quality of life and a suggested treatment of HIV and AIDS. ScientificWorldJournal 2004;4:264-72.
[91] Ventegodt S, Morad M, Merrick J. Clinical holistic medicine: Induction of spontaneous remission of cancer by recovery of the human character and the purpose of life (the life mission). ScientificWorldJournal 2004;4:362-77.
[92] Ventegodt S, Morad M, Kandel I, Merrick J. Clinical holistic medicine: Treatment of physical health problems without a known cause, exemplified by hypertension and tinnitus. ScientificWorldJournal 2004;4:716-24.
[93] Ventegodt S, Morad M, Merrick J. Clinical holistic medicine: Developing from asthma, allergy and eczema. ScientificWorldJournal 2004;4:936-42.
[94] Ventegodt S, Morad M, Press J, Merrick J, Shek D. Clinical holistic medicine: Holistic adolescent medicine. ScientificWorldJournal 2004;4, 551-561.
[95] Ventegodt S, Solheim E, Saunte ME, Morad M, Kandel I, Merrick J. Clinical holistic medicine: Metastatic cancer. ScientificWorldJournal 2004;4:913-35.
[96] Ventegodt S, Morad M, Kandel I, Merrick J. Clinical holistic medicine: a psychological theory of dependency to improve quality of life. ScientificWorldJournal 2004;4:638-48.
[97] Ventegodt S, Merrick J. Clinical holistic medicine: Chronic infections and autoimmune diseases. ScientificWorldJournal 2005;5:155-64.
[98] Ventegodt S, Kandel I, Neikrug S, Merrick J. Clinical holistic medicine: Holistic treatment of rape and incest traumas. ScientificWorldJournal 2005;5:288-97.
[99] Ventegodt S, Morad M, Merrick J. Clinical holistic medicine: Chronic pain in the locomotor system. ScientificWorldJournal 2005;5:165-72.
[100] Ventegodt S, Merrick J. Clinical holistic medicine: Chronic pain in internal organs. ScientificWorldJournal 2005;5:205-10.
[101] Ventegodt S, Kandel I, Neikrug S, Merrick J. Clinical holistic medicine: The existential crisis – life crisis, stress and burnout. ScientificWorldJournal 2005;5:300-12.
[102] Ventegodt S, Gringols M, Merrick J. Clinical holistic medicine: Holistic rehabilitation. ScientificWorldJournal 2005;5:280-7.

[103] Ventegodt S, Andersen NJ, Neikrug S, Kandel I, Merrick J. Clinical holistic medicine: Mental disorders in a holistic perspective. ScientificWorldJournal 2005;5:313-23.
[104] Ventegodt S, Andersen NJ, Neikrug S, Kandel I, Merrick J. Clinical Holistic Medicine: Holistic treatment of mental disorders. ScientificWorldJournal 2005;5:427-45.
[105] Ventegodt S, Merrick J. Clinical holistic medicine: The patient with multiple diseases. ScientificWorldJournal 2005;5:324-39.
[106] Ventegodt S, Clausen B, Nielsen ML, Merrick J. Clinical holistic medicine: Advanced tools for holistic medicine. ScientificWorldJournal 2006;6:2048-65.
[107] Ventegodt S, Clausen B, Merrick J. Clinical holistic medicine: The case story of Anna. I. Long-term effect of childhood sexual abuse and incest with a treatment approach. ScientificWorldJournal 2006;6:1965-76.
[108] Ventegodt S, Clausen B, Merrick J. Clinical holistic medicine: the case story of Anna. II. Patient diary as a tool in treatment. ScientificWorldJournal 2006;6:2006-34.
[109] Ventegodt S, Clausen B, Merrick J. Clinical holistic medicine: The case story of Anna. III. Rehabilitation of philosophy of life during holistic existential therapy for childhood sexual abuse. ScientificWorldJournal 2006;6:2080-91.
[110] Ventegodt S, Merrick J. Suicide from a holistic point of view.ScientificWorldJournal 2005;5:759-66.
[111] Ventegodt S, Clausen B, Omar HA, Merrick J. Clinical holistic medicine: Holistic sexology and acupressure through the vagina (Hippocratic pelvic massage). ScientificWorldJournal 2006;6:2066-79.
[112] Ventegodt S, Clausen B, Merrick J. Clinical holistic medicine: Pilot study on the effect of vaginal acupressure (Hippocratic pelvic massage). ScientificWorldJournal 2006;6:2100-16.
[113] Ventegodt S. [Min brug af vaginal akupressur.] My use of acupressure. Ugeskr Laeger 2006;168(7):715-6. [Danish]
[114] Ventegodt S, Thegler S, Andreasen T, Struve F, Enevoldsen L, Bassaine L, et al. Clinical holistic medicine: Psychodynamic short-time therapy complemented with bodywork. A clinical follow-up study of 109 patients. ScientificWorldJournal 2006;6:2220-38.
[115] Ventegodt S, Thegler S, Andreasen T, Struve F, Enevoldsen L, Bassaine L, et al. Clinical holistic medicine (mindful, short-term psychodynamic psychotherapy complemented with bodywork) in the treatment of experienced impaired sexual functioning. ScientificWorldJournal 2007;7:324-9.
[116] Ventegodt S, Thegler S, Andreasen T, Struve F, Enevoldsen L, Bassaine L, et al. Clinical holistic medicine (mindful, short-term psychodynamic psychotherapy complemented with bodywork) improves quality of life, health and ability by induction of Antonovsky-salutogenesis. ScientificWorldJournal 2007;7:317-23.
[117] Ventegodt S, Thegler S, Andreasen T, Struve F, Enevoldsen L, Bassaine L, et al. Clinical holistic medicine (mindful, short-term psychodynamic psychotherapy complemented with bodywork) in the treatment of experienced physical illness and chronic pain. ScientificWorldJournal 2007;7:310-6.
[118] Ventegodt S, Thegler S, Andreasen T, Struve F, Enevoldsen L, Bassaine L, et al. Clinical holistic medicine (mindful, short-term psychodynamic psychotherapy complemented with bodywork) in the treatment of experienced mental illness. ScientificWorldJournal 2007;7:306-9.
[119] Ventegodt S, Thegler S, Andreasen T, Struve F, Enevoldsen L, Bassaine L, et al. Self-reported low self-esteem. Intervention and follow-up in a clinical setting. ScientificWorldJournal 2007;7:299-305.
[120] Flensborg-Madsen T, Ventegodt S, Merrick J. Sense of coherence and physical health. A Review of previous findings. ScientificWorldJournal 2005;5:665-73.
[121] Flensborg-Madsen T, Ventegodt S, Merrick J. Why is Antonovsky's sense of coherence not correlated to physical health? Analysing Antonovsky's 29-item sense of coherence scale (SOCS). ScientificWorldJournal 2005;5:767-76.
[122] Flensborg-Madsen T, Ventegodt S, Merrick J. Sense of coherence and health. The construction of an amendment to Antonovsky's sense of coherence scale (SOC II). ScientificWorldJournal 2006;6: 2133-9.
[123] Flensborg-Madsen T, Ventegodt S, Merrick J. Sense of coherence and physical health. A cross-sectional study using a new SOC scale (SOC II). ScientificWorldJournal 2006;6:2200-11.
[124] Flensborg-Madsen T, Ventegodt S, Merrick J. Sense of coherence and physical health. Testing Antonovsky's theory. ScientificWorldJournal 2006;6:2212-9.

[125] Flensborg-Madsen T, Ventegodt S, Merrick J. Sense of coherence and health. The emotional sense of coherence (SOC-E) was found to be the best-known predictor of physical health. ScientificWorldJournal 2006;6:2147-57.
[126] Merrick J, Ventegodt S. What is a good death? To use death as a mirror and find the quality in life. BMJ. Rapid Response 2003 Oct 31.
[127] Ventegodt S, Merrick J. Medicine and the past. Lesson to learn about the pelvic examination and its sexually suppressive procedure. BMJ. Rapid Response 2004 Feb 20.
[128] Ventegodt S, Morad M, Merrick J. If it doesn't work, stop it. Do something else! BMJ. Rapid Response 2004 Apr 26.
[129] Merrick J, Morad M, Kandel I, Ventegodt S. Spiritual health, intellectual disability and health care. BMJ Rapid Response 2004 Jul 16.
[130] Ventegodt S, Morad M, Kandel I, Merrick J. Maternal smoking and quality of life more than thirty years later. BMJ Rapid Response 2004 Jul 30.
[131] Merrick J, Morad M, Kandel I, Ventegodt S. Prevalence of Helicobacter pylori infection in residential care centers for people with intellectual disability. BMJ Rapid Response 2004 Jul 23.
[132] Merrick J, Morad M, Kandel I, Ventegodt S. People with intellectual disability, health needs and policy. BMJ Rapid Response 2004 Aug 20.
[133] Ventegodt S, Vardi G, Merrick J. Holistic adolescent sexology: How to counsel and treat young people to alleviate and prevent sexual problems. BMJ Rapid Response 2005 Jan 15.
[134] Ventegodt S. Flensborg-Madsen T, Merrick J. Evidence based medicine in favour of biomedicine and it seems that holistic medicine has been forgotten? BMJ Rapid Response 2004 Nov 11.
[135] Ventegodt S, Merrick J. Placebo explained: Consciousness causal to health. BMJ Rapid Responses 2004 Oct 22.
[136] Ventegodt S, Merrick J. Academic medicine must deliver skilled physicians. A different academic training is needed. BMJ Rapid Response 2004 Oct 9.
[137] Ventegodt S, Morad M, Merrick J. Chronic illness, the patient and the holistic medical toolbox. BMJ Rapid Response 2004 Sep 15.
[138] Ventegodt S, Kandel I, Merrick J. Medicine has gone astray - we must reverse the alienation now. BMJ Rapid Response 2005 Mar 10.
[139] Ventegodt S, Merrick J. The consensus paradigm for qualitative research in holistic medicine. BMJ Rapid Response 2005 Nov 24.
[140] Ventegodt S, Kandel I, Merrick J. Principles of holistic medicine. Philosophy behind quality of life. Victoria, BC: Trafford, 2005
[141] Ventegodt S, Kandel I, Merrick J. Principles of holistic medicine. Quality of life and health. New York: Hippocrates Sci Publ, 2005.
[142] Ventegodt S, Kandel I, Merrick J. Principles of holistic medicine. Global quality of life.Theory, research and methodology. New York: Hippocrates Sci Publ, 2005.
[143] Ventegodt S. Measuring the quality of life. From theory to practice. Copenhagen: Forskningscentrets Forlag, 1996.
[144] Freud S, Breuer J. Studies in hysteria. New York: Penguin Classics, 2004. (Original work published 1893, 1895, 1908).
[145] Weiner DB. The clinical training of doctors. An essay from 1793 by Philippe Pinel. Henry E Sigerist Suppl Bull Hist Med 1980;3:1-102.
[146] Modestin J, Huber A, Satirli E, Malti T, Hell D. Long-term course of schizophrenic illness: Bleuler's study reconsidered. Am J Psychiatry 2003;160(12):2202-8.
[147] Knight RP, Preface. In: Searles HF. Collected papers on schizophrenia. Madison, CT: Int Univ Press, 1965:15-18.
[148] Karon BP, VandenBos G. Psychotherapy of schizophrenia. The treatment of choise. New York: Jason Aronson, 1981.
[149] Quante A, Röpke S, Merkl A, Anghelescu I, Lammers CH. [Psychopharmacologic treatment of personality disorders.] Fortschr Neurol Psychiatr 2008;76:1-10. [German].
[150] Buber M. I and thou. New York: Charles Scribner, 1970.

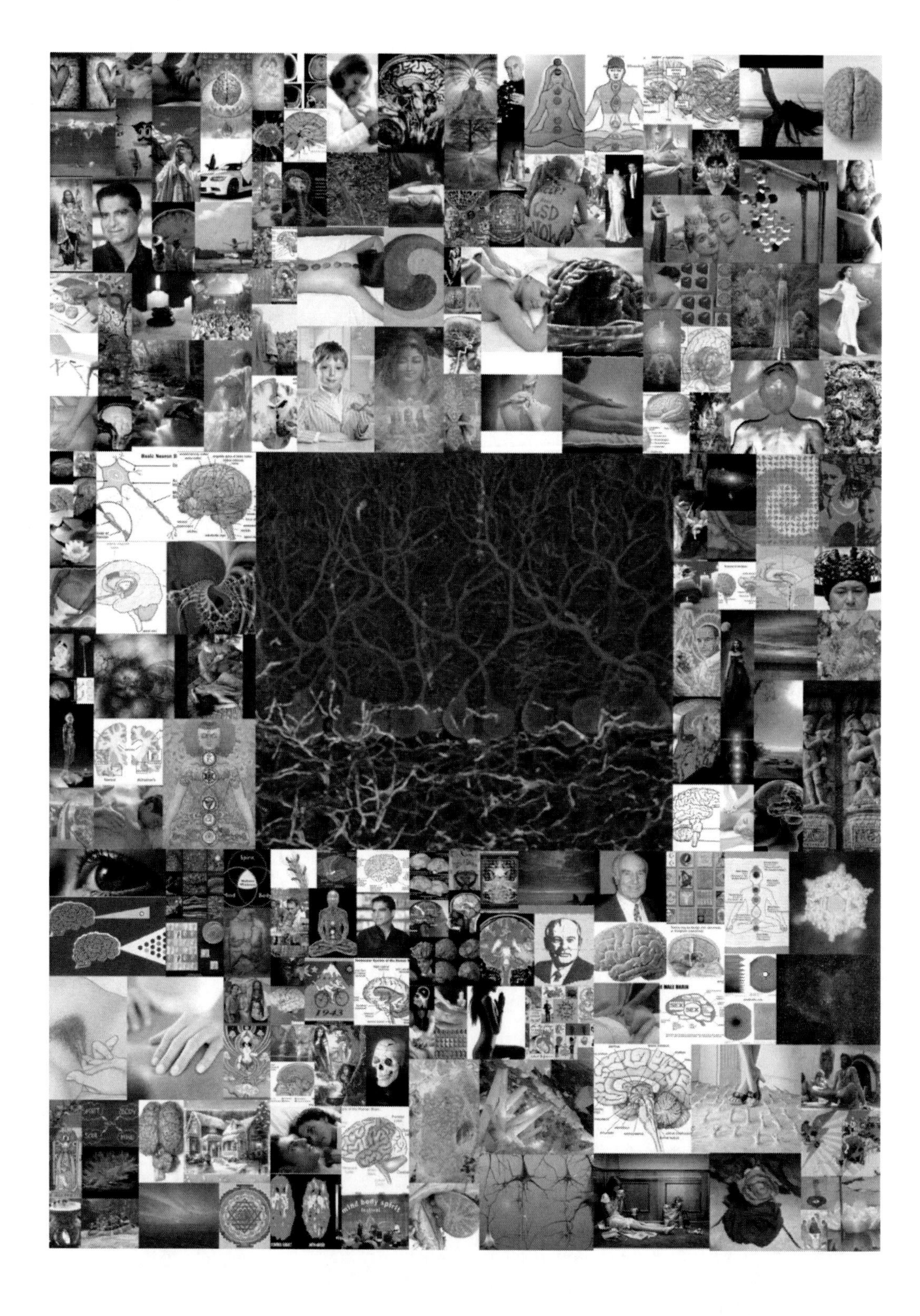
1943
mind body spirit

*Chapter XI*

# Schizophrenia and other psychotic mental diseases

Clinical holistic medicine (CHM) has developed into a system that can also be helpful with mental ill patients. CHM-therapy supports the patient through a series of emotionally challenging, existential and healing crises. The patient's sense of coherence and mental health can be recovered through the process of feeling old repressed emotions, understanding life, self and finally letting go of negative beliefs and delusions, The Bleuler's triple condition of autism, disturbed thoughts, and disturbed emotions that characterizes the schizophrenic patient can be understood as arising from the early defense of splitting, caused by negative learning from painful childhood traumas that made the patient lose sense of coherence and withdraw from social contact. Self-insight gained though the therapy can allow the patients to take their bodily, mental and spiritual talents into use. In the end of therapy the patients are once again living a life of quality centered on their life-mission and they relate to other people in a way that systematically creates value. There are a number of challenges meeting the therapist working with schizophrenic and psychotic patients, from the potential risk of experiencing patient's violence to the obligation to contain the most difficult and embarrassing of feelings, when the emotional and often also sexual content of the patient's unconsciousness becomes explicit. There is a long, well established tradition for treating schizophrenia with psychodynamic therapy and we have found that the combination of bodywork and psychotherapy can enhance and accelerate the therapy and might improve the treatment rate further.

## Introduction

Madness has tormented mankind since its birth and definitely as long back as we have medical recordings. Hippocrates (460-377BCE) devoted attention to mental diseases and used an ingenuous combination of conversational therapy and bodywork as treatment for example of hysteria (from Greek Hystera: Uterus) and other mental conditions (1). As one of his treatments he used pelvic massage (2,3) to "correct the energy of the uterus", but also other provocative and efficient methods of interventions. To avoid the problems of sexual abuse following the use of bodywork and intimacy he invented his famous Hippocratic ethics (1).

Philippe Pinel (1745-1826) (4) at Bicétre in Paris used "moral treatment" for mentally ill patients, and he did that surprisingly successful. According to his statistics about 70% of the patients were healed using the holistic medical principles. With a strong focus on medical ethics, he stressed the respect of the individual and used intensive studies of each single patient through detailed case recordings (4,5). Pinel called his psychiatric therapy for "Traitement moral" and this holistic system represented the first modern attempt at individual psychotherapy. His treatment core values were gentleness, understanding, goodwill and he was opposed to violent methods. He recommended close medical attendance during convalescence, and he emphasized the need of hygiene, physical exercise, and a program of purposeful work for the patient. A number of his therapeutic procedures, including ergo therapy and the placement of the patient in a family group, anticipated modern psychiatric care.

The Swiss psychiatrist Paul Eugen Bleuler (1857-1939) gave birth to the name schizophrenia (earlier named dementia praecox but changed to characterize split mind in Greek)) to describe the splitting in the mental functions between the patient and reality (5). He had three main criterions, or primary symptoms, still being used in today's psychiatry for diagnosing schizophrenia:

- Disturbed thought, especially difficulties in the logic and disorganization of thoughts
- Disturbed emotions, especially the presence of irrelevant feelings and numbness.
- Autism i.e. social withdrawal.

This triad was complemented by a number of secondary symptoms like hallucinations, fixed delusions, catatonia, lack of self-care, and strange ways of speaking and acting. The schizophrenic state was during the last century understood in more and more depth psychodynamically and seen as caused by the mental defense called "splitting", during which a substantial part of the patient's consciousness, emotional and sexual life is repressed (6,7); splitting is a different, more primitive and more radical defense than what we usually call repression in therapy. Spitting was understood psychodynamically as being the emotionally challenged child's psychic survival position. The purpose of assuming the position of splitting was saving the patient's vulnerable core of existence from the threat of destruction by the insensitive contact with parents not meeting the child's sensitive mind and spirit the way it needed to be met. This is not to blame the parents who undoubtedly are doing their best; but some children are extremely sensitive, and some parents are not.

This transformation of an open and vulnerable child into a protective person living in a safe shell of numbness and isolation explained how and why the patient turned herself into a disconnected and severely dysfunctional being. "Fear of dying" – or even panic - is according to the psychodynamic theory the permanent, emotional state of the schizophrenic patient. To cure the schizophrenic patient the therapist must thus offer a "saving" that is perceived as safer than what is offered by the psychotic defense. When the therapist is offering this alternative "safe place" the patient can finally heal by opening up emotionally for the world once again, thus coming back to life and social life. Their might of course be a constitutional factor on the side of the child, like what have been called "karmic traumas" – energetically inherited existential imbalances - that makes such a healing very difficult. Sigmund Freud (1856-1939) (6) and Carl Gustav Jung (1875-1961) (7) saw correctly the psychotic defense as a very early mechanism – happening the first year of life or so or even before then, in the womb – and they were quite pessimistic about addressing this defense in therapy, as it firmly protected the fundamental existence of the being. Jung worked with Bleuler and was more optimistic than Freud in treating psychosis. The neurotic defense mechanisms like repression were seen as a more mature defense mechanism happening later in childhood, and only protecting the content of consciousness, not the container – the existence - itself. Freud believed that only the later were curable by psychoanalysis. Psychodynamic psychotherapists like Harold Frederic Searles (1918-) found in the middle of last century, that the deep existential problems of preventing the loss of self though splitting were actually also curable by psychodynamic psychotherapy, and Searles became famous for curing about 33% of his schizophrenic patients this way; and many more great psychotherapists have been able to cure schizophrenia during the last century (see below under discussion).

Also today psychiatric disorders can be treated by psychodynamic psychotherapy; this kind of therapy has recently in metaanalysis been found superior to standard psychiatric treatment (8-10). Standard psychiatric drug treatment is not curing the patient – and is not claiming to do so either - and it has severe side-effects/adverse effects from the psychopharmacological drugs and from negative implanted philosophy (11), making this treatment a less than perfect medical procedure (12). But it may still be useful in many cases, especially when psychotherapy has failed to help.

Unfortunately psychotherapy with schizophrenic patients can be extremely challenging for the therapist and medical treatment with neuroleptic drugs therefore more attractive and not time-consuming as psychodynamic psychotherapy, holistic therapy and other kinds of psychotherapy that induce recovery and salutogenesis. Only further research can tell us the fraction of patients that can be completely healed; even the most talented of therapists like Searles and Laing had to admit their failure in their attempt of curing schizophrenic patients. There have been critique of research with psychotherapy for schizophrenia, because was mostly done without control groups, but with schizophrenic patients we all know the poor outcome for the patients if not treated, or if treated with biomedicine (antipsychotic drugs like Chlorpromazine) (12), which is exactly why the therapists did not bother to have a control group.

## Etiology of schizophrenia

Today most researchers interpret the findings of a concordance of .25 to .5 in the many monozygotic twin-studies of schizophrenia as proof of a genetic trait and an environmental trait as well (13). Obviously the factor most dominant is the environmental, estimated from the size of the found concordances.

New information about the life as foetus comes from foetal regression, where adult patients and researchers engaged in regression back to the womb; a method practiced for many years by Tibetan Yogis (14), but until recently seen as impossible (15,16) as the foetus has no mature brain – and the early foetus no brain at all. The validity of such experiences has been tested and often the remembered facts were found to be actually correct (15,16), although this is still an issue of debate. The foetus being a conscious being interacting with the world, and actively adapting to the circumstances of life is in severe contrast to the much more mechanical interpretation of embryonic development held by science until recently. If the subjective data about foetal adaptation is found to be valid the twin studies must be reinterpreted. The twin studies are thus neglecting that monozygotic twins are in very close contact to each other in the womb, and that the foetuses are actually aware and communicating and sharing many subjective experiences in the womb also, which might as well as bad genes explain the found concordance.

From the perspective of clinical holistic medicine, where patients go back into the womb very often, and where these experiences are giving meaning and value to the process of existential healing of the most early defense, there is no doubt that environmental factors by far dominates the genetic influence. This is the reason why schizophrenia and other mental illnesses seemingly founded already in the womb in many cases can be healed in holistic existential therapy.

Under all circumstances it is important to stress that the often-heard argument that schizophrenia is in fact an incurable genetic disease documented by the many monozygotic twin studies is not valid; the concordance is much too low to substantiate this view. Data is quite opposite is favour of the view that schizophrenia primarily is a psychosocially induced disturbance, which therefore possibly can be cured by the persisting psychosocial problems from the patient's past being solved. Future clinical research will tell us, if our optimistic interpretation of data is substantiated.

# Diagnostic guidelines (ICD-10, F20 schizophrenia)

In the ICD-10 system the normal requirement for a diagnosis of schizophrenia is that a minimum of one very clear symptom (and usually two or more if less clear-cut) belonging to any one of the groups listed as (a) to (d) below, or symptoms from at least two of the groups referred to as (e) to (h), should have been clearly present for most of the time during a period of one month or more. Conditions meeting such symptomatic requirements but of duration less than one month (whether treated or not) should be diagnosed in the first instance as acute schizophrenia-like psychotic disorder and are classified as schizophrenia if the symptoms persist for longer periods.

a) thought echo, thought insertion or withdrawal, and thought broadcasting;
b) delusions of control, influence, or passivity, clearly referred to body or limb movements or specific thoughts, actions, or sensations; delusional perception;
c) hallucinatory voices giving a running commentary on the patient's behaviour, or discussing the patient among themselves, or other types of hallucinatory voices coming from some part of the body;
d) persistent delusions of other kinds that are culturally inappropriate and completely impossible, such as religious or political identity, or superhuman powers and abilities (e.g. being able to control the weather, or being in communication with aliens from another world);

e) persistent hallucinations in any modality, when accompanied either by fleeting or half-formed delusions without clear affective content, or by persistent over-valued ideas, or when occurring every day for weeks or months on end;
f) breaks or interpolations in the train of thought, resulting in incoherence or irrelevant speech, or neologisms;
g) catatonic behaviour, such as excitement, posturing, or waxy flexibility, negativism, mutisme, and stupor;
h) "negative" symptoms such as marked apathy, paucity of speech, and blunting or incongruity of emotional responses, usually resulting in social withdrawal and lowering of social performance; it must be clear that these are not due to depression or to neuroleptic medication;
i) a significant and consistent change in the overall quality of some aspects of personal behaviour, manifest as loss of interest, aimlessness, idleness, a self-absorbed attitude, and social withdrawal.

## Diagnostic criteria (DSM-IV code 295 schizophrenia)

The DSM-IV system is basically focusing on the same symptoms, but we are using a slightly different system:

*A. Characteristic symptoms:* Two (or more) of the following, each present for a significant portion of time during a one month period (or less if successfully treated):

- delusions
- hallucinations
- disorganized speech (e.g., frequent derailment or incoherence)
- grossly disorganized or catatonic behaviour
- negative symptoms, i.e., affective flattening, alogia, or avolition

Note: Only one Criterion A symptom is required if delusions are bizarre or hallucinations consist of a voice keeping up a running commentary on the person's behaviour or thoughts, or two or more voices conversing with each other.

*B. Social/occupational dysfunction*: For a significant portion of the time since the onset of the disturbance, one or more major areas of functioning such as work, interpersonal relations, or self-care are markedly below the level achieved prior to the onset (or when the onset is in childhood or adolescence, failure to achieve expected level of interpersonal, academic, or occupational achievement).

*C. Duration:* Continuous signs of the disturbance persist for at least 6 months. This 6-month period must include at least 1 month of symptoms (or less if successfully treated) that meet Criterion A (i.e., active-phase symptoms) and may include periods of prodromal or residual symptoms. During these prodromal or residual periods, the signs of the disturbance may be manifested by only negative symptoms or two or more symptoms listed in Criterion A present in an attenuated form (e.g., odd beliefs, unusual perceptual experiences).

*D. Schizoaffective and mood disorder exclusion:* Schizoaffective disorder and mood disorder with psychotic features have been ruled out because either 1) no major depressive, manic, or mixed episodes have occurred concurrently with the active-phase symptoms; or 2) if mood episodes have occurred during active-phase symptoms, their total duration has been brief relative to the duration of the active and residual periods.

*E. Substance/general medical condition exclusion*: The disturbance is not due to the direct physiological effects of a substance (e.g., a drug of abuse, a medication) or a general medical condition.

Relationship to a pervasive developmental disorder: If there is a history of Autistic disorder or another pervasive developmental disorder, the additional diagnosis of schizophrenia is made only if prominent delusions or hallucinations are also present for at least a month (or less if successfully treated). As both diagnostic systems use almost the same pathognomonic criteria, it has been quite easy to establish the diagnosis with great certainty for almost a century.

## Clinical Holistic Medicine (CHM) and schizophrenia

In CHM schizophrenia is seen as the most extreme state of lack of sense of coherence (17-25). The purpose of CHM is rehabilitating the sense of coherence through healing somatoform and psychoform dissociation and rehabilitation of the patients physical, emotional, mental and spiritual contact with other people though the channels of body and mind. To obtain this polyvalent effect the standard short-term psychodynamic psychotherapy (STPP) - traditionally focusing on the patient's emotional mind and sexuality - is complemented with bodywork (of Marion Rosen type) (26) and philosophy of life (27-36).

CHM is using the life mission theory (25,37-42) to understand the degeneration of the self into the ego, the shadow, the evil side of man, the loss of libido and talents though the repression of painful emotions, and the loss of existential coherence though the loss of energy, meaning, light and joy (25). CHM uses an expanded toolbox[43] and four central healing principles (44-46):

Induce healing of the whole existence of the patient (also called salutogenesis) (17,18,45,46) and not only his/her body or mind. The healing often includes goals like recovering purpose and meaning of life by improving existential coherence and ability to love, understand and function sexually.

Adding as many resources to the patient as possible (6,7,15-18,45,46), as the primary reason for originally repressing the emotionally charged material was lack of resources - love, understanding, empathy, respect, care, acceptance and acknowledgement - to mention a few of the many needs of the little child. The principle was also to use the minimal intervention necessary by first using conversational therapy, then in addition philosophical exercises if needed, then adding bodywork or if needed adding role plays, group therapy and finally when necessary in a few cases, referring to a psychiatrist for psychotropic intervention. If the patient was in somatic or psychiatric treatment already at the beginning of the therapy, this treatment was continued with support from the holistic therapist.

Using the similarity principle that seems to be a fundamental principle for all holistic healing (45,46). The similarity principle is based on the belief that what made the person sick originally will make the patient well again, when given in the right, therapeutic dose.

This principle leads to often dramatic events in the therapy and to efficient and fast healing, but seems to send the patient into a number of crises that must be handled professionally (47-49). The scientific background for a radical and fast healing using the similarity principle is analyzed in (50-55).

Using Hering's Law of Cure (50-55) supporting the patient going once again through all the disturbances and diseases – in reverse order - that brought the patient to where he or she is now.

Other important axioms of Hering's Law of Cure is that the disease goes from more to less important organs, goes from the inside out, and goes from upside down. The scientific rationale for the last three axioms is less clear than for the first: the patient must go back his time-line to integrate all the states and experiences s/he has met on her/his way to disease. Going back in time is normally done though spontaneous regression in holistic existential therapy.

Using these tools and principles many physical, mental, sexual and existential problems can be addressed (1-10,46-48,57-81) with satisfactory results (82-86). Even severe mental problems can be alleviated (4,5,85) and in several cases patients with schizophrenia have been cured (see cases below) (5,85,87,88), but we still need research to document the effect of CHM with a large group of well-diagnosed, schizophrenic patients. As the patients we have been working with might be in the more healthy part of the schizophrenic spectrum (see the cases below) we have been warned that many schizophrenic patients will be more difficult to cure.

## Clinical holistic treatment of schizophrenia and other psychotic diseases

While many of the psychiatric diseases can be efficiently treated with short-term psychodynamic psychotherapy, schizophrenia still seems to challenge the psychodynamic psychotherapist. The most difficult aspect of the therapy is how to engage the patient in the often quite unpleasant therapy.

The autistic aspect of schizophrenia makes it difficult to get into contact at all; the severe emotional disturbances makes it difficult to get into a normal relationship with the patient, and the severe thought disturbances makes it difficult to talk in a coherent and meaningful way and to make a therapeutic contract with the patient. The patient's hallucinations make it difficult to share a common reality; delusions gives birth to strange behaviour and idiosyncratic logic; apathy, paucity of speech, and blunting or incongruity of emotional responses results in general social withdrawal and lowering of social performance often leaving the patient without any resources and thus taking the patient completely out of the "game of life".

So where to start? The goal is to help the patient back into the world as a contributing person; the practical solution of clinical holistic medicine is using a "the triple handle": the patient is contacted though body, mind and total being (spirit) at the same time.

The therapy uses whatever aspect the patient offers, for getting into contact and inviting a proper therapeutic response. The fundamental goal of the existential therapy is always to induce salutogenesis, or existential healing. Existential healing happens when the patient intents to heal, and gets the resources needed for the healing process from the outside at the same time. During the process of healing, the patient will heal in three dimensions:

- The outer world – healing relations and ability of function
- The inner world – healing emotions, philosophy of life and existential problems
- The presence - healing the psychoform and somatoform dissociation through contact, communication and development of the vital sense of coherence.

The therapy must have a balanced focus on these three dimensions at all times.

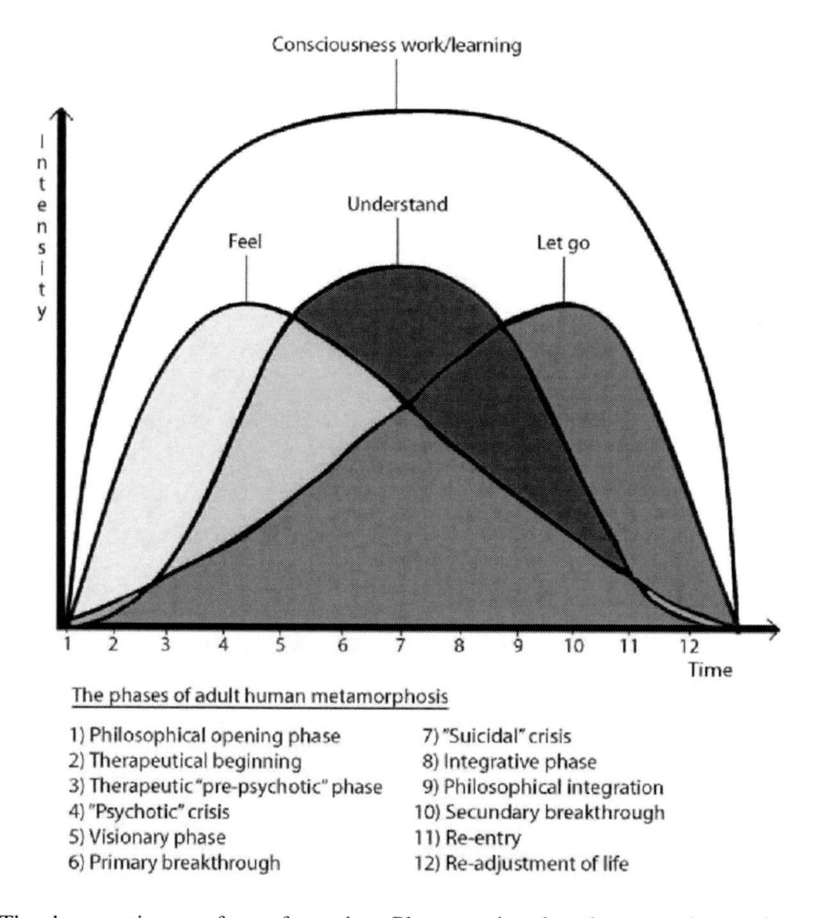


Figure 1. The therapeutic arc of transformation. Please notice that there are three existential crises connected to the process of healing from schizophrenia: loss of old, safe self and survival mechanism (giving up the splitting) – often (re)experienced by the patient as a psychic death (number 4) in the figure); the visionary phase often called the healing crisis and often experienced as "holy madness" by the patient (number 5 and 6); and the most intense, existential crisis of "to be or not to be" – often experiences as a suicidal crises by the patient (number 7), where the basic value of life is considered, and where the patient finally must choose life as it is (78).

# A standard course of clinical holistic therapy

With severely mentally ill patients, the existential healing is happening according to the metaphor of metamorphosis (78): The patient is like a caterpillar, getting into the pupae stage to remember her true nature and transform, and finally reappearing likes the butterfly. The phases of the existential healing seen though this metaphor is depicted in figure 1, which has been explained in an earlier chapter.

Please notice that the patient supported by holistic therapy is neither getting psychotic, mad, nor suicidal in the crises mentioned in the legend of figure 1. The names refer to the subjective experience of the phases of healing, not to the patient's external and objective behaviour.

Actually, the patient is normally coming back to life during these crises, but the emotional intensity demands the most intense support and holding, often by several therapists at a time. The use of the concepts in CHM is thus very different from the use of the same concepts in standard psychiatry, as the concepts refer to the subjective experience, not to the objective symptoms.

When it comes to the most ill schizophrenic patients it might be impossible to give the holding and support needed at all times, so it might be that we actually see psychotic relapses during therapy with this group of patients; such relapses might also be understood as a habitual pattern of defensive behaviour, and as a re-experiencing and reintegrating of earlier psychotic events.

# Key concepts

## A. Personal development of quality of life and insight in self

To engage a severely mentally ill patient in therapy the fundamental metaphor must be easily understood and appealing. The concept of personal development is doing the job for most patients. The rehabilitation of the patient's character has been alpha and omega since Hippocrates (1).

## B. Body-mind-spirit-existence (wholeness)

Holistic therapy makes it possible for the therapist to work with the whole patient, not only his mind. To define the therapy as holistic will open up for the therapist's use of bodywork, philosophical exercises etc. that immediately mobilizes patient-resources that cannot be activated within the standard frame of psychodynamic psychotherapy.

## C. Purpose of life – good and evil (41)

To engage the patient in a deep self-exploration looking for the hidden purpose of life is often very helpful with the mentally ill patient. To explore the shadow – the good purpose reversing into the evil intent often troubling the patient – might be the door to a common understanding of the world, the illness and the therapy – the later as the way out of the underworld, in which the patent finds himself caught.

### D. Clinical holistic medicine: Holding and processing

Love and support is necessary for the patient to relax, lean in, and assimilate the offered resources to get the process of healing going. The picture of the therapy as the therapist keeping a firm grip of the patient in one hand, and beating him with the other – the good and the evil parent in one – is often giving much sense to the patient.

### E. Spontaneous regression, symbolic processing, death-rebirth, foetal regression, re-experiencing conception

When the patient receives the resources needed for existential healing he will go back to the painful moments of childhood where he repressed large part of his consciousness to survive (the trauma causing the patients splitting). We call this process for spontaneous regression. It can take the patient all the way back to his first years of life, to his birth, even into the womb and all the way back to conception. Even if this gives no sense for a sceptical mind, this is what the patients often experience in therapy, as first noticed by Grof (15,16) and before that by the tradition of Tibetan Buddhism (14) and other ancient mystery schools. The re-experience of conception often gives a strong feeling of direction in life, and of primary talent (the life mission) (25,37-42).

### F. Rehabilitation of patient's talents of sex, consciousness and love

The primary talents of the patient is related to body, mind and spirit – and thus to sexuality, consciousness, and love (39). Many researchers in the treatment of schizophrenia has been focusing on rehabilitation of the patients sexuality; Wilhelm Reich, Harold F Searles and many other outstanding therapist believed that the main etiology to schizophrenia and most other mental diseases was the patient's unconscious repression of genital sexuality. We believe that the ability to love and understand is as important for mental health as the ability to function sexually.

### G. From isolation and meaninglessness to contribution and sense of coherence

One extremely important issue in CHM is the rehabilitation of the sense of coherence. This is achieved by rehabilitation of the patient's constructive attitude and behaviour towards other people and the surrounding world. Using the talent for being of value to other is the essence of love, and when the patient is able to love and contribute, (s)he is often well again.

## H. Philosophy of life – from negative, destructive and delusions to rational and constructive understanding

Rehabilitating the patient's positive and constructive, natural philosophy of life and rational thoughts is the most important condition for a permanent cure (5). The negative philosophy is actually a sum of hundreds of negative decisions though life, each holding on to a negative emotion from a painful life event. In the therapy, as the emotional charge is removed from the personal history, a constructive and positive philosophy of life is slowly reappearing.

## I. The metaphor of metamorphosis – psychic death, transformation, and re-entry in the world

The schizophrenic patient's flow of consciousness is most often filled with negative issues like death, illness, rotten flesh, urine and faces, perverted sex, incest, homosexuality, rape, sadomasochism, paedophilia, violence, all kinds of evilness and torture, darkness and death. The acceptance of all these elements and the rational explanation of these elements dominating position in the patient's mind are often experienced as a great relief.

The therapist being familiar with all these emotionally difficult subjects and accepting them allows the patient to share for the first time in his or her life the true content of the stream of consciousness.

These elements have been classical elements of the traditions of Tantra (14,89,90) and other mystery schools; but most people do not accept to talk about them, even when they are present in there experiential life, as they are a strong taboo of contemporary western culture and society. To allow the patient to engage fully in the exploration of the shadow side of modern man and western culture is often a major key to healing.

## J. The healing crisis, hole madness, and crazy wisdom

With hundreds of thousands of hit in a yahoo.com or google.com search, these concepts are well integrated in contemporary spiritual culture. Originally coming from the orient, most people engaged in serious, spiritual development now know them. They signify the wisdom coming from within and materializing itself though dreams and visions in states of expanded consciousness.

These states are introduced by meditation, holotropic breath work, foetal regression, or other intense self-explorative techniques. Most unfortunately, many psychiatrists do not know them, and to not recognize when the patient has entered a healing crises that is an obligatory part of any recovery from schizophrenia.

Instead of supporting the patient in the vital project of self-exploration these doctors take the patient "down" from the expanded state of consciousness with antipsychotic drugs, thus arresting the spontaneous healing taking place.

### K. Wounded healer

The only way a therapist can truly help his patient is by letting him be the tool for the patient's healing. To do that he must admit that he is only a human being himself; he must admit that he has all human flares and faults himself; he must admit that he is also a wounded child, and not perfect yet; he is also in the process of human development and in that sense very much in the same position as the patient. Only by sharing the common human conditions, and being together in a true fellowship, can the therapist give sufficient support and holding for the patient to heal the core of his existence.

### L. Confronting the evil in whatever form

We are as evil as we are good. We pretend that we are good, or we repress our evil side to our shadow, but when we are true and honest we must admit, that only by choosing the good and abandoning the evil, can we become decent and ethical human beings. Owing the evil is mandatory for the schizophrenic patient, as splitting of the evil side of man is the most common kind of splitting. Secondary is the splitting of the body and sexuality, or of the divine, spiritual aspect of the patient's being.

### M. Negative decisions and axiomatic thinking

A trauma always consists of an unbearable feeling and a life-denying, negative decision. This decision is a generalized justification that works as an axiomatic basis for the interpretation of the patient's world. These negative decisions is behind the delusions that the patient presents, and only by taking the patient all the way back to the fundamental emotional pain of the trauma fixating the negative believe, can the patient get rid of his delusions.

Table 1(78) is a list of the most important negative and life-denying sentences that was released during the therapy, when the patient healed her borderline condition. The sentences were the essence of the gestalts that was integrated in the therapy; they are both feelings and thoughts at the same time, making them extremely to the point of the experience.

### N. The fundamental conditions of existence (the "philosophical existentials")

Every person is alive and therefore going to die, which create anxiety; every person is autonomous and therefore basically alone; and every person is intending to contribute in love, and therefore failing and suffering. These three existential pains are inevitable, and every conscious person on Earth must bare these fundamental conditions for being a human being. This must be thoroughly understood by the patient, who normally thing that this is unique and horrible conditions that God gave this pour soul.

**Table 1. The 25 most importance sentences a borderline patient did let go of in holistic therapy (CHM); while letting go of these decisions she healed her existence and recovered from a severely dysfunctional state. The traumas were sexual abuse in her childhood (78)**

| |
|---|
| 1. Nobody likes me |
| 2. I don't want to know it |
| 3. I can't stay anywhere |
| 4. I am out in the space |
| 5. This is unreal |
| 6. I am empty |
| 7. I am hollow |
| 8. It is not me |
| 9. I can do nothing |
| 10. I do not need you |
| 11. I need nobody |
| 12. I cannot do that |
| 13. I am a failure |
| 14. There is no room for me |
| 15. I am nothing |
| 16. It is absurd |
| 17. She is a schizophrenic |
| 18. I am a schizophrenic |
| 19. I do not deserve to live |
| 20. Why didn't they kill me? |
| 21. I get smashed up |
| 22. I go to pieces |
| 23. She is going to kill me |
| 24. He is going to kill me |
| 25. They are going to kill me |

## O. Precautions

To make psychodynamic therapy with CHM a success there are certain issues of crucial importance:

1) Avoid high age. The older the patient, the more difficult the therapy.
2) Avoid institutionalization. The longer time at an institution, the more difficult the therapy.
3) Avoid pharmaceutical drugs. The higher the dose and the longer time treated, the more difficult the therapy. If the patient is already a psychiatric patient on antipsychotic drugs, who wishes a CHM-treatment, this situation must be handled carefully. For the CHM-therapy to be efficient patients need their full intellectual capacity; as they often experience the antipsychotic drugs as sedating they will often insist on coming of the antipsychotic drugs. We find this reasonable and suggest that it happens gradually, with the patients well supported, in a number of well-controlled

steps. Sometimes the patients want to get of the drugs right away which might make them re-enter their original psychosis; this can be very therapeutic, but only if there are sufficient therapeutic resources available (several therapists and holders 24hours/7day a week). Most often in our experience the patients who wants to get of the drugs do not have compliance and only pretend to take the drugs, making this problem much less that it might seem.

4) Avoid giving a psychiatric diagnosis if possible. The more the patient thinks of herself as "schizophrenic", the more difficult the therapy. If they already have a diagnosis, this must be carefully explained as something temporary and not something final.
5) Avoid negative, philosophical implants. The more hopeless the patient believes her situation to be, the more difficult the therapy.
6) Handle the transference of love and sexuality with great care. The more the patient feels rejected and judged, the more difficult the therapy.
7) Handle the acute psychosis with patients and love. The more severe the trauma from losing control to psychosis is, the more difficult is future therapy.
8) Prevent suicide attempts. The more attempts, the more difficult the therapy.
9) Prevent self-mutilating, self-abuse, humiliation, and loss of: friends and social network, social reality like school, family, self-worth, and self-respect. The deeper the patient falls, the less resources and the more difficult the therapy. One efficient way to do this is by having a person (a "mentor" or a "sponsor") entering into a close, intimate, supportive relation with the patient, for a while being his or her "best friend".

## Case stories

*Psychotic illness in a 7-year-old boy caused by implanted philosophy and cured in one hour (5)*

A 7-year-old boy was taken into therapy, because he day-and-night washed his face and hands every 30 minutes, obsessively. He went furious if somebody stopped him doing this. VandenBos (5) discovered during a one hour session that cured the boy that a doctor had implanted the understanding that the nerves was worms living under his skin. Just clearing the misunderstanding cured the boy. If VandenBos had not examined the boy and cleared this up he would have been taking to a psychiatric ward, and the normal procedure and the trauma of the hospitalization in itself could easily had given symptoms that would have confirmed the tentative diagnoses of schizophrenia. This could easily have turned the child into a chronic patient as VandenBos concluded[5]. If only all cases were this easy!

*Schizophrenic 30-year-old male cured by three years of holistic therapy (CHM).*

30-year-old man who had lived a protected life on a small island. From early childhood he had lived with his grandparents, as his own parents could not raise him. When he came to the clinic he had for years suffered from emotional blunting and an almost complete withdrawal from other people (autism); he had severe delusions of living in outer space combined with strongly peculiar obsessive, catatonic behaviour (standing fixated on top of telephone boxes to be close to other people) combined with the symptoms of subjective depersonalization and de-realization. At the time he started therapy he considered committing suicide, but was also very scared of dying (ambivalence). He was severely visually hallucinated. He was thinking according to his own personal logic. He sometimes used prostitutes, which he mostly paid to talk with him, which was his only contact to the other sex. On the quality of life scale (QOL5) he rated himself as 4 (bad; 1-5, five being bottom of scale); he was rating his self-evaluated mental health as "poor" (4 on the five point Likert scale).

This patient who had persistent hallucinations (e), catatonic behaviour (g), negative symptoms (h), significant and consistent change in personal behaviour, and social withdrawal (i) was diagnosed /F20 Schizophrenia/ according to ICD-10. He was presumably catatonic schizophrenic, but this diagnosis was not used.

He was in the beginning of the CHM-therapy only treated philosophically, as philosophical discussions was the only contact possible with this patient; the patient was given books to read and then the content discussed with the therapist (SV). The books were about philosophy of life, like Buber[91], and Chopra[92]. The patient was clearly intelligent (IQ not measured) and this resource was used. In the next, psychodynamic phase of the therapy, he came into contact with his feelings and went through the existential crisis that is standard with CHM (see figure 1) and was now given the challenging exercises to confront his enormous anxiety. He had to visualize that the anxiety was a fire where he was burned and purified. We did this successfully. Then he was supported in confronting his visual hallucinations, which he also managed to do.

The next theme was supporting him in confronting his problems with women and sexuality. He let go of his use of prostitutes and used his sexual drive to go to town and meet and talk to women; after months of demanding, behavioral training he finally managed to behave socially acceptable on a dance floor, and finally he got a girlfriend and a semi-normal sexual life.

After four month of therapy one hour a week, and intensive writings of dozens of full pages in the form of a patients diary, the patient was able to use the concepts from therapy and from the books he has been reading in his thinking; and for the first time in his life he had a valid language for his strange, alienated perceptions. This made him reflect upon himself and he realized how sick he really was: "Today I was surprised to realize that I really have hallucinations…I jumped into a state of death, with no ability at all to express my sense of I-Thou".

The middle phase of therapy consisted of holistic bodywork (a female holistic physiotherapist) to help him; she managed to take the patient back to the most painful part of early childhood, where the patient were abandoned by his mother (and father), and in healing these old, deep wounds on the patient's soul, he finally came back into normal, emotional contact (induction of salutogenesis through the parallel healing of psychoform and somatoform dissociation).

The third and final part of the therapy was focusing on supporting the patient in creating a new philosophy of life that allowed him to step into character and use his bodily, mental and spiritual talents (25,42).

The CHM-case record for this patient is close to 100 pages, most of them written by the patient. They demonstrate the complete transformation in the patient's logic, value system, relationship with himself and the world, and sexuality. He is not yet able to love other people in a normal way, but he is still recovering, and there is no doubt that his sense of coherence is being rehabilitated. At the end of therapy three years after he started, he rated his QOL5 as 3 (intermediate) and his self-evaluated mental health as "good" (2 on the five point Likert scale). He had no longer hallucinations (symptom e), his catatonic behaviour was gone (g), his negative symptoms gone (h), his significant and consistent change in personal behaviour and social withdrawal (i) was radically improved. Thus he did no longer fit the diagnosis of /ICD10-F20 Schizophrenia/ (or DSM-IV Code 295). The patient was thus cured after about 40 sessions (one every third week) of CHM-therapy during three years. He continued in therapy for another year to improve his general ability, and after that he went to university to take his MSc in computer science, where he did well.

> *Schizophrenic 15-year-old male cured by two years of holistic therapy (CHM).*
>
> This 15-year old boy was brought to the Research Clinic for Holistic Medicine by his parents, who were not satisfied with the results from several years of psychiatric treatment with neuroleptic drugs and hospitalization at an institution for violent young mentally ill patients. The parents believed that the drugs did not help him, that he got too much medicine, which sedated him without curing him, as they did not see any improvement as time went by.
>
> He had been extremely violent in school, clearly psychotic and living in strong delusions of being another person, a German soldier from the Second World War, which life he clearly remembered. The things he told from his personal story were strongly worrying; amongst other things he had been just about to kill a friend at school, of which he was rather proud – it proved that he was the strong Nazi-soldier he believed himself to be. He was hallucinated and saw his father as an English pilot he remembered that he killed during the war.
>
> We accepted to take him into CHM-therapy and the municipality accepted to pay for the therapy (yearly cost for the institution was about 150,000 Euro, the cost of treatment in our clinic about 4,000 Euro a year). According to ICD-10 he was clearly having the following symptoms:
>
> (d) persistent delusions that are culturally inappropriate
> (e) persistent visual hallucinations occurring every day for months on end
> (h) "negative" symptoms such as blunting and incongruity of emotional responses
> (i) a significant and consistent change in the overall quality of personal behaviour

According to ICD-10 his diagnosis was thus /F20 Schizophrenia/. In the beginning of the therapy the patient was very vulnerable and weak in the emotional contact; he went through a big transformation process and astonishingly ended up on his feet as a healthy young man who is doing well socially and at school. He stopped the medicine during the first months of therapy by himself, without sharing is with anybody, and obviously without needing it any more.

In the therapy evilness was the big theme, and after months of confrontation of his shadow (his evil side) he ended up by choosing to be good and letting go of his idea of being the German warrior. After this fundamental shift in his personal philosophy, he was able to slowly regain empathy and emotional contact; he went back to school where he is doing really fine and caching up on the three years he missed. After a few episodes of moderate violence (fighting with the other boys) he managed to get his anger and furry under control, and continues to developed into a well-functioning boy, that is fitting in and being appreciated by the other kids. He got a girlfriend, which is very good for his self-esteem and feeling of being a young man, growing up and participating in society. He is now of great help to his family, and his progress highly appreciated.

In the holistic therapy using also bodywork the patient's psychoform and somatoform dissociations were healed and his sense of coherence slowly recovered. After two years and about 40 sessions he was out of regular therapy, but he continued for follow-up sessions every six months. About a year after the therapy ended he got the following statement from his teacher at school:

"PATIENT NAME has in relation to diligence and cooperation been doing satisfactorily work. He has been positive and very engaged in the subjects. In the class room PATIENT NAME has contributed creating a good and positive atmosphere as a good listener and friend. PATIENT NAME has furthermore good relations to the school staff. The school therefore gives him the best recommendations."

His delusions, hallucination, incongruity emotional responses, and behavioural disturbances including his tendency to violence have now completely gone. Thus he did no longer fit with the diagnosis of /ICD10-F20 Schizophrenia/ (or DSM-IV Code 295).

## Challenges for the therapist

Working with schizophrenic patients gives the therapist all the challenges you can with for – and a little more. Only if you are up to an intense project of accelerated self-development and an exploration into your own shadow for deep self-insight, will you find it really rewarding to work with this group of patients. Below is listed the challenges that we have met in our work with the patients.

All symptoms and symbols are meaningful – the therapist must contain his confusion, because in the end all questions will be answered, but in the most surprising ways.

The sexual content of the patients unconscious will be explicit– most traumatic events shared by the patient refers to real events, whether it being incest or rape (5) and you must be worth your salt as a therapist when the patient brings this to the sessions.

*Implanted philosophy:* The most important gift the therapist can give his patient is his optimism about the patient's ability to heal and recover (5); often you can hardly believe that the patient has a chance, but you must choose to believe it.

Never expect your patient to be grateful or to acknowledge improvements. When a problem is gone – it is out of the patients mind forever. So keep a thorough case report and do not expect patients to remember their progress or even to thank you for curing them when they are cured (5).

The healthier the patient gets in the process, the more troubled will the patient's feelings and emotions be. An example from (5) is a girl that starts completely unable to have sex, and after successful therapy starts complaining about her not liking her new boyfriend much, and not getting too much pleasure from sex. She is not grateful at all for her being able to have the boyfriend now but only angry over things that are not right and perfect yet. This is clearly a patient healing. Only by keeping a good case record, this progress can be appreciated by the therapist.

The patient being more emotionally labile, angry, expressive and difficult is a good sign of the patient healing. Most therapists – as most parents – do not really appreciate people getting more powerful, selfish, and demanding. But it is a fine sign of individuation. Emotional crisis will get more and more intense and more and more frequent. That is the patient coming back to life, which is always painful. Often the awakening sexuality will give the patient strong sexual feelings and a most uncomfortable and embarrassing behaviour, especially when the patient is transferring sexuality on the therapist. This is not the patient getting sicker but the patient getting into a developmental state similar to retarded puberty, and the sexuality of the patient must not be condemned or repressed it the therapist wants the patient to recover.

The patient's borders are often transgressed and badly defined. Most patients have never had a private room in their life, and the establishment of such a sacred, personal space is a necessity for the patient to recover his identity. To support the patient in having such a space, the therapist must accept the patient to have secrets.

*Counter transferences are often difficult.* The schizophrenic patient is often living in a self-made hell that we do not want to look into; when we do so our empathy courses us unbearable pain. Especially sharing the position of feeling reduced from being a person to being something like a mistreated animal, or even a thing without life and existence, puts us in severe agony. The patient's defense will make the patient do everything to hinder that we get close to the patient, so very often the patient will make himself dirty, ugly, repelling etc., just to make us keep an emotional distance to him. Some patients use urine, faces, saliva, dirty cloths etc. to make themselves less appealing. Psychotic patients presents their emotional, sexual etc. material in the most raw and least socially acceptable form for the same reason: To prove to themselves that we do not like them at all – the same way they felt rejected and not loved by their parents.

*Risking murder and suicide.* Psychotic patients do not have the inhibitions that normal people have. Sometimes they kill themselves, and sometimes they kill others. The psychology of a murder is often a patient that cannot accept angry impulses (cannot contain conscious anger), and represses these impulses till the day he explodes (5). Often sexuality and jealousy are central issues here. Most schizophrenic patients are not dangerous at all, but the therapist should use his intuition and common sense and be very careful, when the patient feels like a "bomb" of repressed anger, and is living in a conflict involving jealousy.

Most patients, whether psychotic or borderline, consider committing suicide during the therapy (5). Actually the suicidal crisis must be seen as an important part of the therapy, because this is when the patient for the first time in life really chooses life. Fortunately the consideration is hardly ever leading to the action of committing suicide, but the danger of the patient committing suicide must be considered in every consultation, and if suicidal thoughts are present, the issue must be directly addressed, to support the patient in taking the learning from the crisis, and preventing suicide.

Suicide, when actually committed, is often materializing the desperate intent of revenge. The calculation is that if the patient kills himself, the person(s) who failed the patient will be really sorry! Most often suicidal attempts are nothing but a cry for help – the young girl takes four sleeping pills and knows she will be found with the suicide letter in her hand. Much more seriously endangered is the 60-years old, male and recently retired patient that demonstrates the "presuicidale syndrome"(93).

It is very important to notice that research has shown that ECT (electroconvulsive therapy) is not preventing suicide, but just postpones it (94). The prescription of antipsychotic drugs is very dangerous in the case of a suicide threat, as everybody knows that drugs are often used to commit suicide; drugs are also taking the patient into depression enhancing the emotional drive against suicide (94).

*Risking violence from the patient.* Therapists are often exposed to threats and even at rare occasions to violence, when working on schizophrenic patients. Karon (5) described a patient putting a pin into her knee during a session, in the intent of making the therapist hate him. For most schizophrenic patients love and kindness is had to stand; hatred and anger are better, and emotionally cold rejection and even total lack of interest is making the patient feel safe.

*Mastering controlled fail of the patient.* The reason is that most schizophrenic patients comes from severely dysfunctional families, where they have survived without getting the love and close contact that is a normal part of other children's upbringing. The ability of the therapist to fail the patient intentionally, using the principle of similarity, is a central condition for being able to cure. Most therapists engage themselves in their patients; and when they are starting to know them they are often also coming to like them. In this case the holding is appropriate, and processing must follow. Here the therapist must shift between being the good father/mother of the patient, and the evil father/mother. Many therapists find this shifting necessary for supporting the schizophrenic patient most difficult.

*Containing self-mutilation.* Often the schizophrenic patients are self-destructive, and this must be contained by the therapist. When this is directly addressed, the reason for the impulses is often understood and self-mutilations stops. Karon described a self-mutilating patient that cut his arm using broken glass from a glass bulb[5]. Karon used the occasion to give the patient credit for stopping before the artery was cut: "I am proud of you. You stopped cutting yourself before somebody else had to stop you" (5). This direct confrontation without any judgment made the patient stop his self-mutilation.

*Patient that will not eat.* Karon and VandenBos (5) recommended psychotherapy during a meal as the key to solving this problem.

*Sleeping disorders.* Karon and VandenBos (5) recommended full accept of the state as solution, and recommended the patient not to sleep but just to lay down for eight hours of resting – without getting up during the night. Most patients argue that this is very boring, and the answer is to acknowledge the boredom, and reassure the patient that he will be able to function the next day.

*Illegal drugs.* Most schizophrenics are not attracted to heroin or other similar drugs, but if they are hallucinated, they can be very interested in hallucinogenic drugs that can enhance the hallucinations and give the patient insight in the nature and hidden courses of the hallucinations; regular use of high doses of hallucinogens are to be considered self-destructive (5) and the therapist should warn the patient against the negative consequences of abuse, like bad trips (drug-traumas) and flash backs (5).

## Discussion

Schizophrenia is today often regarded as the most difficult disease to treat with psychotherapy, especially when the patient is in a psychotic state, or hospitalized (95). Normally, therefore, the schizophrenic patient is treated with a drug, and only when the patient is back in a "normal" and communicative state of being, can additional psychotherapy be introduced.

Unfortunately only 1 in 4 or less reacts well to for example chlorpromazine and one in two gets serious physical side effects (12). The drug is also suspected to provoke severe mental adverse-effects with dysphoria, depression and even the feeling of "being like a zombie" (96). In addition to that, a spontaneous over-mortality of up to 150% has recently been documented by the Danish Health Authorities for specific subgroups (97).

The standard psychiatric treatment is known not to cure schizophrenia, but only to reduce some of its symptoms, and schizophrenia is considered by most psychiatrists to be a chronic and incurable disease. The standard psychiatric treatment is thus a rather imperfect treatment for schizophrenia, and alternatives must be sought. Luckily the last decade has given us documentation of psychodynamic psychotherapy being efficient with mental diseases[8-10] and presumably also with schizophrenia (5,85,87,88).

Psychotherapy in patients with schizophrenia has been considered more difficult than the treatment of any other group of mental illnesses, due to the triad of autism, emotional "flattening" and not correctable delusions. When the contact with the patient is very poorly anchored in mind, feeling, and body, as we see it in patients with severe somatoform and psychoform dissociation, the possibility to have an impact on a patient is rather limited. If the patient is psychotic, and not oriented in time, space and own data, this becomes even harder. Seen from the therapist's perspective, there is no "handle" to get hold on the patient and start turning him back towards reality.

To solve this problem, we have expanded short-term psychodynamic psychotherapy with bodywork and philosophy of life exercises (47-49), giving the therapist a possibility to get in contact with the patient at a physical, mental and spiritual level at the same time. The triple grip of the patient allows us to work with even the most psychotic patient, although therapeutic progress is not always visible in the beginning of the therapy. We have observed in the patients that come to our clinic that three things are associated to a good outcome of therapy: the younger the patient is, the shorter time a patient has spent in a psychiatric ward, the shorter time the patient has been on antipsychotic drugs, and the shorter time the patient has been ill, the easier it is to help. We have worked with 10 insufficiently diagnosed schizophrenic/schizotypical patients and about 30 borderline patients (44) and have noticed a certain path of healing for these patients that often takes a quite dramatic form, when treated with clinical holistic medicine, with a quite number of severe existential crises before healing existentially (see figure 1).

We have been working on the schizophrenic patients directly with the deluded thoughts, the flattened emotions and the autistic withdrawal from the world. We have found that all these symptoms characterizing the schizophrenic patients can in most cases quite easily be traced back to severely dysfunctional family patterns of the patient's childhood. Especially the method of spontaneous regression, where taking the patient into foetal regression, has made is possible to include the prenatal adaptation to the future family, which has given many of the missing pieces to a full psychodynamic understanding of schizophrenia. These adaptations also seem to be able to explain the concordance seen in the twin studies with schizophrenic patients, stressing the environmental factors and thus giving an alternative hypothesis to the hypothesis of genetic courses of schizophrenia.

The patient is often found in a severely dysfunctional state of being, with very few if any stable intimate, personal, confidential contacts. So helping the patient back to life is basically about inducing salutogenesis by rehabilitating sense of coherence in two directions – inwards, towards life, and outwards, towards other people and the surrounding world. To induce the recovery of schizophrenia, the first thing to be done is to give the schizophrenic patient the optimal holding they need, to go back to confront old childhood traumas. In the therapy we normally give them two "new" parents: a male and a female therapist, who during therapy act as if they were the patient's "good" and "bad" parents. One of the therapists is good, while the other therapist evil, taking the patient back using the principle of similarity, while giving the patient all the loving and caring support needed for the existential healing.

We have found that as soon as we are able to engage the patient in the therapeutic contract, the therapy is starting to work. We have found that one in two of the schizophrenic patients (the limitation is our small sample) was cured during one year of holistic therapy. Unfortunately the limited number is not sufficient for statistical analysis and the diagnosis were not made strictly according to an international system like ICD10 or SDM-IV, so we are now conducting another experiment including a larger number of patients and more well-defined international diagnostic criteria.

Dissociation is a well-established phenomenon [DSM IV, 98-102] occurring in people who have experienced some form of trauma. Trauma can be defined as anything that overwhelms our resources (99). According to the Diagnostic and Statistical Manual for Mental Disorders, Fourth Edition (DSM-IV; American Psychiatric Association, 1994), the essential feature of dissociation is a disruption of the normal integrative functions of consciousness, memory, identity, and perception of the environment. Much of the research on dissociation emerged from the identification of Post-Traumatic Stress Disorder as a distinct condition. Van der Kolk (98) identified core symptoms of PTSD as intrusions (thoughts, dreams, flashbacks), hyper arousal and numbing. Dissociation is a real, biological phenomena arising from trauma, and both somatoform and psychoform dissociation must be healed to cure schizophrenia and other psychotic mental disorders.

It is still a matter of discussion if traumas are the underlying cause of schizophrenia; our success in healing a few schizophrenic patients by healing their traumas definitely points in this direction.

During the last two centuries thousands of therapists have succeeded to cure a fraction of their schizophrenic patients; we know that Philippe Pinel and his students with their moral therapy cured patients, but as the diagnosis schizophrenia (or dementia praecox) was not available yet, we do not know the fraction of cured schizophrenic patient. When data on the treatment of schizophrenia became available we see that 33% were cured and 33% radically improved, but the rest only little improvement or not helped by psychotherapy (Harold Searles statistics are documented in ([103], the introduction). Similar results were produced by a number of remarkable therapist, like Jung (1875-1961)(7), Adler (1870-1937)(104), Abraham (1877-1925)(105), Federn (1871-1950)(106), Harry Stack Sullivan and Frida Fromm Reichmann further developed by Will (1961)(107) and Searles (1965)(108), Schilder (1935)(109), Rosenfeld (1965)(110), Segal (1950)(111), Fairbairn (1954)(112), Guntrip (1969)(113), Perry (1961)(114), Lidz (1973)(115), Kernberg (1975,1976)(116,117), Volkan (1976)(118), Sechehaye (1951)(119), Rosen (1953)(120), Eissler (1952)(121), Arlow and Brenner (1964)(122), Giovacchini (1979)(123), Arieti (1974)(124), Bellak (1979)(125), Gendlin (1967)(126), Prouty (1976)(127), Gunderson and Mosher (1976)(128), and Karon and VandenBos (1981)(5). But even before Pinel and the psychotherapists the Hippocratic doctors healed the hysteric and mentally ill patients for millennia with holistic medicine.

In spite of this strong and scientifically well-established tradition many physicians today have come to believe, that schizophrenia cannot be treated with psychotherapy, which has been discussed by Karon and VandenBos (5). It seems that many physicians believe that it is very difficult and demands special skills, knowledge, talents and training to make therapy with schizophrenic patients available. Karon and VandenBos argued that this is not the case, since everybody who cares about people and knows elementary psychotherapy can treat schizophrenic patients, and although these patients can be very difficult, some of them are easy to help, and almost nobody is completely impossible to help (5).

# Conclusion

It is not new that psychodynamic psychotherapy and holistic medicine can help cure schizophrenia and other psychotic mental disorders. In one study Searles treated a group of 18 of the most heavy, chronically ill schizophrenics with duration of illness of in average 9,2 years, and 2,3 years of hospitalization on average before entrance into the study. After therapy 33,3% were cured ("remarkably improved" and out of hospital) and further 38,9% were "remarkably improved", but still hospitalized (103). Searles kept records of 600 patients for his research and continued to be optimistic throughout his life. It is generally believed that the earlier the treatment starts the better will be the therapeutic results. Based on the available data we estimate that schizophrenic patients can actually be cured by intensive holistic therapy, if they are treated right at onset of disease.

But to work with these "heavy" patients the therapist must be prepared to invest his whole existence and he must expect to be challenged at all levels of existence. To maximize the therapeutic effect of psychodynamic psychotherapy it must be turned into the system of clinical holistic medicine (CHM), also using bodywork and philosophy of life. CHM has been developed though the last two decades to treat even severely mentally ill patients, like schizophrenia.

There are many different factors to get hold of and a lot of theory to master before a therapist can treat schizophrenic patients easily. As a therapist you need to acknowledge the gift of a daily challenge. You need to appreciate the gift of not getting gratefulness in return for a most demanding and even exhausting job. You need to like to work with the human shadow, looking deep down into the evil, the sexual, the mystery, and the divine side of life. We need therapists and researchers to engage in the development of CHM, because we owe the patient a treatment that cures them, not just a treatment that alleviates some patients of the symptoms and give many more patients side effects. If you can love even the sickest person, if you can see all the illnesses you meet in your patient in yourself too, if you want to develop yourself and obtain wisdom, then working with schizophrenic patients might be the job of your dreams.

We find that holistic, psychodynamic treatment (CHM) is the cure of choice for schizophrenia, as the psychopharmacological treatment has proved less efficient with many side effects. We therefore recommend further research in scientific holistic therapy and its development.

# References


[1] Jones WHS. Hippocrates. Vol. I–IV. London: William Heinemann, 1923-1931.

[2] Ventegodt S, Clausen B, Omar HA, Merrick J. Clinical holistic medicine: Holistic sexology and acupressure through the vagina (Hippocratic pelvic massage). ScientificWorldJournal 2006;6:2066-79.

[3] Ventegodt S, Clausen B, Merrick J. Clinical holistic medicine: Pilot study on the effect of vaginal acupressure (Hippocratic pelvic massage). ScientificWorldJournal 2006;6:2100-16.

[4] Weiner DB. The clinical training of doctors. An essay from 1793 by Philippe Pinel.. Henry E Sigerist Suppl Bull Hist Med 1980;3:1-102.

[5] Karon BP, VandenBos G. Psychotherapy of schizophrenia. The treatment of choise. New York: Jason Aronson, 1981.

[6] Jones E. The life and works of Sigmund Freud. New York: Basic Books, 1961.

[7] Jung CG. Man and his symbols. New York: Anchor Press, 1964.

[8] Leichsenring F, Rabung S, Leibing E. The efficacy of short-term psychodynamic psychotherapy in specific psychiatric disorders: a meta-analysis. Arch Gen Psychiatry 2004;61(12):1208-16.

[9] Leichsenring F. Are psychodynamic and psychoanalytic therapies effective? A review of empirical data. Int J Psychoanal 2005;86(Pt 3):841-68.

[10] Leichsenring F, Leibing E. Psychodynamic psychotherapy: a systematic review of techniques, indications and empirical evidence. Psychol Psychother 2007;80(Pt 2):217-28.

[11] Ventegodt S, Kandel I, Merrick J. Clinical holistic medicine: How to recover memory without "implanting" memories in your patient. ScientificWorldJournal 2007;7:1579-589.

[12] Adams CE, Awad G, Rathbone J, Thornley B. Chlorpromazine versus placebo for schizophrenia. Cochrane Database Syst Rev 2007;18(2):CD000284.

[13] Sullivan PF, Kendler KS, Neale MC. Schizophrenia as a complex trait: evidence from a meta-analysis of twin studies. Arch Gen Psychiatry 2003;60(12):1187-92.

[14] Sambhava P, Thurman RA, Pa KG. The Tibetan book of the dead. New York: Bantam, 1994.

[15] Grof S. LSD psychotherapy: Exploring the frontiers of the hidden mind. Alameda, CA: Hunter House, 1980.

[16] Grof S. Psychology of the future. Albany, NY: State Univ New York Press, 2000.

[17] Antonovsky A. Health, stress and coping. London: Jossey-Bass, 1985.

[18] Antonovsky A. Unravelling the mystery of health. How people manage stress and stay well. San Franscisco: Jossey-Bass, 1987.

[19] Flensborg-Madsen T, Ventegodt S, Merrick J. Sense of coherence and physical health. A Review of previous findings. ScientificWorldJournal 2005;5:665-73.

[20] Flensborg-Madsen T, Ventegodt S, Merrick J. Why is Antonovsky's sense of coherence not correlated to physical health? Analysing Antonovsky's 29-item sense of coherence scale (SOCS). ScientificWorldJournal 2005;5:767-76.

[21] Flensborg-Madsen T, Ventegodt S, Merrick J. Sense of coherence and health. The construction of an amendment to Antonovsky's sense of coherence scale (SOC II). ScientificWorldJournal 2006;6: 2133-9.

[22] Flensborg-Madsen T, Ventegodt S, Merrick J. Sense of coherence and physical health. A cross-sectional study using a new SOC scale (SOC II). ScientificWorldJournal 2006;6:2200-11.

[23] Flensborg-Madsen T, Ventegodt S, Merrick J. Sense of coherence and physical health. Testing Antonovsky's theory. ScientificWorldJournal 2006;6:2212-9.

[24] Flensborg-Madsen T, Ventegodt S, Merrick J. Sense of coherence and health. The emotional sense of coherence (SOC-E) was found to be the best-known predictor of physical health. ScientificWorldJournal 2006;6:2147-57.

[25] Ventegodt S, Flensborg-Madsen T, Andersen NJ, Merrick J. Life mission theory VII: Theory of existential (Antonovsky) coherence: a theory of quality of life, health and ability for use in holistic medicine. ScientificWorldJournal 2005;5:377-89.

[26] Rosen M, Brenner S. Rosen method bodywork. Accessing the unconscious through touch. Berkeley, CA: North Atlantic Books, 2003.

[27] Hermansen TD, Ventegodt S, Rald E, Clausen B, Nielsen ML, Merrick J. Human development I. Twenty fundamental problems of biology, medicine and neuropsychology related to biological information. ScientificWorldJournal 2006;6:747-59.
[28] Ventegodt S, Hermansen TD, Nielsen ML, Clausen B, Merrick J. Human development II. We need an integrated theory for matter, life and consciousness to understand life and healing. ScientificWorldJournal 2006;6:760-6.
[29] Ventegodt S, Hermansen TD, Rald E, Flensborg-Madsen T, Nielsen ML, Clausen B, Merrick J. Human development III. Bridging brain-mind and body-mind. Introduction to "deep" (fractal, poly-ray) cosmology. ScientificWorldJournal 2006;6:767-76.
[30] Ventegodt S, Hermansen TD, Rald E, Flensborg-Madsen T, Nielsen ML, Clausen B, Merrick J. Human development IV. The living cell has information-directed self-organization. ScientificWorldJournal 2006;6:1132-8.
[31] Ventegodt S, Hermansen TD, Flensborg-Madsen T, Nielsen ML, Clausen B, Merrick J. Human development V: Biochemistry unable to explain the emergence of biological form (morphogenesis) and therefore a new principle as source of biological information is needed. ScientificWorldJournal 2006;6:1359-67.
[32] Ventegodt S, Hermansen TD, Flensborg-Madsen T, Nielsen M, Merrick J. Human development VI: Supracellular morphogenesis. The origin of biological and cellular order. ScientificWorldJournal 2006;6:1424-33.
[33] Ventegodt S, Hermansen TD, Flensborg-Madsen T, Rald E, Nielsen ML, Merrick J. Human development VII: A spiral fractal model of fine structure of physical energy could explain central aspects of biological information, biological organization and biological creativity. ScientificWorldJournal 2006;6:1434-40.
[34] Ventegodt S, Hermansen TD, Flensborg-Madsen T, Nielsen ML, Merrick J. Human development VIII: A theory of "deep" quantum chemistry and cell consciousness: Quantum chemistry controls genes and biochemistry to give cells and higher organisms consciousness and complex behavior. ScientificWorldJournal 2006;6:1441-53.
[35] Ventegodt S, Hermansen TD, Flensborg-Madsen T, Rald E, Nielsen ML, Merrick J. Human development IX: A model of the wholeness of man, his consciousness and collective consciousness. ScientificWorldJournal 2006;6:1454-9.
[36] Hermansen TD, Ventegodt S, Merrick J. Human development X: Explanation of macroevolution — top-down evolution materializes consciousness. The origin of metamorphosis. ScientificWorldJournal 2006;6:1656-66.
[37] Ventegodt S. The life mission theory: A theory for a consciousness-based medicine. Int J Adolesc Med Health 2003;15(1): 89-91.
[38] Ventegodt S, Andersen NJ, Merrick J. The life mission theory II. The structure of the life purpose and the ego. ScientificWorldJournal 2003;3:1277-85.
[39] Ventegodt S, Andersen NJ, Merrick J. The life mission theory III. Theory of talent. ScientificWorldJournal 2003;3:1286-93.
[40] Ventegodt S, Andersen NJ, Merrick J. The life mission theory IV. Theory on child development. ScientificWorldJournal 2003;3:1294-1301.
[41] Ventegodt S, Andersen NJ, Merrick J. The life mission theory V. Theory of the anti-self (the shadow) or the evil side of man. ScientificWorldJournal 2003;3:1302-13.
[42] Ventegodt S, Kromann M, Andersen NJ, Merrick J. The life mission theory VI. A theory for the human character: Healing with holistic medicine through recovery of character and purpose of life. ScientificWorldJournal 2004;4:859-80.
[43] Ventegodt S, Clausen B, Nielsen ML, Merrick J. Clinical holistic medicine: Advanced tools for holistic medicine. ScientificWorldJournal 2006;6:2048-65.
[44] Ventegodt S, Thegler S, Andreasen T, Struve F, Enevoldsen L, Bassaine L, et al. Clinical holistic medicine: Psychodynamic short-time therapy complemented with bodywork. A clinical follow-up study of 109 patients. ScientificWorldJournal 6, 2220-2238.
[45] Ventegodt S, Andersen NJ, Merrick J. Holistic Medicine III: The holistic process theory of healing. ScientificWorldJournal 2003;3: 1138-46.

[46] Ventegodt S, Andersen NJ, Merrick J. Holistic Medicine IV: Principles of the holistic process of healing in a group setting. ScientificWorldJournal 2003;3:1294-1301.
[47] Ventegodt S, Kandel I, Merrick J. Principles of holistic medicine. Philosophy behind quality of life. Victoria, BC: Trafford, 2005.
[48] Ventegodt S, Kandel I, Merrick J. Principles of holistic medicine. Quality of life and health. New York: Hippocrates Sci Publ, 2005.
[49] Ventegodt S, Kandel I, Merrick J. Principles of holistic medicine. Global quality of life.Theory, research and methodology. New York: Hippocrates Sci Publ, 2006.
[50] Antonella R. Introduction of regulatory methods. Systematics, description and current research. Graz: Interuniversity College, 2004.
[51] Blättner B. Fundamentals of salutogenesis. Health promotion (WHO) and individual promotion of health guided by resources. Graz: Interuniversity College, 2004.
[52] Endler PC. Master's program for complementary, psychosocial and integrated health sciences. Graz: Interuniversity College, 2004.
[53] Endler PC. Working and writing scientifically in complementary medicine and integrated health sciences. Graz: Interuniversity College, 2004.
[54] Kratky KW. Complementary medicine systems. Comparison and integration. New York, Nova Sci, 2008.
[55] Pass PF. Fundamentals of depth psychology. Therapeutic relationship formation between self-awareness and casework. Graz: Interuniversity College, 2004.
[56] Spranger HH. Fundamentals of regulatory biology. Paradigms and scientific backgrounds of regulatory methods. Graz: Interuniversity College, 2004.
[57] Ventegodt S, Morad M, Merrick J. Clinical holistic medicine: Holistic treatment of children. ScientificWorldJournal 2004;4:581-8.
[58] Ventegodt S, Morad M, Merrick J. Clinical holistic medicine: Problems in sex and living together. ScientificWorldJournal 2004;4: 562-70.
[59] Ventegodt S, Morad M, Hyam E, Merrick J. Clinical holistic medicine: Holistic sexology and treatment of vulvodynia through existential therapy and acceptance through touch. ScientificWorldJournal2004; 4:571-80.
[60] Ventegodt S, Flensborg-Madsen T, Andersen NJ, Morad M, Merrick J. Clinical holistic medicine: A Pilot on HIV and Quality of Life and a Suggested treatment of HIV and AIDS. ScientificWorldJournal 2004;4:264-72.
[61] Ventegodt S, Morad M, Merrick J. Clinical holistic medicine: Induction of spontaneous remission of cancer by recovery of the human character and the purpose of life (the life mission). ScientificWorldJournal 2004;4:362-77.
[62] Ventegodt S, Morad M, Kandel I, Merrick J. Clinical holistic medicine: Treatment of physical health problems without a known cause, exemplified by hypertension and tinnitus. ScientificWorldJournal 2004;4:716-24.
[63] Ventegodt S, Morad M, Merrick J. Clinical holistic medicine: Developing from asthma, allergy and eczema. ScientificWorldJournal 2004;4:936-42.
[64] Ventegodt S, Morad M, Press J, Merrick J, Shek DTL. Clinical holistic medicine: Holistic adolescent medicine. ScientificWorldJournal 2004;4:551-61.
[65] Ventegodt S, Solheim E, Saunte ME, Morad M, Kandel I, Merrick J. Clinical holistic medicine: Metastatic cancer. ScientificWorldJournal 2004;4:913-35.
[66] Ventegodt S, Morad M, Kandel I, Merrick J. Clinical holistic medicine: a psychological theory of dependency to improve quality of life. ScientificWorldJournal2004;4:638-48.
[67] Ventegodt S, Merrick J. Clinical holistic medicine: Chronic infections and autoimmune diseases. ScientificWorldJournal 2005;5: 155-64.
[68] Ventegodt S, Kandel I, Neikrug S, Merrick J. Clinical holistic medicine: Holistic treatment of rape and incest traumas. ScientificWorldJournal 2005;5:288-97.
[69] Ventegodt S, Morad M, Merrick J. Clinical holistic medicine: Chronic pain in the locomotor system. ScientificWorldJournal 2005;5:165-72.

[70] Ventegodt S, Merrick J. Clinical holistic medicine: Chronic pain in internal organs. ScientificWorldJournal 2005;5:205-10.
[71] Ventegodt S, Kandel I, Neikrug S, Merrick J. Clinical holistic medicine: The existential crisis – life crisis, stress and burnout. ScientificWorldJournal 2005;5:300-12.
[72] Ventegodt S, Gringols M, Merrick J. Clinical holistic medicine: Holistic rehabilitation ScientificWorldJournal 2005;5:280-7.
[73] Ventegodt S, Andersen NJ, Neikrug S, Kandel I, Merrick J. Clinical holistic medicine: Mental disorders in a holistic perspective. ScientificWorldJournal 2005;5:313-23.
[74] Ventegodt S, Andersen NJ, Neikrug S, Kandel I, Merrick J. Clinical holistic medicine: Holistic treatment of mental disorders. ScientificWorldJournal 2005;5:427-45.
[75] Ventegodt S, Merrick J. Clinical holistic medicine: The patient with multiple diseases. ScientificWorldJournal 2005;5:324-39.
[76] Ventegodt S, Clausen B, Merrick J. Clinical holistic medicine: The case story of Anna: I. Long term effect of child sexual abuse and incest with a treatment approach. ScientificWorldJournal 2006;6:1965-76.
[77] Ventegodt S, Clausen B, Merrick J. Clinical holistic medicine: the case story of Anna. II. Patient diary as a tool in treatment. ScientificWorldJournal 2006;6:2006-34.
[78] Ventegodt S, Clausen B, Merrick J. Clinical holistic medicine: The case story of Anna. III. Rehabilitation of philosophy of life during holistic existential therapy for childhood sexual abuse. ScientificWorldJournal 2006;6:2080-91.
[79] Ventegodt S, Merrick J. Suicide from a holistic point of view. ScientificWorldJournal 2005;5:759-66.
[80] Ventegodt S. [Min brug af vaginal akupressur.] My use of acupressure. Ugeskr Laeger 2006;168(7):715-6. [Danish]
[81] Ventegodt S, Clausen B, Omar HA, Merrick J. Clinical holistic medicine: Holistic sexology and acupressure through the vagina (Hippocratic pelvic massage). ScientificWorldJournal 2006;6:2066-79.
[82] Ventegodt S, Thegler S, Andreasen T, Struve F, Enevoldsen L, Bassaine L, et al. Clinical holistic medicine (mindful, short-term psychodynamic psychotherapy complemented with bodywork) in the treatment of experienced impaired sexual functioning. ScientificWorldJournal 2007;7:324-9.
[83] Ventegodt S, Thegler S, Andreasen T, Struve F, Enevoldsen L, Bassaine L, et al. Clinical holistic medicine (mindful, short-term psychodynamic psychotherapy complemented with bodywork) improves quality of life, health, and ability by induction of Antonovsky-salutogenesis. ScientificWorldJournal 2007;7:317-23.
[84] Ventegodt S, Thegler S, Andreasen T, Struve F, Enevoldsen L, Bassaine L, et al. Clinical holistic medicine (mindful, short-term psychodynamic psychotherapy complemented with bodywork) in the treatment of experienced physical illness and chronic pain. ScientificWorldJournal 2007;7:310-6.
[85] Ventegodt S, Thegler S, Andreasen T, Struve F, Enevoldsen L, Bassaine L, et al. Clinical holistic medicine (mindful, short-term psychodynamic psychotherapy complemented with bodywork) in the treatment of experienced mental illness. ScientificWorldJournal 2007;7:306-9.
[86] Ventegodt S, Thegler S, Andreasen T, Struve F, Enevoldsen L, Bassaine L, et al. Self-reported low self-esteem. Intervention and follow-up in a clinical setting. ScientificWorldJournal 2007;7:299- 305.
[87] Mosher LR. Evaluation of psychosocial treatments. In: Gunderson, JG, Mosher LR, eds. Psychotherapy of schizophrenia. New York: Aronson, 1975:253-8.
[88] Mosher LR. (1975) Psychotherapy research. In: Gunderson, JG, Mosher LR, eds. Psychotherapy of schizophrenia. New York: Aronson, 1975:243-52.
[89] Trungpa C. Crazy wisdom. Berkeley, CA: Dharma Ocean Series, Shambhala Publ, 1969..
[90] Feuerstein G. Hole madness spirituality, crazy-wise teachers and enlightenment. New York: Hohm Press, 2001.
[91] Buber M. I and thou. New York: Charles Scribner´s Sons, 1970.
[92] Chopra D. Quantum healing. Exploring the frontiers of mind body medicine. New York: Bantam Books, 1990.
[93] Polewka A,Maj JC,Warchol K, Groszek B. [The assessment of suicidal risk in the concept of the presuicidal syndrome, and the possibilities it provides for suicide prevention and therapy--review] Przegl Lek 2005;62:399-402. [Polish]

[94] Avery D, Winokur G. Mortality in depressed patients treated with electro convulsive therapy and antidepressants. Arch Gen Psychiatry 1976;33:1029-37.

[95] Malmberg L, Fenton M. Individual psychodynamic psychotherapy and psychoanalysis for schizophrenia and severe mental illness. Cochrane Database Syst Rev 2001;3:CD001360.

[96] The Swedich Council of Technology Assessment in Health Care. Treatment with antipsychotic drugs [Behandling med neuroleptika.] Stockholm: SBU-Report 133/1 and 133/2, 1997. [Swedish]

[97] Lindhardt A, et al. The use of neurolectic drugs among patients 18-64 years old with schizophrenia, mania or bipolar affective mental disorder [Forbruget af antipsykotika blandt 18-64 årige patienter med skizofreni, mani eller bipolar affektiv sindslidelse"]. Copenhagen: Danish Natl Board Health, 2006. [Danish]

[98] van der Kolk B, McFarlane A, Weisaeth L, eds. Traumatic stress: The effects of overwhelming experience on mind, body, and society. New York: Guilford, 1996.

[99] Levine P, Frederick A. Waking the tiger. Healing trauma. Berkeley, CA: North Atlantic Books, 1997.

[100] Nijenhuis ERS. Somatoform dissociation: Major symptoms of dissociative disorders. J Trauma Dissociation 2000;1(4):7-32.

[101] Rothschild B. The body remembers. The psychophysiology of trauma and trauma treatment. New York: WW Norton, 2000.

[102] Shapiro F. Eye movement desensitization and processing.Basic principles. Protocols and procedures. 2nd ed. London: Guildford, 2001.

[103] Searles HF. Preface. In: Searles HF. Collected papers on schizophrenia. Madison, CT: Int Univ Press, 1965:15-18.

[104] Adler A. The practice and theroy of individual psychology. London: Routledge Kegan Paul, 1925.

[105] Abraham K, Abraham H. Clinical papers and essays on psycho-analysis. London: Maresfield Reprints, 1979.

[106] Federn P. Ego psychology and the psychoses. New York: Basic Books, 1953.

[107] Will OA. Process, psychotherapy, and schizophrenia. New York; Basic Books, 1961.

[108] Searles HF. Collected papers on schizophrenia. Madison, CT: Int Univ Press, 1965.

[109] Schilder P. The image and appearance of the human body. London: Kegan Paul, 1935.

[110] Rosenfeld HA. Psychotic states: A psycho-analytical approach. Madison, CT: Int Univ Press, 1965.

[111] Segal H. Some aspects of the analysis of a schizophrenic. Int J Psycho Analysis 195031, 268-278.

[112] Fairbairn RWD. An object-relations theory of the personality. Oxford: Basic Books, 1954.

[113] Guntrip H. (1968) Schizoid phenomena, object relations and the self. Madison, CT: Int Univ Press, 1968.

[114] Perry JW. Image, complex, and transference in schizophrenia. Psychotherapy of the psychoses. New York: Basic Books, 1961:90-123.

[115] Lidz T. The origin and treatment of schizophrenic disorders. Madison, CT: Int Univ Press, 1990.

[116] Kernberg OF. Borderline conditions and pathological narcissism. New York: Jason Aronson, 1975.

[117] Kernberg OF. Object relations theory and clinical psychoanalysis. New York: Jason Aronson, 1976.

[118] Volkan VD. Primitive internalized object relations. Madison, CT: Int Univ Press, 1976.

[119] Sechehaye MA. Symbolic realization. Madison, CT: Int Univ Press, 1951.

[120] Rosen JN. Direct analysis (selected papers). New York: Grune Stratton, 1953.

[121] Eissler KR. Remarks on the psychoanalysis of schizophrenia. In: Brody EB, Redlich FC, eds. Psychotherapy with schizophrenics. Madison, CT: Int Univ Press, 1952:130-67.

[122] Arlow JA, Brenner C. Psychoanalytic concepts and the structural theory. Oxford: Int Univ Press, 1964.

[123] Giovacchini PL. Treatment of primitive mental states. New York: Jason Aronson, 1979.

[124] Arieti S. Interpretation of schizophrenia, 2nd ed. New York: Basic Books, 1974.

[125] Bellak L. Disorders of the schizophrenic syndrome. New York: Basic Books, 1979.

[126] Gendlin ET. Therapeutic procedures in dealing with schizophrenics. In: Rogers CR, ed. The therapeutic relationship and its impact. A study of psychotherapy with schizophrenics. Madison, WI: Univ Wisconsin Press, 1967:369-400.

[127] Prouty G. Pre-therapy: a method of treating pre-expressive retarded and psychotic patients. Psychotherapy 1976;1:290-4.

[128] Gunderson JG, Mosher LR. Psychotherapy of schizophrenia. New York: Jason Aronson, 1975.

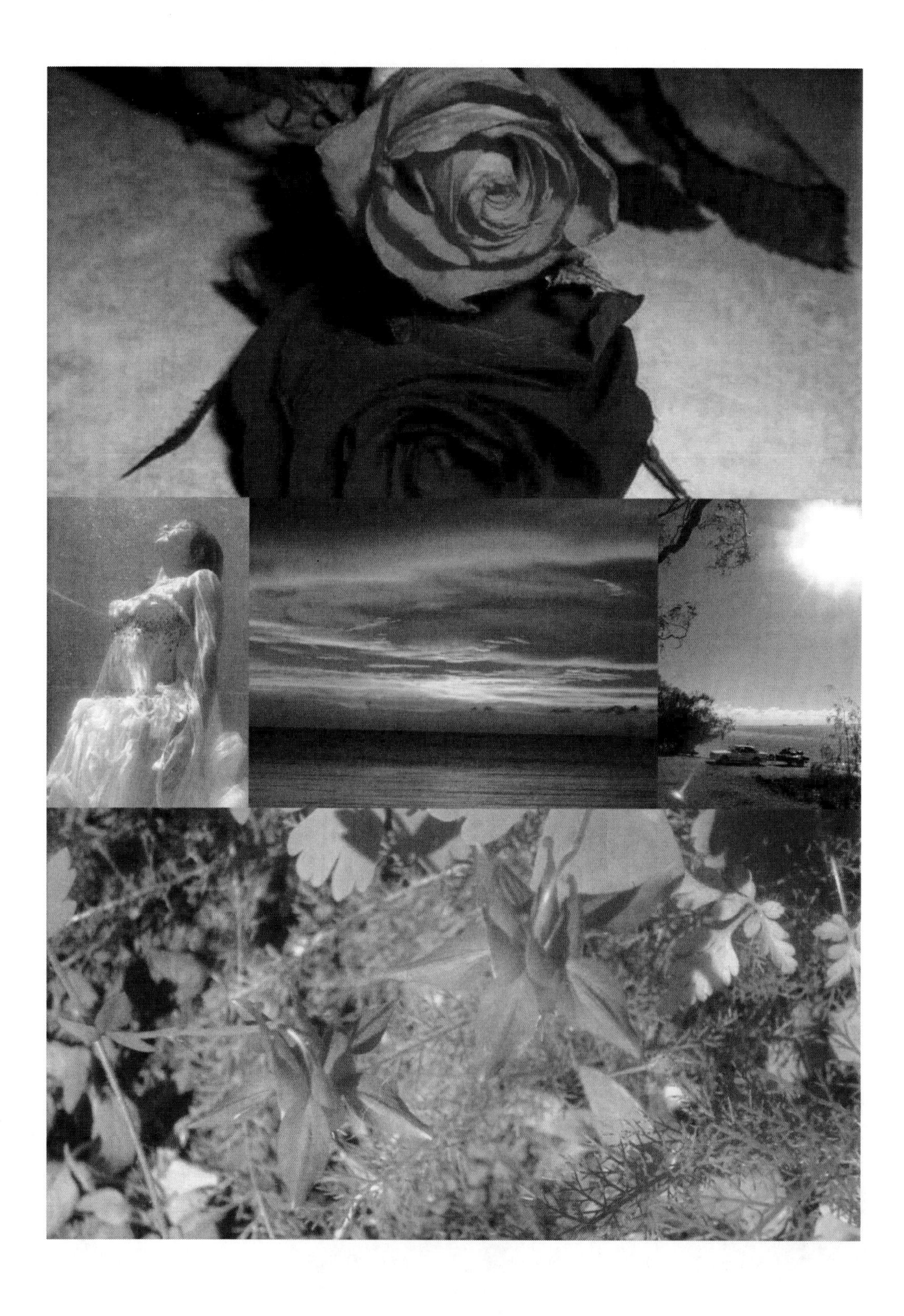

*Chapter XII*

# Clinical research

Clinical research in holistic medicine needs the endpoints shown to be the best predictors of future health and survival. We know that such endpoints are self-evaluated health and self-evaluated quality of life. Fortunately these endpoints are extremely easy to collect with small questionnaires that only take a few minutes to fill out for the patient (like QOL1, QOL5 and QOL10)(1-4), meaning that every physician or therapist can easily conduct clinical research and also use the measurements by such questionnaire for quality assurance of his clinic and the therapists working there.To be sure that such research will be up to standard we have made the Open Source Protocol that can be used by everybody (5).

An important research question is if the clinical results are temporary or permanent and in order to answer this question we have developed a special research design called the "square curve paradigm" (6). This is also easy to use; it simply says that you need to measure your patients before and after intervention, and then again sufficiently long time after to be sure that the results of therapy is lasting. We recommend at least one year before follow up. When we did such a study in our clinic (7) we noticed that the clinical results were not only lasting, but also improved over time. It seems like the holistic treatment is able to heal the patient and also teach the patient how to continue growing and learning. This is a very encouraging finding, which has also been found by other researchers.

So, when you start treating your patients with holistic medicine, give them the QOL10 questionnaire before and after treatment and calculate the QOL1, QOL5 and QOL10 scores before and after to learn how much your patients have improved – it can be used free of charge for all non-commercial clinical research. Notice also the specific areas, where your patients have improved and the areas where improvement has been less positive. If the patients end up at a lower stage that the beginning point and no serious progressive illness like cancer can explain that, you might have ended therapy prematurely, which is also important to notice. It is normal that the patient will have a healing crisis with lower marks in the middle of the therapy. This is also where some patients have a tendency to drop out of treatment. If you suspect that your patient is in a crisis you can have him or her answering the questionnaire at that point in time, and the ratings will show this right away. So there are many practical applications of scientific measuring.

We always measure the patient with QOL10 before therapeutic intervention to set goals for the treatment. It is easy to remember such goals and very easy to see, if they are accomplished. Naturally all measurements and goals are noted in the case record.

We have also noticed that when people are related in time and space and grounded existentially your rating of the patient and the patients' own rating will often be very similar. If there is a large discrepancy this is a good subject for a talk in order to help the patient to be more down to earth and centred.

## References


[1] Lindholt JS, Ventegodt S, Henneberg EW. Development and validation of QOL5 for clinical databases. A short, global and generic questionnaire based on an integrated theory of the quality of life. Eur J Surg 2002;168(2):107-13.

[2] Ventegodt S, Merrick J, Andersen NJ. Measurement of quality of life IV: Use of the SEQOL, QOL5, QOL1 and other global and generic questionnaires. ScientificWorldJournal 2003;3:992-1001.

[3] Ventegodt S, Merrick J, Andersen NJ. Measurement of quality of life V: How to use the SEQOL, QOL5, QOL1 and other and generic questionnaires for research. ScientificWorldJournal 2003;3:1002-14.

[4] Ventegodt S, Andersen NJ, Merrick J. QOL10 for clinical quality-assurance and research in treatment-efficacy: Ten key questions for measuring the global quality of life, self-rated physical and mental health, and self-rated social-, sexual and working abulity. J Altern Med Res 2009;1(2):113-22.

[5] Ventegodt S, Andersen NJ, Kandel I, Merrick J. The open source protocol of clinical holistic medicine. J Altern Med Res 2009;1(2): 129-44.

[6] Ventegodt S, Andersen NJ, Merrick J. The square-curve paradigm for research in alternative, complementary and holistic medicine: a cost-effective, easy and scientifically valid design for evidence based medicine. ScientificWorldJournal 2003;3:1117-27.

[7] Ventegodt S, Thegler S, Andreasen T, Struve F, Enevoldsen L, Bassaine L, Torp M, Merrick J. Clinical holistic medicine: Psychodynamic short-time therapy complemented with bodywork. A clinical follow-up study of 109 patients. ScientificWorldJournal 2006;6:2220-38.

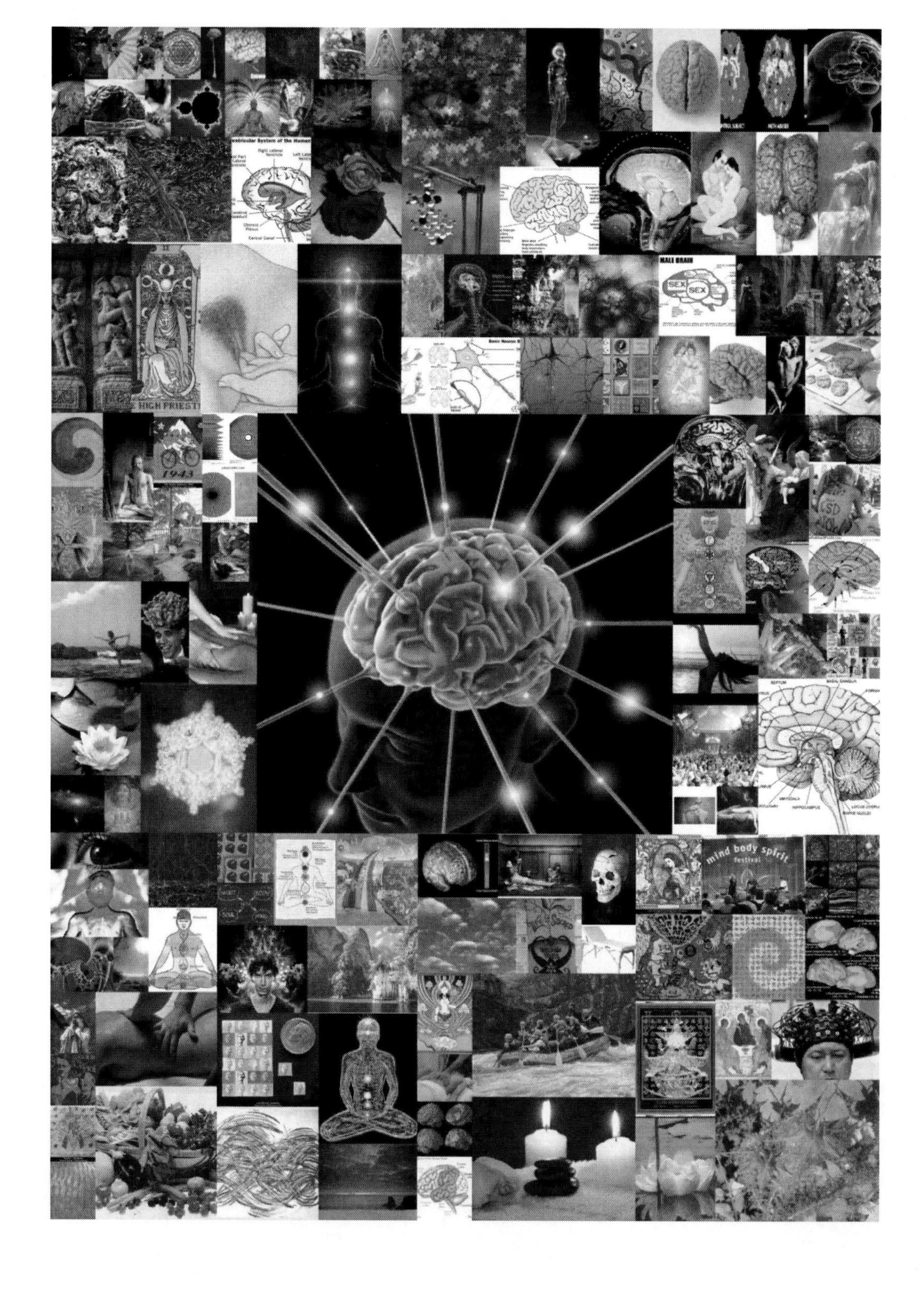

mind body spirit
festival
SEX
SEX
1943

*Chapter XIII*

# Research in evidence-based holistic medicine

Evidence-based holistic medicine means that the treatment efficacy and safety are thoroughly documented by clinical research. Research in holistic medicine needs to have the same quality as biomedical research protocols. The lack of research expertise and national organs to regulate this kind of research and assure its quality has lead us to develop the concept "Open Source Research Protocol", where all important procedures, treatment techniques, ethical considerations, documentation standards, systems for quality assurance, including instruments for measurement of effect like questionnaires that have been published in peer-reviewed scientific journals (see table 1) (1).

**Table 1. The peer-reviewed journals that have published the research protocols and scientific papers on quality of life research and clinical holistic medicine**

- Arch Sex Behaviour (sexology) (Medline/PubMed)
- BMJ (medicine) (Medline/PubMed)
- Child Care Health Dev (paediatrics) (Medline/PubMed)
- Eur J Surg (surgery) (Medline/PubMed)
- Int J Adolesc. Med Health (adolescent medicine, Pediatrics) (Medline/PubMed)
- Int J Child Health Human Dev (pediatrics, human development) (PsycINFO, PubMedCentral)
- Int J Disabil Hum Dev (disability, human development) (PsycINFO)
- Ital J Pediatr (pediatrics, adolescent medicine)
- J Altern Med Res (alternative medicine)
- J Coll Physicians Surg Pak (Medicine) (Medline/PubMed)
- J Compl Integr Medicine (alternative medicine) (Medline/PubMed)
- J Pediatric Adolesc Gynecol (gynecology, pediatrics) (Medline/PubMed)
- J Pain Management (medicine) (PsycINFO, PubMedCentral)
- Med Sci Monit (medicine) (MedLine/PubMed)
- Oral Health Prev Dent (dentistry) (Medline/PubMed)
- South Med J (medicine) (Medline/PubMed)
- Social Indicators Research (sociology) (PsycINFO)
- ScientificWorldJournal (medicine) (Medline/PubMed)
- Ugeskrift for Læger (medicine) (Medline/PubMed)

The publication of all aspects of the protocol and the research that resulted has made it possible to have an excellent standard of research. We also believe that by publishing all part of the protocol and receiving critique from internationally recognized scientific journals have avoided much of the bias that all research obviously contain.

The research papers have been arranged according to several systematic categories according to the headlines and topics listed in table 2. The general title of the papers is mentioned in the title of the paper to make it easy to identify all papers of a series.

**Table 2. The most important series of papers that constitute the research protocol in clinical holistic medicine**

- QOL methodology describes the method used to measure quality of life used with the Quality of Life Survey Study at the Copenhagen University Hospital (Rigshospitalet), Denmark.
- QOL philosophy describes the philosophy behind our work with quality of life presented in the books "Quality of life. To seize the meaning of life and get well again" (1995), "Life philosophy that heals. Quality of life as medicine" (1999), "Consciousness-based medicine" (2003) and "Principles of Holistic Medicine. Philosophy behind quality of life" (2005). These are publications describing the philosophy on which the entire project is based.
- QOL theory covers the related life and human points of view described theoretically.
- QOL questionnaires are the questionnaires used in the Quality of Life Survey Study and later studies.
- QOL results are results from the Quality of Life Survey Study.
- Theories of existence are new theories on quality of life and the human nature described coherently and concisely.
- Holistic medicine describes our research program for the holistic-medical project ? a new research paradigm for researching alternative and holistic medicine and a theory for process of holistic healing.
- QOL as medicine describes results from the treatment of patients suffering from various chronic diseases, like chronic pains, alcoholism and Whiplash Associated Disorders.
- Clinical holistic medicine describes how to deal with the variety of problems presented by the patients in the medical clinic using holistic medicine.
- Human development is a series of papers to address a number of unsolved problems in biology today. First of all, the unsolved enigma concerning how the differentiation from a single zygote to an adult individual happens has been object for severe research through decades. By uncovering a new holistic biological paradigm that introduces an energetic-informational interpretation of reality as a new way to experience biology, these papers try to solve the problems connected with the events of biological ontogenesis from a single cell involvement in the fractal hierarchy, to the function of the human brain and "adult human metamorphosis".
- Quality of working life research is a series of paper that addresses the fundamental needs for happiness and efficiency the working situation. This applies to physicians and therapists as well as other occupations. The series of paper analyses how we can develop in our job, and continue to learn and grow, and avoid the routine and boredom that in the end forces us to compromise with quality and patience.

# Research in clinical holistic medicine

On both a formal and informal way research and clinical practice in holistic medicine has been performed for several thousands of years (1-8) and in the last century two huge movements have put this old knowledge into use: psychoanalysis (9) and psychodynamic therapy (10,11) (most importantly STPP or short term psychodynamic psychotherapy) (12,13) going through the mind on the one hand and through the body on the other. Bodywork developed through most importantly Reich (14), Lowen (15) and Rosen (16) with sexual therapy along the tantric tradition (17). A third road, but much less common path has been directly though the spiritual reconnection with the world (18,19).

Our international research collaboration became interested in existential healing from the data that originated from the Copenhagen Perinatal Birth Cohort 1959-61. Almost 20 years ago we were conducting epidemiological research on quality of life, closely examining the connection between global quality of life and health for more than 11,000 people in a series of huge surveys (20) using large and extensive questionnaires. We found that quality of life, mental and physical health, and ability of social, sexual and working ability seemed to be caused primarily by the consciousness and philosophy of life of the person in question.

In Denmark where we have conducted the research, almost all patients that had complementary medical treatment of the holistic, existential type, had tried biomedical treatment first, and after this often several complementary and alternative types of treatment, before they entered our research protocol. In one study, the patients had their problems and suffering for 8.9 years (mean) (1).

**Table 3. Treatment success rate when all treatment failures (non-responders), drop-outs of the survey, and dropouts of treatment are taken as non-responders. Patient's own experience as measured self-rated with the questionnaire QOL10, and the patient is taken as cured if the state of the measured factor was bad or very bad before treatment and not bad after treatment (and one year after treatment, statistically, using the square curve paradigm). The data comes from clinical studies covering the holistic treatment of 600 patients. (CHM: Clinical holistic medicine. (21-26) (HMS: Holistic manual sexology (27). HMS-D: Holistic manual sexology – Dodson's method for treating chronic anorgasmia) (28)**

| | |
|---|---|
| Physical illness (CHM) | 39%(p=0.05) (21) |
| Mental illness (CHM) | 57% (p=0.05) (22) |
| Low quality of life (CHM) | 56% (p=0.05) (23) |
| Low self-esteem (CHM) | 61% (p=0.05) (24) |
| Low working ability (CHM) | 52% (p=0.05) (25) |
| Sexual dysfunction(CHM) | 42% (p=0.05) (26) |
| Sexual dysfunction (HMS) | 56% (p=0.05) (27) |
| Sexual dysfunction (HMS-D) | 93% (p=0.05) (28) |

As nothing had helped these patients before they came to our clinic, we find it justified to use them as their own controls. Quite remarkably we have been able to help every second of the patients independent of the type of problem they have presented, and independent of the seriousness of the problem (see table 3) (21-28). In our recent protocols we have only included patients, who experienced their problem as "bad" or "very bad" on a five point Likert scale (1).

We have used a new research paradigm called the "square curve paradigm" that documents the lasting effect of an immediate significant improvement that comes simultaneously with the process of existential healing of the patient – the process that we call Antonovsky-salutogenesis (1).

One of the great concerns in our project has been to cover also the philosophical, methodological, and interdisciplinary aspects of the research, which has led to many series of papers. We have also found it extremely important to find the dimensions we need to intervene on to help the patients in many different research designs to avoid the bias from one specific research strategy.

Therefore the prospective cohort design has been extremely important in our research and we have developed a unique concept of recording the case, including measuring before and after the treatment with validated quality of life and health questionnaire, which has allowed us to monitor every side effect and unexpected event during the treatment.

## Quality assurance

The strategy for data collection and quality assurance in the clinic has been developed since 2004 (1). We are using a questionnaire (QOL10) measuring global quality of life (QOL1, QOL5), self-rated mental and physical health, self-rated social, sexual and working ability, self-rated I-strength, self-rated self-esteem (relation to self) and relation to partner and friends.

We measure before treatment, after treatment (three month) and again one year after the treatment has been completed. The complete lack of side or adverse effects from ethical and professionally conducted consciousness-based medicine has been documented through a systematic review of the literature (1,29).

## Ethical aspects

The rationale for treating with clinical holistic medicine is naturally its high efficacy compared with the complete lack of adverse/side effects. Hippocrates' ethics "primum non nocera", "first do no harm", is fully respected in clinical holistic medicine, but not always adapted or possible in biomedicine. Scientific holistic medicine has had its highly developed ethics already from its first days, when it was created as a science by Hippocrates and his students.

We have carefully considered all ethical aspects relevant for today's practice of holistic medicine and holistic sexology and have participated in the development of the ethical rules of the International Society of Holistic Health that organize holistic medical practitioners worldwide (1).

## Informed consent

The most important aspect of ethical conduct is full information to the patient and the openness of the protocol with public and scientific publications that will give every patient the possibility to see exactly what the principles, procedures, results, and side effects of the treatment are. An important aspect of communication and decision making by the patients is the selection of material for reading by the patient and also verbally explained to the patient, before initiating the treatment and making the therapeutic contract. The patient filling in the questionnaire and the other papers related to the treatment is legally taken as a written consent. As not every patient is able to read scientific papers, we have also published easy-to-read books on quality of life philosophy, clinical holistic medicine and the results from the research, which have been included as a part of the research protocol. In the Research Clinic for Holistic Medicine in Copenhagen, we also have one page of written patient information giving just the core information and we have put a summary of the research on our homepage (www.livskvalitet.org). For researchers we have collected the most important papers in a series of books on principles of holistic medicine (30-33).

Before treatment in holistic medicine the patient should be informed about the course of the treatment in general terms and it is recommended to also receive a written contract for the treatment signed by the patient.

## Political and financial aspects

Fortunately national authorities as well as international experts have recently started to recognize the clinical, holistic medicine as scientific and efficient. Recently the Interuniversity College, Graz, has graduated a number of therapists with the master degree on the basis of their research work in clinical holistic medicine (1), making Austria the first country to officially acknowledge clinical holistic medicine as a scientific complementary-medical treatment system. In USA the conflicts between biomedicine and complementary medicine (CAM including holistic medicine) has often reached the court system and the supreme court of California has in the last decade realized this and systematically judged in support of the practitioners of CAM and holistic medicine in these conflicts.

## References

[1] Ventegodt S, Andersen NJ, Kandel I, Merrick J. The open source protocol of clinical holistic medicine. J Altern Med Res 2009;1(2), 129-44.
[2] Antonella R. Introduction of regulatory methods. Graz, Austria: Interuniversity College, 2004.
[3] Blättner B. Fundamentals of salutogenesis. Graz, Austria: Interuniversity College, 2004.
[4] Endler PC. Master program for complementary, psychosocial and integrated health sciences Graz, Austria: Interuniversity College, 2004.
[5] Endler PC. Working and writing scientifically in complementary medicine and integrated health sciences. Graz, Austria: Interuniversity College, 2004.
[6] Kratky KW. Complementary medicine systems. Comparison and integration. New York, Nova Sci, 2008.

[7] Pass PF. Fundamentals of depth psychology. Therapeutic relationship formation between self-awareness and casework Graz, Austria: Interuniversity College, 2004.
[8] Spranger HH. Fundamentals of regulatory biology. Paradigms and scientific backgrounds of regulatory methods Graz, Austria: Interuniversity College, 2004.
[9] Jones E. The life and works of Sigmund Freud. New York: Basic Books, 1961.
[10] Jung CG. Man and his symbols. New York: Anchor Press, 1964.
[11] Jung CG. Psychology and alchemy. Collected works of CG Jung, Vol 12. Princeton, NJ: Princeton Univ Press, 1968.
[12] Leichsenring F, Rabung S, Leibing E. The efficacy of short-term psychodynamic psychotherapy in specific psychiatric disorders: a meta-analysis. Arch Gen Psychiatry 2004;61(12):1208-16.
[13] Leichsenring F. (2005) Are psychodynamic and psychoanalytic therapies effective? A review of empirical data. Int J Psychoanal 2005;86(Pt 3):841-68.
[14] Reich W. [Die Function des Orgasmus]. Köln: Kiepenheuer Witsch 1969. [German]
[15] Lowen A. Honoring the body. Alachua, FL: Bioenergetics Press, 2004.
[16] Rosen M, Brenner S. Rosen method bodywork. Accessing the unconscious through touch. Berkeley, CA: North Atlantic Books, 2003.
[17] Anand M. The art of sexual ecstasy. The path of sacred sexuality for western lovers. New York: Jeremy P Tarcher/Putnam, 1989.
[18] Antonovsky A. Health, stress and coping. London: Jossey-Bass, 1985.
[19] Antonovsky A. Unravelling the mystery of health. How people manage stress and stay well. San Francisco: Jossey-Bass, 1987.
[20] Ventegodt S, Flensborg-Madsen T, Andersen NJ, Nielsen M, Mohammed M, Merrick J. Global quality of life (QOL), health and ability are primarily determined by our consciousness. Research findings from Denmark 1991-2004. Soc Indicator Res 2005;71:87-122.
[21] Ventegodt S, Thegler S, Andreasen T, Struve F, Enevoldsen L, Bassaine L, Torp M, Merrick J. Clinical holistic medicine (mindful, short-term psychodynamic psychotherapy complemented with bodywork) in the treatment of experienced physical illness and chronic pain. ScientificWorldJournal 2007;7:310-6.
[22] Ventegodt S, Thegler S, Andreasen T, Struve F, Enevoldsen L, Bassaine L, Torp M, Merrick J. Clinical holistic medicine (mindful, short-term psychodynamic psychotherapy complemented with bodywork) in the treatment of experienced mental illness. ScientificWorldJournal 2007;7:306-9.
[23] Ventegodt S, Thegler S, Andreasen T, Struve F, Enevoldsen L, Bassaine L, Torp M, Merrick J. Clinical holistic medicine (mindful, short-term psychodynamic psychotherapy complemented with bodywork) improves quality of life, health, and ability by induction of Antonovsky-salutogenesis. ScientificWorldJournal 2007;7:317-23.
[24] Ventegodt S, Thegler S, Andreasen T, Struve F, Enevoldsen L, Bassaine L, Torp M, Merrick J. Self-reported low self-esteem. Intervention and follow-up in a clinical setting. ScientificWorldJournal 2007;7:299-305.
[25] Ventegodt S, Andersen NJ, Merrick J. Clinical holistic medicine in the recovery of working ability. A study using Antonovsky salutogenesis. Int J Disabil Hum Dev 2008;7(2):219-22.
[26] Ventegodt S, Thegler S, Andreasen T, Struve F, Enevoldsen L, Bassaine L, Torp M, Merrick J. Clinical holistic medicine (mindful, short-term psychodynamic psychotherapy complemented with bodywork) in the treatment of experienced impaired sexual functioning. ScientificWorldJournal 2007;7:324-9.
[27] Ventegodt S, Clausen B, Merrick J. Clinical holistic medicine: Pilot study on the effect of vaginal acupressure (Hippocratic pelvic massage). ScientificWorldJournal 2006;6:2100-16.
[28] Struck P, Ventegodt S. Clinical holistic medicine: Teaching orgasm for females with chronic anorgasmia using the Betty Dodson method. ScientificWorldJournal 2008;8:883-95.
[29] Ventegodt S, Merrick J. A review of side effects and adverse events of non-drug medicine (non-pharmaceutical CAM): Psychotherapy, mind-body medicine and clinical holistic medicine. J Compl Integr Medicine 2009, In press.
[30] Ventegodt S, Kandel I, Merrick J. Principles of holistic medicine. Philosophy behind quality of life. Victoria, BC: Trafford, 2005.
[31] Ventegodt S, Kandel I, Merrick J. Principles of holistic medicine. Quality of life and health. New York: Hippocrates Sci Publ, 2005.

[32] Ventegodt S, Kandel I, Merrick J. Principles of holistic medicine. Global quality of life.Theory, research and methodology. New York: Hippocrates Sci Publ, 2005.
[33] Ventegodt S, Merrick J. Sexology from a holistic point of view. A textbook of classic and modern sexology. New York: Nova Science, 2010.

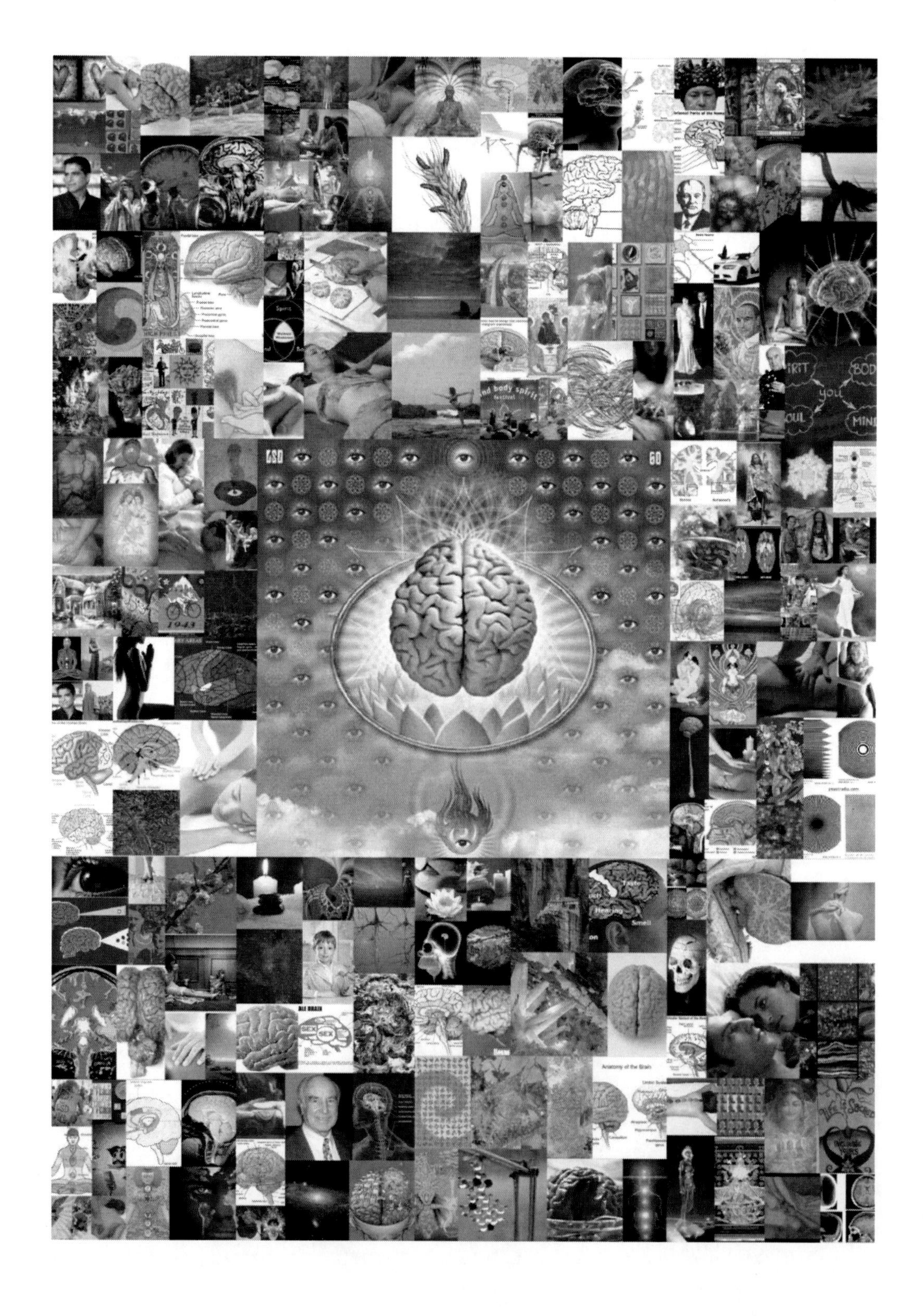
1943
Hearing
Smell
Anatomy of the Brain

*Chapter XIV*

# Sometimes you need to stop what you usually do

In Denmark and other countries with socialized biomedicine about one in four has a chronic mental illness that cannot be cured by biomedical drugs. Sometimes we need to stop doing what we usually do, when it does not work. This seemingly being the most difficult thing a physician can do! May we suggest that we expand the range of the physician's activities with other toolboxes than the biomedical, so that we can find something new to do, when what we usually do does not work? If the NNT (number needed to treat) of the best working drug or operation is say 5, 10, 20 or even often higher, rendering only a small fraction of our patients (5-20% of them) helped by our medical intervention?

Remembering the old humoristic definition of insanity and its treatment: "to continue doing what we always have done, expecting new results", we on the other hand suggest that the physician should be open-minded to other kinds of treatment and perspectives on health and disease. In fact we actually want the modern physician to be multi-paradigmatic.

All medical work is based on the intention of doing good, either improving the health, the quality of life, or the ability of functioning – or a combination. Independently of the good intention coming from the physician, the medical work is always bound to some medical theory or a frame of interpretation. Hence the different paradigms (1) - giving a number of different perceptions, hypothesis, diagnoses, actions and reactions. Just compare how we construct our consciousness in general life and in science (2,3).

The process of healing is – as life itself - often fairly complicated. The course of the disease, the healing process, personal development, learning and coping in connection with a disease is highly individual. The modern physician is often multi-paradigmatic as he must be to serve many different types of people in many different existential circumstances. He basically has the three, very different sets of technologies or "toolboxes" at his disposal, derived from three different medical paradigms:

- Classical, manual medicine, where the hands – used with the best and most humane intentions – constitute the main tools. It dates back to Hippocrates and Greek antiquity (4,5).

- Biomedicine, which came into widespread use around 1950, born paradigmatically along with the discovery of penicillin, where biomedicine has a focus on body chemistry and physiology (5).
- Holistic medicine – scientific, consciousness-oriented mind-body medicine - which originally was invented by Hippocrates and his students but is now appearing in a modern, scientific version as a new and increasingly popular trend with many family physicians in the western world. It draws on a variety of healing processes, philosophies and systems, taken in the original or modified form from the pre-modern cultures. The most important thinkers influencing holistic medicine in Europe today is great physicians and philosophers like Jung (6,7), Maslow (8), Antonovsky (9,10), Frankl (11), Fromm (12), Goleman (13,14), Sartre (15), Kiekegaard (16) and Allart (17). The holistic approach focus on the person as a whole, where this wholeness, soul or total existence is thought to be able to heal from its very totality – becoming "whole again", when the wholeness is partly or completely lost (18-27).

Depending on the perspective, or paradigm, very different things might happen to the patient, when treated by the physician, where the signs and symptoms of development or progress of health and disease is interpreted very differently. If you go to a homeopathic doctor, which for example is fairly common in Germany, it is seen as a good sign, if the treatment makes you feel worse for a while (28-31), but if you consult a biomedical doctor, then medicine is expected to make you feel better almost at once. If you consult a holistic doctor working according to the holistic process theory and the life mission theory (5,26,27), you would normally expect a very different path, even when occasionally confronting painful old traumas. The reason for this is that the earliest existential wounds normally are the toughest to overcome, but the more resources you have, the more severe wounds on your soul, you will manage to confront and heal.

In lack of a better term we have called the extended medical science, integrating these three different paradigms and their three strands of tools and methods for bio-psycho-social, holistic medicine. It is really medicine based on biological science in its widest sense – i.e. based on *the science of life*.

## Consciousness-based medicine

In the search for the best way to make a new medical clinical practice to serve the new type of patients we now see in our western society (the critical and knowledgeable patient or the patient focused on personal or spiritual development), we have worked with three different approaches to the new medicine:

Quality of life as medicine: Focusing on human feelings and emotions, we have combined bio-medicine with a number of complementary therapies, like Rosen body work, classical Chinese acupuncture and gestalt psychotherapy. We have called this holistic approach "quality of life as medicine". The combined treatment have the intention of inducing existential healing and encompasses three phases, which is popularly described as: "Feel, understand, and let go": Feel the blockages in body and mind, behind your health problems and symptoms, understand the life- denying conclusions you reached then which created them, and let go of these decisions once you are ready to assume responsibility and be your true, responsible self again. The team of physician and alternative therapist complementing each other working under medical supervision, could be the most efficient way to induce existential healing, in spite of the differences in professional language, culture and paradigm.

Meaning of life as medicine: focusing on the purpose of life, meaning of life, life mission and talent. Focusing on the hidden potentials, on the beauty and magnificence of the soul and on the power of our existential choices, gives many patients faith and a fast healing progress. When the existential theories, the QOL philosophy and theories, and the QOL concepts are explained to the patients and internalized, patients gradually find themselves, and return to a natural state of being, comparable in some aspects to the state in which they were born with a certain purpose of life, and certain great talents to be used. The life mission theory simply states, that denying your meaning in life leads you to illness, unhappiness and poor performance, while recovering your purpose of life depends on finding and working for your purpose of life.

Love as medicine: Based on the concept of genuine human relationships and the power of unconditional love and acceptance, we have worked with the spiritual gift of love and the healing power of this in what we have designated an experimental, social utopia (18). When patients belong to a small community with true companionship, contact and emotional surplus, their way to recovery seems to be much shorter. The problem with social utopia is, that it is very difficult to create and even more difficult to control. One of the preconditions seems to be that the participants do not have sex with each other, as this disturbs the possibility of intimacy in the group setting.

Although consciousness-based medicine supports individuals in their personal development; therapy and the patient-physician relationship can never replace a vibrant reality lived with those most important to them. It is the conquest of a good personal world to live in, which can bring wholeness and healing. Quite simply, an individual can only realize the meaning and purpose of life in a social context. This purpose is what we are meant to be and with this gift we will be able to give to others. This can only happen most fully in intimate relationships, full of trust and love. A huge body of evidence has been collected on the connection between health and survival, and love and intimacy (19).

Many medical doctors seem to be unable to work with therapists not scientifically trained, and many therapists do not like to be directed by a medical doctor, which makes the approach very difficult. Problems of this kind in the treatment team do not help the patients, as we have painfully experienced in our own clinical practice.

As human beings we are often limited to loving only a few percentages of our fellow men, at least before we develop the general ability of love and serve all. This is an issue that often naturally grows to a larger fraction, as we grow older, more wise, spacious and containing, as we understand that love might be a leading concept in medicine. Maybe even the strongest of the three concepts for inducing existential healing. Since such an approach for many seems unnatural, we are for all practical purposes left with the second approach in order for the modern physician to use the "new medicine", which really seems to be very similar to the classical holistic medicine.

Interestingly, the three approaches mentioned above express to what degree the physician is willing to come close with the patient. This mirrors the intention of the physician towards his patient. In a) the physician has the intent of helping the patient to heal, in b) he has the intent of personally giving a gift to the patient from the bottom of his heart and in c) the physician has the intention to let the patient be a part of his life, in true appreciation of the magnificence of this unique soul in front of him. We believe that most physicians of our time, who search their soul will find that the intentions of b) are an appropriate ambition for their work. The physician, who truly can give the holding (8,9) and processing in order to come close to his patient's needs, will always be loved and respected by his patients.

## What makes a physician excellent?

What will make a physician excellent are his good intentions, his deep knowledge and developed skills. In order to assist his patient to a successful treatment and help his patient, the physician is only excellent, when the good intentions result in the patient being adequately helped. The patient is helped when one of the following two conditions is fulfilled:

- The patient gets what he wants: quality of life in some aspect or globally, health in some aspect or globally, or ability of functioning in some aspect or globally – or a combination of these.
- The physician gets what he wants: the broken leg healed or the disease treated or prevented.

So the situation is fairly complex, and much is depending on the physician choosing the right medical paradigm or toolbox. It is not easy to tell, what a good medical treatment is, unless:

- you understand the paradigm chosen, and look at the patient from inside it.
- you keep track of all the subjective, objective factors and events involved in the process of healing through time.
- you have a valid way of testing the end result of the treatment.

All this is more or less complicated depending on the paradigm with the subjective paradigm the easiest to demonstrate. This makes it surprisingly easy to make research and quality improvement in the holistic medical clinic, introducing existential healing according to the holistic process theory, and surprisingly difficult to document effect of the biomedical treatments, because of the objective approach. This later approach needs a difficult set-up with control groups in the Cochrane design to be valid.

## An example of the three medical paradigms at work: Low back pain (20)

To make things simple here we will not look at schizophrenia, but on physical pain, which torments a surprising large number of mentally ill patients.

A patient comes to the physician with low back pain. If the physician uses manual medicine, he will examine the patient carefully to exclude the need of surgery; he works with his hands on the patient, helping the patient to be more relaxed, less tense and less in pain. Most fine body workers or chiropractors can remove a normal low back pain within an hour. When the cause in the body is understood and removed, the job is done. If the pain returns, so must the patient. If he gets a bad discus (a slipped disc) and a severe problem later with compression of the spinal nerves it is not related to this treatment.

If the physician is working according to biomedicine, he will examine the patient carefully to exclude the need of surgery, and if the problem is not serious he will mobilize the patient, and use the painkillers necessary for this. He will talk about prevention, avoiding heavy lifting or poor working postures. If the cause of the pain is understood this is fine, but mostly the low back pain has no objective cause and this is no obstacle for giving the treatment. When the patient is well again after the mobilization – it normally takes a couple of days – the job is done.

If the physician is working with conscious-based medicine he will first examine the patient carefully to exclude the need of surgery. He will then, together with the patient, look for the cause of the illness in the patient's consciousness and sub-consciousness – difficult feelings repressed and placed in the longissimus thoraces muscles and other muscles. He will talk to the patient, give "holding" and processing, and inspire him to a more honest and joyful living. When the cause in the (un)consciousness is understood and removed, and the pain is gone, the job is done.

It is not that any of these medical paradigms are better or worse that the other. The excellent physician mastering what we call the "new bio-psycho-social, holistic medicine" uses the most efficient way to help every patient, giving him or her exactly what is needed under the circumstances. So, if it does not work, stop the treatment and try something else.

# References

[1] Kuhn TS. The structure of scientific revolutions. Int Encyclopedia Unified Sci 1962;2:2.
[2] Gadamer H. Truth and method. New York: Continuum, 2003.
[3] Chalmers A. What is this thing called science? Buckingham: Open Univ Press, 1999.
[4] Hanson AE. Hippocrates: Diseases of Women. Signs 11975;2:567-84.
[5] Ventegodt S, Morad M, Merrick J. Clinical holistic medicine: Classic art of healing or the therapeutic touch. ScientificWorldJournal 2004;4:134 -47.
[6] Jung CG. Man and his symbols. New York: Anchor Press, 1964.
[7] Jung CG. Psychology and alchemy. Collected works of CG Jung. Princeton, NJ: Princeton Univ Press, 1968.
[8] Maslow AH. Toward a psychology of being. New York: Van Nostrand, 1962.
[9] Antonovsky A. Health, stress and coping. London: Jossey-Bass, 1985.
[10] Antonovsky A. Unravelling the mystery of health. How people manage stress and stay well. San Franscisco: Jossey-Bass, 1987.
[11] Frankl V. Man´s search for meaning. New York: Pocket Books, 1985.
[12] Fromm E. The art of living. New York, Harper Collins, 2000.
[13] Goleman DL. Emotional intelligence. New York: Bantam, 1995.
[14] Goleman DL. Destructive emotions. New York: Mind Life Inst, 2003.
[15] Sartre JP Being and nothingness. London: Routledge, London, 2002.
[16] Kierkegaard SA. The sickness unto death. Princeton, NJ: Princeton Univ Press, 1983.

[17] Allardt E. To have, to love, to be – about welfare in the Nordic countries. Lund: Argos, 1975. [Swedish].
[18] Ventegodt S. Consciousness-based medicine. Copenhagen: Forskningscenterets Forlag, 2003. [Danish].
[19] Ornish D. Love and survival. The scientific basis for the healing power of intimacy. New York: Harper Collins, 1999.
[20] Ventegodt S, Morad M, Merrick J. Clinical holistic medicine: The "new medicine", the multi-paradigmatic physician and the medical record. ScientificWorldJournal 2004;4:273-85.

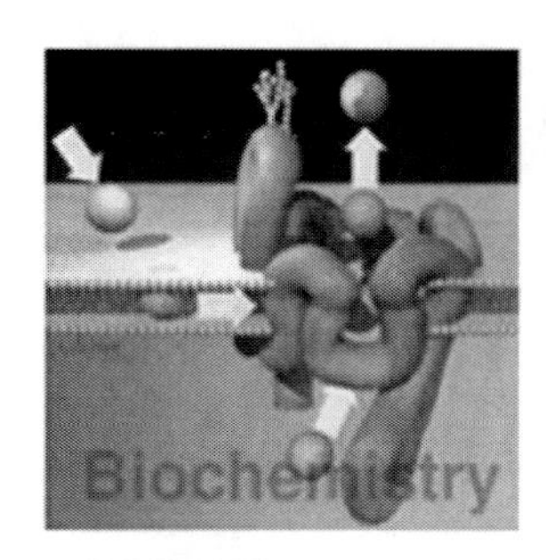
Biochemistry

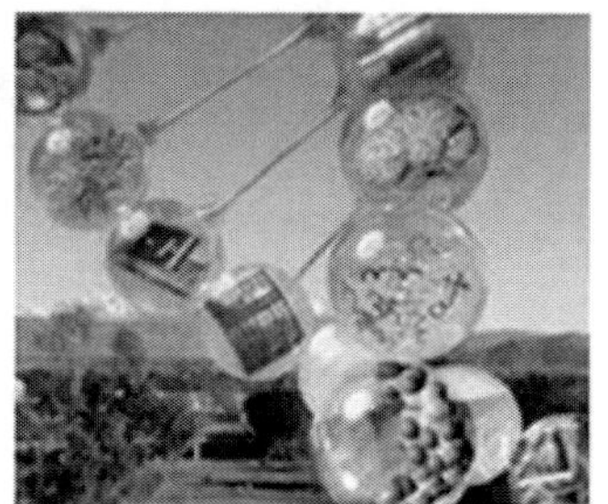

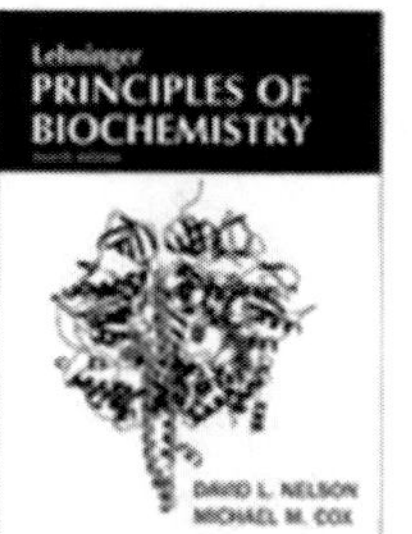
Lehninger
PRINCIPLES OF
BIOCHEMISTRY
DAVID L. NELSON
MICHAEL M. COX

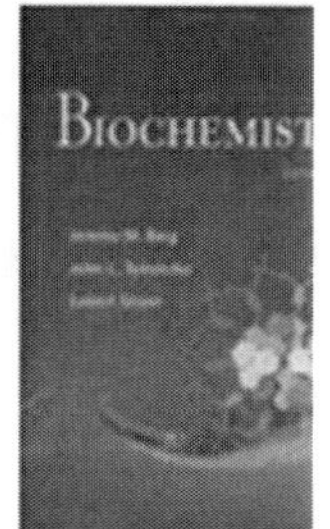
BIOCHEMIST

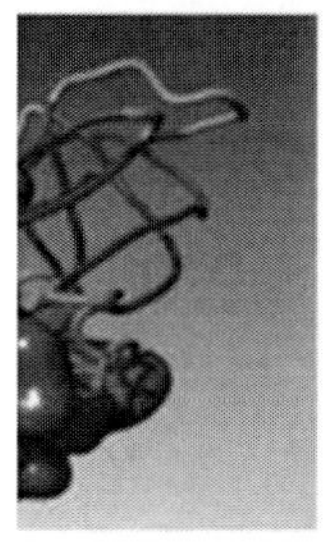

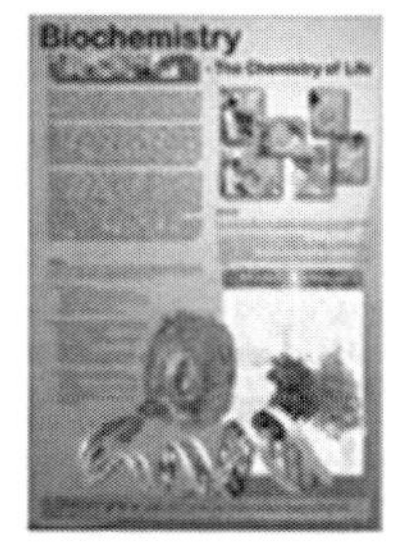
Biochemistry
- The Chemistry of Life

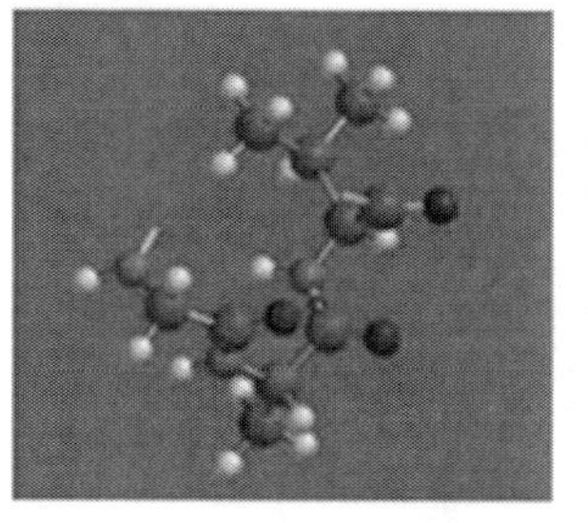

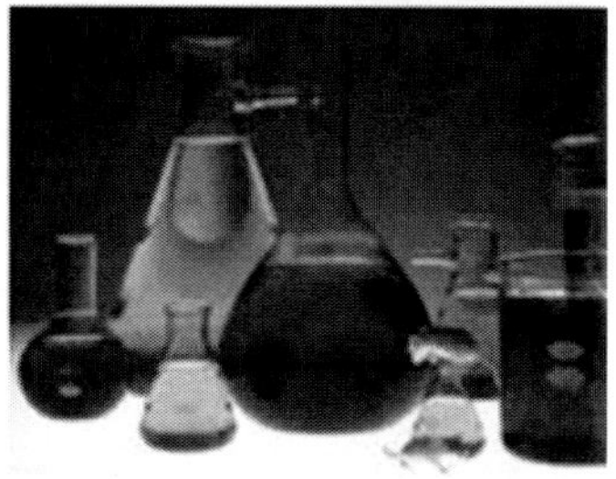

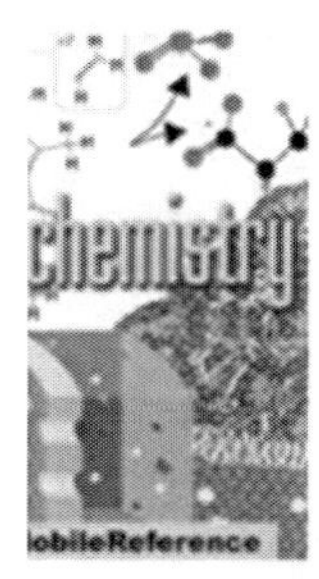

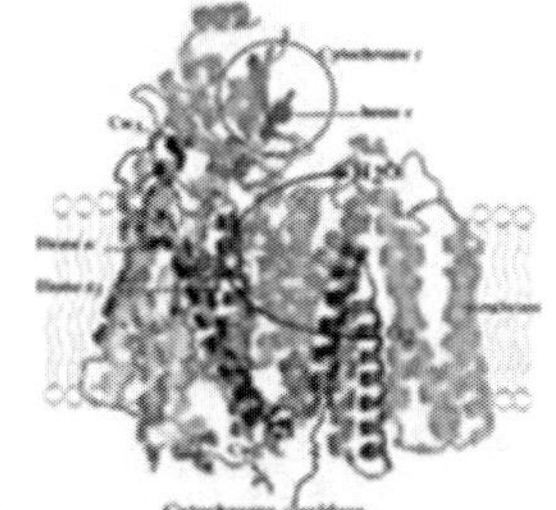
Cytochrome c oxidase

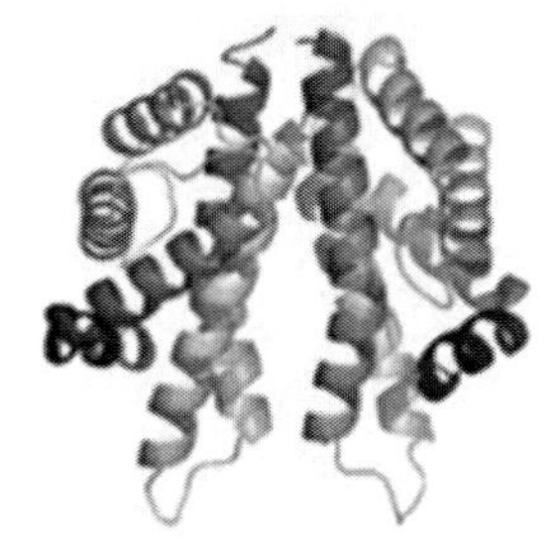

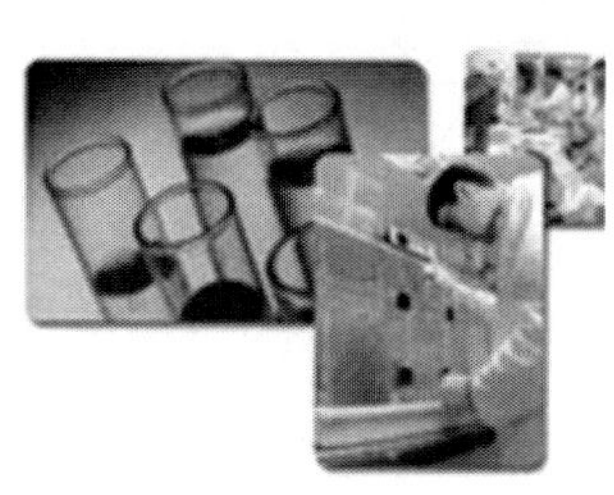

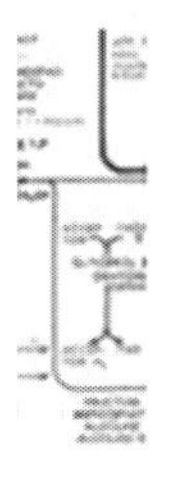

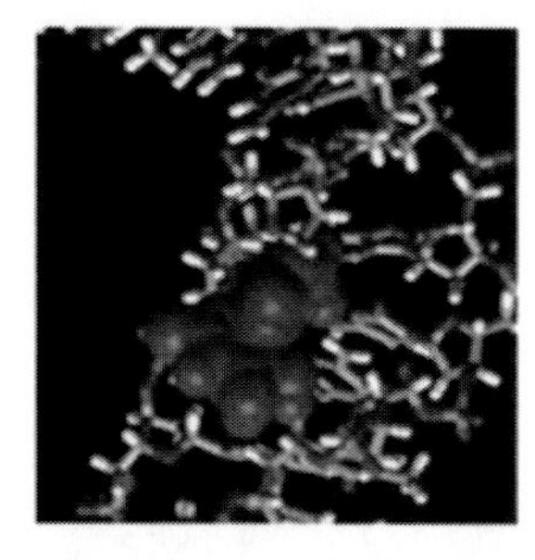

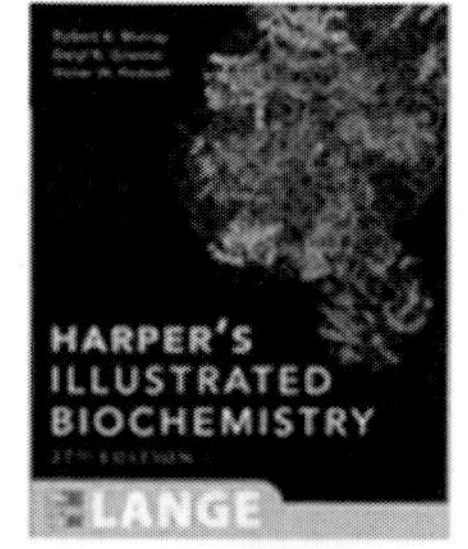
HARPER'S
ILLUSTRATED
BIOCHEMISTRY
LANGE

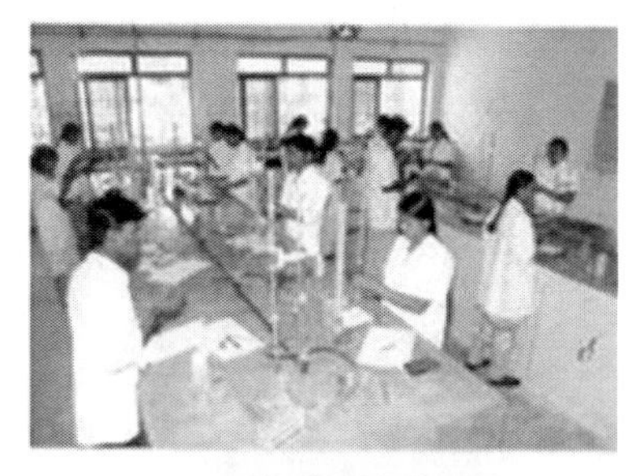

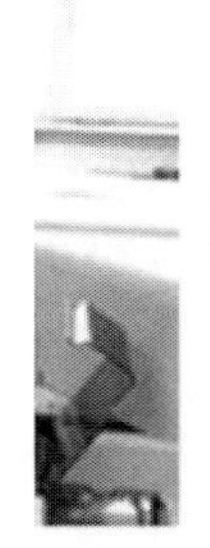

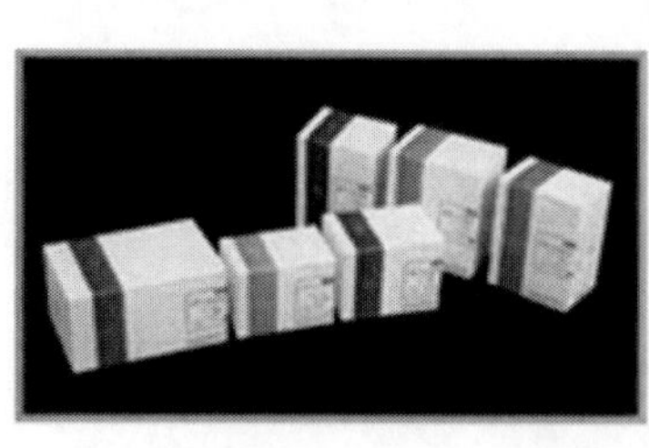

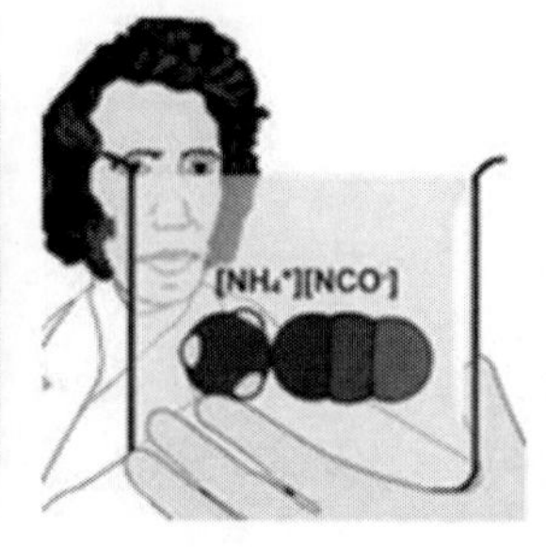
$[NH_4^+][NCO^-]$

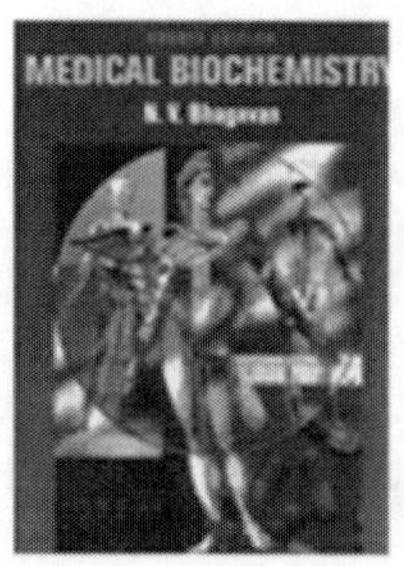
MEDICAL BIOCHEMISTRY
N. V. Bhagavan

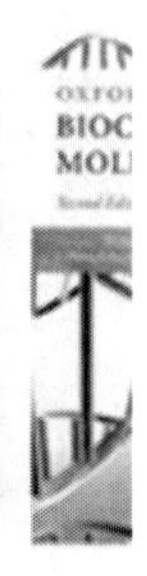

*Chapter XV*

# A critical analysis of Cochrane meta-analyses of the therapeutic value of anti-psychotic drugs

About 5% of people in the developed world are prescribed anti-psychotic drugs. The scope of this chapter is to evaluate the positive and negative effects of anti-psychotic drugs, when treating the psychotic, mentally ill patient in comparison with placebo. We conducted a meta-analysis of the Cochrane protocols on anti-psychotic drugs, which included all randomized clinical trials, where anti-psychotics have been tested in comparison with placebo. The primary outcomes of treatment of interest to the study were: Mental health (or "mental state"), cooperativeness (or "behaviour"), a hybrid measure of mental health, cooperativeness and hallucinatory behaviour (or "global state"), relapse of primarily un-cooperativeness or hallucinatory behaviour (or "relapse") as well as adverse effects. The study included analyses of dichotomous data using fixed effects relative risk (RR), an estimation of the 95% confidence interval (CI) as well as a calculation of the number needed to treat (NNT) and the number needed to harm (NNH). All significant NNHs were summed to estimate the sum of total NNH. The results showed, that anti-psychotic drugs improved mental health (NNT=50). It was also found that uncooperative behaviour (NNT=4) and "relapse" (NNT=4) was reduced, and that "global state" was improved (NNT=7). Anti-psychotic drugs were shown to have many adverse effects (total NNH=0.67) and the different types of anti-psychotic drugs had similar positive and negative effects. Anti-psychotic drugs did not cure or improve mental health for patients with psychotic or mental illness, as the small, positive effect found could be explained by the bias. The drugs have many severe adverse effects.

## Introduction

According to the World Health Organization (WHO), 400 million people suffer from a severe mental illness (1). In Denmark, the yearly consumption of anti-psychotic drugs equals 6% of the population or about 300,000 people with an annual expense of 122 million EURO (2).

Some studies have recently shown that anti-psychotic drugs are of miniature efficiency, when treating children, patients with learning disabilities, as well as other groups of patients (3-5). Alongside these findings, a tendency towards attributing an increase of importance to patient narratives concerning a less positive impression of the treatment with anti-psychotic drugs has emerged (6,7) and mentally ill patients are known to frequently have discontinued the treatment. A significant part of the explanation is the patients' experiences of the treatment with anti-psychotic drugs as being less than perfect (8,9). Some researchers have even suggested that anti-psychotic drugs mainly work by reducing salience of ideas and perceptions, and thus doubt the positive effect of the drugs on the patient's mental health (10). Other researchers have suggested that non-drug therapy might be better for the patients in the long run (11). All of this has created an interest to re-evaluate the positive and negative effects of anti-psychotic drugs.

The ideal study would be an all-including meta-analysis of the positive and negative effects of all the anti-psychotic drugs in the treatment of the psychotic mental illnesses in general. But such a study has been considered difficult to complete, among other reasons due to the non-uniform quality of many of the studies, and because of the diversity of effect and adverse effects among the different types of anti-psychotic drugs. However during the last decade, many studies of the positive and negative effects of the anti-psychotic drugs vs. placebo have been thoroughly analyzed in a large number of Cochrane meta-analyses (12-88). Moreover, recently a large Cochrane study documented that all the different types of anti-psychotic drugs shared similar qualities in regards to beneficence, non-beneficence or even harmful qualities (13). As an effect of that, a significant step towards overcoming the obstacles hindering such a general meta-analysis seems to have been taken, thus making this current study possible.

The present chapter is a meta-analysis of the effect on anti-psychotic drugs in general for the psychotic mental illnesses in general. As the recent Cochrane study on the effects of the different antipsychotic drugs indicated that mental health ("mental state") did not improve significantly (13), a central research question of interest is therefore, if there is a positive treatment effect on mental health with the use of anti-psychotic drugs.

## Cochrane collaboration

Cochrane Collaboration software for preparing and maintaining Cochrane reviews (Review Manager), and the basic review and meta-analysis principles recommended by the Cochrane Collaboration (89,90,91) were used in this study. The methodological quality of the studies was independently assessed by at least two authors. The data was extracted by two reviewers. We searched Medline/PubMed and the Cochrane Library (CENTRAL) for all Cochrane reviews including studies investigating the effects of anti-psychotic drugs versus placebo for all illnesses, and these studies formed the basis of the study at hand. Only randomized controlled trials were included, while quasi-randomized studies were excluded. All participants were people with a diagnosis of schizophrenia or other types of psychotic mental illness, irrespective of age, sex or severity of illness.

The search allowed us to include data from 127 studies on the positive effect of anti-psychotic drugs including 16,646 patients and data from 556 studies on the adverse effects, which included 74,369 patients in the present analysis. As inclusion necessitated at least a Category B on The Cochrane Handbook rating of allocation, a similar number of studies were excluded. The reason for reviewing studies based on quantitative methods only was the lack of quantitative research in the field.

## Types of intervention

Any of the following: High dose (Chlorpromazine, Thioridazine), middle dose (Zuclupenthixol, Peraphenazine), low-dose (Fluphenazine, Haloperidole, Sulpiride, Pimozide, Penfluridol), or atypical, (Risperidone, Aripiprazole, Quetiapine, Amisulpride, Olanzapine, Sertindole, Ziprasidone). Thus including any dose or mode of administration (oral or by injection).Any dose or mode of inactive placebo.

## Types of outcome measures

Mental health (psychotic symptoms or "mental state"): Clinical significant response (short and medium term: 0 days – 6 month)

Behaviour (un-cooperative/disturbed/deteriorated/hallucinatory): Clinical significant response (medium term: 6 weeks – 6 month)

Global state (Hybrid measures of mental health and uncooperative or hallucinatory behaviour): Clinical significant response (short and medium term: 0 days – 6 month)

Relapse (as defined in the clinical trials, often of un-cooperative or hallucinatory behaviour): Clinical significant response (long term: 6 month to 2 years)

Adverse effects (see Table 1): (short and medium term: 0 days – 6 month).

## Methodological quality

*Randomization:* A fairly low percentage (about 10% of the studies) described the methods used to generate random allocation. For most studies, it did not seem completely clear that bias was minimized during the allocation procedure. About 40% reported that the participants allocated to each treatment group were estimated to be similar.

*Blinding:* About 50% gave a description of their attempts to make the investigation double-blind.

*Treatment withdrawals:* The description of those who left the study early was in general unclear or sometimes absent.

*Outcome reporting:* Studies frequently presented both dichotomous and continuous data in graphs, or reported statistical measures of probability (p-values). This diminished the possibility to acquire raw data for a synthesis. It was also common to use p-values as a measure of association between intervention and outcomes instead of showing the strength of the association. Although p-values are influenced by the strength of the association, they also depend on the sample size of the groups. Frequently, continuous data were presented without providing standard deviations/errors (about 60% of trials) or no data were presented at all (about 20% of trials). Thus a lot of possibly informative data were not at hand; we estimated that half of the information was lost here. Many studies used the Brief Psychiatric Rating Scale (BPRS) that contains data related to quality of life like “anxiety”, “emotional withdrawal”, “guilt feelings”, “blunted affect”, “depression”, “tension” and “anergia”, but these subjective data were not analyzed in any Cochrane studies, and is therefore not included in the present study.

*Overall quality:* The quality of trials as measured in the previous version of the review varied (mean using the Jadad Scale was about 3.5). Inclusion necessitated at least a Category B on the Cochrane Handbook rating of allocation. Practically no studies reached Category A, so all data must be considered to be prone to a moderate degree of bias.

### Meta-analytical calculations

The meta-analysis was done in line with recommendations from the Cochrane Collaboration and the Quality of Reporting of Meta-analyses guidelines (89,90,91). The randomized-analyzed endpoints used in the Cochrane reviews were used to group studies according to the above-mentioned outcomes. Funnel plots were made for each outcome and to summarize the effect, relative risks (RR) and risk differences (RD) were calculated, and the number needed to treat (NNT) and number needed to harm (NNH) was calculated from RDs. To combine data in this meta-analysis the fixed effects model was used.

We did not apply weighting for study quality, since we did not have any empirical basis for doing so. The pooled NNH that combined all adverse effects into one measure was calculated as the inverse of the added inverse NNHs of all significant adverse effects (see Table 1). We avoided counting the same adverse effect twice, by grouping similar side effects into one group.

## What we found

Adding together all anti-psychotic drugs into the same meta-analysis we found data to favour anti-psychotic drugs according to: mental health (clinical significant response on psychotic symptoms or mental state) (n=8,407, 53 RCTs, RR 0.87, CI 0.81-0.94), NNT 50; cooperativeness (n=1085, 9 RCTs, RR 0.52, CI 0.45-0.61), NNT 4; clinical significant response in “global impression” (n=5,453, 47 RCTs, RR 0.76, CI 0.73-0.80), NNT 7; and long-term relapse (primarily of hallucinatory or un-cooperative behaviour) (n=1,701, 18 RCTs, RR 0.58, CI 0.53-0.64), NNT 4.

The NNT estimates varied substantially according to the different outcomes. Hence, the NNT for relapse and cooperativeness were 4 and 4 respectively, while the NNT for a clinical significant response to mental health (psychotic symptoms or mental state) was 50. Sub-dividing the meta-analysis into different categories of drugs showed the same pattern, with relapse and cooperativeness being the outcomes with the lowest NNT for all kinds of drugs and clinical significant responses to mental health (psychotic symptoms or mental state) having a substantially higher NNT.

## Adverse effects

Adding together all anti-psychotic drugs we found data to favour placebo treatment according to a number of adverse effects. Table 1 shows the adverse effects that we found statistically significant for at least one group of antipsychotic drugs.

**Table 1. Number needed to harm (NNH) according to type of antipsychotic drug and adverse effects (estimation of the NNHs of middle-dose typicals and atypicals was not possible due to lack of data)**

| | **NNH High-dose typicals** | **NNH Low-dose typicals** | **NNH All antipsychotic drugs** |
|---|---|---|---|
| **1. Photosensitivity** | **7.9** (6.2-11.0) | No studies | **7.9** (6.2-11.0) |
| **2. Eye problems** | **6.5** (4.9-9.8) | Not significant | **6.5** (4.9-9.6) |
| **3. Low blood pressure** | **10.2** (7.7-15.4) | Not significant | **14.6** (11.6-19.8) |
| **4. Constipation** | **18.5** (12.2-38.7) | **8.8** (4.6-96.9) | **26.0** (17.9-47.5) |
| **5. Dry mouth** | **9.5** (7.5-13.1) | **8.5** (5.0-26.3) | **10.8** (9.1-13.3) |
| **6. Weight gain** | **3.6** (2.4-5.4) | **9.1** (5.7-22.3) | **14.9** (11.6-20.7) |
| **7. Salivation and drooling** | **40.7** (24.4-132.6) | **13.9** (8.9-32.2) | **40.9** (27.3-80.7) |
| **8. Peripheral oedema** | No studies | No studies | **9.4** (5.7-26.9) |
| **9. Dystonia** | **25.7** (17.3-49.7) | **8.3** (5.0-25.4) | **21.9** (14.9-41.3) |
| **10. Parkinsonism** | **8.8** (6.8-12.7) | **3.1** (2.4-4.4) | **13.4** (9.8-21.2) |
| **11. Tremor** | **15.8** (9.5-48.3) | **9.6** (6.6-17.7) | **21.2** (16.3-30.4) |
| **12. Rigidity** | **12.0** (7.8-26.4) | **3.7** (2.9-5.3) | **11.1** (8.3-17.0) |
| **13. Weakness including asthenia** | **6.1** (4.0-12.9) | No studies | **13.8** (9.6-24.5) |
| **14. Sleepiness and sedation** | **4.2** (3.7-5.0) | **7.7** (5.5-12.0) | **7.0** (6.3-7.9) |
| **15. Fits (loss of consciousness)** | **38.2** (19.0 - ¥) | Not significant | **35.8** (18.8-389.2) |
| **16. Liver problems** | **11.8** (7.2-31.9) | Not significant | **9.9** (6.3-23.9) |
| **17, Urinary problems** | **52.1** (26.2-3977.3) | Not significant | **25.5** (17.7-45.8) |
| **18. Blurred vision** | Not significant | **12.0** (7.0-40.7) | **62.4** (27.7-247.4) |
| **19. Thick speech or speech disorder** | Not significant | Not significant | **15.3** (9.9-33.9) |
| **20. General movement disorder** | Not significant | **7.0** (3.5-292.6) | **24.3** (17.4-39.9) |
| **21. Dizziness** | No studies | Not significant | **20.8** (14.4-37.6) |
| **22. Akathisia** | Not significant | **7.8** (5.2-15.5) | Not significant |
| **ALL (added together)** | **0.60** (0,43-0.98) | **0.58** (0.38-1.23) | **0.67** (0.49-1.09) |

It is important to notice that while most of the adverse effects might be seen as less burdensome than the mental illness they intent to cure, i.e. weight gain, some of the adverse effects must be considered serious threats to the patients' health, like liver problems, Parkinsonism, and general movement disorders. Adding up all side effects showed a NNH of 0.67 (0.49-1.09), meaning that every patient treated with an antipsychotic drug was likely to get adverse effects. High-dose typicals (NNH=0.60; 0.43-0.98) and low-dose typicals (NNH=0.58; 0.38-1.23) showed similar low NNHs; an estimation of the total NNH of middle-dose typicals and atypicals was not possible due to lack of data.

### Heterogeneity

The studies varied regarding type of inclusion criteria, anti-psychotic drugs and outcomes. In order to reduce the heterogeneity, it is common practice in Cochrane studies to exclude trials that differ much. In this study we included all studies irrespective of the heterogeneity in order to avoid bias. In addition to fixed effect model we also used a random effects model, but this did not change the results much.

## Discussion

Two per cent of the mentally ill patients treated with anti-psychotic drugs improved their mental health ("mental state") (NNT=50); as we included all studies the effect tested for was a small, but significant clinical effect. A significant bias of all data can easily explain this small effect, Therefore it is not correct to claim based on these data that mentally ill patients can be cured. Uncooperative behaviour and relapse of hallucinatory behaviour was significantly reduced in a quarter of the patients prescribed anti-psychotic drugs (NNT=4), but this is likely to be due to a pacifying effect of the drug, in a way poisoning the patients. In accordance with this interpretations we found adverse effects to be very common (total NNH=0.67).

We aimed to use long-term data for the effects of anti-psychotic drugs, as many patients have them prescribed for a relatively long period (sometimes several years). Long-term data for "relapse" was found, but very few long-term studies were found in order to investigate the other outcomes. For "behaviour" and "global impression", only short- and medium-term data was found, and for "mental state" and "adverse effect" a finding of primarily short-term data complemented with little medium-term data took place. In order to make the present analysis it was necessary to include short, medium and long-term data in order to uphold the validity of this study, There are some indications that the positive effects diminish over time; "global impression" thus falls from NNT=4 (short-term) to NNT=7 (middle-term) (4), but there were no long-term data. Based on the experience gained from performing this study, the research group recommends that long-term data should be collected in future testing of anti-psychotic drugs. In addition, many of the original outcome measures of the studies were non-theory-based hybrid measures that included both mental health and behaviour (i.e. the Brief Psychiatric Rating Scale, BPRS). These hybrid measures have been grouped together and relabelled "global impression" in the Cochrane studies, but their significance is not clear.

The interpretation of the NNH values found is debatable as the different types of anti-psychotic drugs have different profiles of adverse effects. The aim of the present analysis of the adverse effects was not to establish the single NNH numbers, which are better established in the tests of the different groups of anti-psychotic drugs one by one, but to establish the total NNH, which expresses the likelihood to get one or more side effects using any type of anti-psychotic drug. In spite of the different profiles, the non-beneficial or harmful effects of the different types of anti-psychotic drugs seem to be of similar intensity in this data interpretation. We do not know if some of the adverse effects are statistically correlated, but this is likely to be the case. If that is the case, then the total NNH is calculated too small. A moderate correlation of 0.1 would change the NNH to about 1. There is an on-going methodological debate about the concepts of "number needed to treat" and "number needed to harm" (92,93), but we do not find the arguments against these concepts presented convincing, and before better concepts are developed, we should not abandon the few effective tools we have to evaluate the clinical value of drugs. Abandoning the NNTs and NNHs would make it quite impossible to evaluate the products of the pharmaceutical industry in metaanalysis, which we obviously need to do, the antipsychotic drugs being an example of this urgent need.

There are several problems with the study inclusion criteria:a) Why look at only placebo controlled trials? Although active controlled trials are not that numerous in antipsychotic trials, nevertheless they would methodologically still provide usable comparisons between individual compounds. b) Why only look at randomized trials? - although they are accepted as the 'best design these trials will almost never be actually designed as safety trials, as they nearly always have efficacy as their primary objective. Often trials - even otherwise good ones - are poor at systematically reporting all safety data. They also tend not to be large enough to be powered to look at rare events, even when aggregated in a meta-analysis across studies. They are also known in many different clinical areas to generally select an atypical subset of the treatable population into the RCT. We found it problematic that many of the early studies did not allow the efficacy result from a study to be extracted (e.g. just a P-value was given). It is pointless having an optimized search algorithm, if then the data cannot be extracted. This might have serious implications for the robustness of the findings.

We found only 127 studies (~17,000 patients) to be of sufficient quality to be included, but 556 studies on adverse events (~70,000 patients). The reason for this is that the drugs four times as often were tested against each other than against placebo. This fact should not induce bias.

There was a 'general heterogeneity' in the old trials (different drugs, different designs, different adverse effects signals, different population, differing quality etc). One could fairly argue that the quality of the studies was so poor in general and bias so large that the "Cochrane-type metaanalysis" are in fact completely meaningless. This position might be philosophically correct, but will render us completely without tools for evaluating the therapeutic effects of any drugs, giving the pharmaceutical industry power to float the market with inefficient and harmful drugs, so we do not want to go there.

Research has not been thorough, when it comes to the studies of global quality of life, sexual or social functioning, so we have drawn our conclusions based on rather incomplete data. We have assumed that because the early studies of the effect of antipsychotic drugs showed that quality of life, social and sexual functioning were significantly reduced, the pharmaceutical industry simply avoided these measures in the later research, the same way as they avoided all long term measures for adverse effects, This assumption might be wrong and we encourage researchers more resourceful than our group to investigate this.

The Cochrane studies did not test the effect of anti-psychotic drugs against "active placebo" (94), which is another more serious source of bias (95). We recommend that all future studies of mind-altering pharmaceutical drugs be tested this way, or even better against the optimal, alternative non-drug CAM treatment for the relevant disorder (96).

There are people who do not believe in vitamin C for scurvy, antibiotics for infection, blood transfusions etc. There are also people not believing in antipsychotic drugs. We do not consider our self "non-believers". We just want to base treatment of mentally ill patients on evidence. And we find no evidence that antipsychotic drugs improve patient's mental state or mental health.

Should we conclude from our review that we need more efficacious medication with fewer adverse events? No, Fifty years of intensive research not documenting any progress obviously shows that we are going the wrong way using strongly poisonous drugs as medicine for the mentally ill. This project cannot be saved by improving the drugs. It is a wrong project, presumably based on the wrong understanding of mental disorder.

The most problematic side of the present finding is that many psychiatrists and patients seem to function well with the antipsychotic drugs, so how could these drugs not be helpful? Our answer is that a close and supportive relationship between patient and physician IS helpful; if drugs are the only acknowledged treatment among psychiatrists the gifted and skilful psychiatrist will use the drugs as the anchor of treatment and build rapport, hope and mutual understanding around this treatment. Even if the antipsychotic drug only has harmful effects the treatment using such drugs could still be very beneficial. But statistics talks its own language: Such positive outcomes might exist but they are very rare; most patients are only harmed by the drugs. This is what should be learned from this study.

What is the relevance of combining studies of antipsychotics from all illnesses? How does this further our understanding or guide treatment decisions compared to existing meta-analyses of antipsychotics restricted to single diagnoses? Well, this mirrors well the complex daily reality of psychiatrists that will get all these different kinds of psychotic mentally ill patients, that all will be treated very much the same way: With antipsychotic drugs. The rationale of adding all studies together is to evaluate the value of the modern psychiatric practice using antipsychotic drugs. What the results shows us is that we do not help a significant fraction of the patients, if any at all. This shows us, that we need a fundamentally new kind of psychiatry.

Their conclusion that you have to treat only a single (0.6) patient to give them side effects is sadly, according to the reviewers of this paper, not far from clinical practice. One could argue that by including studies from decades ago, this study does not reflect modern practice where tolerability and the minimization of side effects while optimizing outcome is a key clinical objective. Well, Adams et al (13) showed us that the new drugs did not work better than the old ones. While we do not want to ignore the difficult clinical and ethical questions of risk to benefit ratio, and of values in health, for this to be a relevant argument, there should be improvement of patient's mental health (mental state, including hallucinations etc.). Our finding in this regard was very clear: Antipsychotic drugs do not improve mental health in any way. It only reduces hallucinatory behaviour, presumably because of there obviously sedating and poisoning effects.

In general reviewers that we have send this chapter to, of which there has been many, agreed that antipsychotic drugs has very limited value to the patients; to quote one reviewer: "It has been extensively demonstrated that antipsychotic drugs have very limited efficacy, fail to treat many aspects of the illness such as negative symptoms and cognition, and that patients experience frequent adverse effects." The question is if this meta-analysis does move knowledge forward. We think it does. We think that it makes this general knowledge so clear that it is time to look for other ways in general than drugs to treat mentally ill patients. We need to go back in time and use the more "old-fashioned" kinds of psychotherapy and bodywork that has helped so many patients just half a century ago. We need to return to mind-body medicine. We need to understand that the doctor is the tool, not some more or less toxic drugs. Basically, what we learn from this review chapter, is that psychiatry has been going the wrong way for half a century, and that it is timely to realize this and go back to what worked without harming the patient – the classical Hippocratic non-drug medicine.

Interestingly the statistical reviewer of the Lancet (where this chapter was send as a scientific paper) accepted the final version of the paper, its methods and its conclusions. It was rejected by two of three clinicians who would not accept to let go of the use of antipsychotic drugs; the third clinical reviewer accepted the paper. Allow us to quote the reviewer briefly: "Reviewer #5: THE LANCET-D-08-00436R2" wrote: "Statistical review. Comments for the authors: This is a major improvement on the previous version. The statistical methods used now seem appropriate largely throughout." In the end the paper was rejected and used in a shorter version as a chapter in this book.

## Conclusion

In this meta-analysis, data from 127 studies on the positive effect of anti-psychotic drugs including 16,646 patients has been interpreted in the first general meta-analysis on the effect of antipsychotic drugs. The statistical analysis showed, that the anti-psychotic drugs actually did improve mental health ("mental state") compared with placebo (NNT=50). As we have included all outcomes, large and small, we know that this effect is very small indeed, as one in fifty gets a small improvement. We also know that all data is moderately biased, but we find that the small effect can be easily explained by the bias. We therefore did not find the antipsychotic drugs to improve the mental state of mentally ill patients. The study showed that the patients' "behaviour" seems to be significantly improved due to a reduction in un-cooperativeness and "relapse" seems to improve due to less hallucinatory behaviour (NNT=4).

These effects can be explained from a pacifying effect of the drugs coming from a general poisoning of the patient. "Global state", a hybrid measure of unclear significance, was also improved. The anti-psychotic drugs had many adverse effects (total NNH=0.67), but this should probably be corrected to total NNH=1 as we expect some correlation between adverse effects. All types of anti-psychotic drugs had in general similar levels of positive and negative effects. Thus an overall conclusion of this data interpretation is that the anti-psychotic drugs included in this study did not improve mental health. Taken together with the shown extent of the side effects following the use of such medicine, the treatment of psychotic, mentally ill patients with anti-psychotic drugs cannot be considered rational.

## References

[1] Janca A. World and mental health in 2001. Curr Psychiatry Rep 2001;3(2):77-8.

[2] Gunnersen SJ. Statistical Yearbook 2007. Copenhagen: Statistics Denmark, 2008.

[3] Editorial. Children and psychiatric drugs: disillusion and opportunity. Lancet 2008;372(9645):1194.

[4] Sikich L, Frazier JA, McClellan J, Findling RL, Vitiello B, Ritz L, et al. Double-blind comparison of first- and second-generation antipsychotics in early-onset schizophrenia and schizo-affective disorder: Findings from the treatment of early-onset schizophrenia spectrum disorders (TEOSS) study. Am J Psychiatry 2008; 165:1420-31.

[5] Yawar A. The doctor as human being. J R Soc Med 2005;98(5):215-7.
[6] Goff man E. Asylums. London: Penguin, 1991.
[7] Thornicroft G, Tansella M, Becker T, et al. The personal impact of schizophrenia in Europe. Schizophr Res 2004; 69: 125–32.
[8] Whitaker R. Mad in America. New York: Basic Books, 2002
[9] Lieberman JA, Stroup TS, McEvoy JP, et al. Effectiveness of anti-psychotic drugs in patients with chronic schizophrenia. N Engl J Med 2005;353:1209–23.
[10] Kapur S. Psychosis as a state of aberrant salience: a framework linking biology, phenomenology, and pharmacology in schizophrenia. Am J Psychiatry 2003;160:13–23.
[11] Bola JR, Mosher LR. Treatment of acute psychosis without neuroleptics: 2-year outcomes from the Soteria project. J Nerv Ment Dis 2003;191:219–29.
[12] Abhijnhan A, Adams CE, David A, Ozbilen M. Depot fluspirilene for schizophrenia. Cochrane Database Syst Rev 2007;(1):CD001718.
[13] Adams CE, Awad G, Rathbone J, Thornley B. Chlorpromazine versus placebo for schizophrenia. Cochrane Database Syst Rev 2007;(2):CD000284.
[14] Amato L, Minozzi S, Pani PP, Davoli M. Anti-psychotic medications for cocaine dependence. Cochrane Database Syst Rev 2007;(3):CD006306.
[15] Arunpongpaisal S, Ahmed I, Aqeel N, Suchat P. Anti-psychotic drug treatment for elderly people with late-onset schizophrenia. Cochrane Database Syst Rev 2003;(2):CD004162.
[16] Bagnall A, Lewis RA, Leitner ML. Ziprasidone for schizophrenia and severe mental illness. Cochrane Database Syst Rev 2000;(4):CD001945.
[17] Bagnall A, Fenton M, Kleijnen J, Lewis R. Molindone for schizophrenia and severe mental illness. Cochrane Database Syst Rev 2007;(1):CD002083.
[18] Ballard C, Waite J. The effectiveness of atypical anti-psychotics for the treatment of aggression and psychosis in Alzheimer's disease. Cochrane Database Syst Rev 2006;(1):CD003476.
[19] Basan A, Leucht S. Valproate for schizophrenia. Cochrane Database Syst Rev 2004;(1):CD004028.
[20] Belgamwar RB, Fenton M. Olanzapine IM or velotab for acutely disturbed/agitated people with suspected serious mental illnesses. Cochrane Database Syst Rev 2005;(2):CD003729.
[21] Binks CA, Fenton M, McCarthy L, Lee T, Adams CE, Duggan C. Pharmacological interventions for people with borderline personality disorder. Cochrane Database Syst Rev 2006;(1):CD005653.
[22] Carpenter S, Berk M, Rathbone J. Clotiapine for acute psychotic illnesses. Cochrane Database Syst Rev 2004;(4):CD002304.
[23] Chakrabarti A, Bagnall A, Chue P, Fenton M, Palaniswamy V, Wong W, Xia J. Loxapine for schizophrenia. Cochrane Database Syst Rev 2007;(4):CD001943.
[24] Chua WL, de Izquierdo SA, Kulkarni J, Mortimer A. Estrogen for schizophrenia. Cochrane Database Syst Rev 2005;(4):CD004719.
[25] Coutinho E, Fenton M, Quraishi S. Zuclopenthixol decanoate for schizophrenia and other serious mental illnesses. Cochrane Database Syst Rev 2000;(2):CD001164.
[26] Cure S, Rathbone J, Carpenter S. Droperidol for acute psychosis. Cochrane Database Syst Rev 2004;(4):CD002830.
[27] David A, Adams CE, Eisenbruch M, Quraishi S, Rathbone J. Depot fluphenazine decanoate and enanthate for schizophrenia. Cochrane Database Syst Rev 2005;(1):CD000307.
[28] David A, Quraishi S, Rathbone J. Depot perphenazine decanoate and enanthate for schizophrenia. Cochrane Database Syst Rev 2005;(3):CD001717.
[29] DeSilva P, Fenton M, Rathbone J. Zotepine for schizophrenia. Cochrane Database Syst Rev 2006;(4):CD001948.
[30] Dinesh M, David A, Quraishi SN. Depot pipotiazine palmitate and undecylenate for schizophrenia. Cochrane Database Syst Rev 2004;(4):CD001720.
[31] Duggan L, Brylewski J. Anti-psychotic medication versus placebo for people with both schizophrenia and learning disability. Cochrane Database Syst Rev 2004;(4):CD000030.
[32] Duggan L, Fenton M, Rathbone J, Dardennes R, El-Dosoky A, Indran S. Olanzapine for schizophrenia. Cochrane Database Syst Rev 2005;(2):CD001359.

[33] El-Sayeh HG, Morganti C. Aripiprazole for schizophrenia. Cochrane Database Syst Rev 2006;(2):CD004578.
[34] Elias A, Kumar A. Testosterone for schizophrenia. Cochrane Database Syst Rev 2007;(3):CD006197.
[35] Fenton M, Rathbone J, Reilly J, Sultana A. Thioridazine for schizophrenia. Cochrane Database Syst Rev 2007;(3):CD001944.
[36] Gibson RC, Fenton M, Coutinho ES, Campbell C. Zuclopenthixol acetate for acute schizophrenia and similar serious mental illnesses. Cochrane Database Syst Rev 2004;(3):CD000525.
[37] Gilbody SM, Bagnall AM, Duggan L, Tuunainen A. Risperidone versus other atypical anti-psychotic medication for schizophrenia. Cochrane Database Syst Rev 2000;(3):CD002306.
[38] Gillies D, Beck A, McCloud A, Rathbone J, Gillies D. Benzodiazepines alone or in combination with anti-psychotic drugs for acute psychosis. Cochrane Database Syst Rev 2005;(4):CD003079.
[39] Hartung B, Wada M, Laux G, Leucht S. Perphenazine for schizophrenia. Cochrane Database Syst Rev 2005;(1):CD003443.
[40] Hosalli P, Davis JM. Depot risperidone for schizophrenia. Cochrane Database Syst Rev 2003;(4):CD004161.
[41] Huf G, Alexander J, Allen MH. Haloperidol plus promethazine for psychosis induced aggression. Cochrane Database Syst Rev 2005;(1):CD005146.
[42] Hunter RH, Joy CB, Kennedy E, Gilbody SM, Song F. Risperidone versus typical anti-psychotic medication for schizophrenia. Cochrane Database Syst Rev 2003;(2):CD000440.
[43] Jayaram MB, Hosalli P, Stroup S. Risperidone versus olanzapine for schizophrenia. Cochrane Database Syst Rev 2006;(2):CD005237.
[44] Jesner OS, Aref-Adib M, Coren E. Risperidone for autism spectrum disorder. Cochrane Database Syst Rev 2007;(1):CD005040.
[45] Joy CB, Adams CE, Rice K. Crisis intervention for people with severe mental illnesses. Cochrane Database Syst Rev 2006;(4):CD001087.
[46] Joy CB, Adams CE, Lawrie SM. Haloperidol versus placebo for schizophrenia. Cochrane Database Syst Rev 2006;(4):CD003082.
[47] Kennedy E, Kumar A, Datta SS. Anti-psychotic medication for childhoodonset schizophrenia. Cochrane Database Syst Rev 2007;(3):CD004027.
[48] Kumar A, Strech D. Zuclopenthixol dihydrochloride for schizophrenia. Cochrane Database Syst Rev 2005;(4):CD005474.
[49] Leucht S, Hartung B. Benperidol for schizophrenia. Cochrane Database Syst Rev 2005;(2):CD003083.
[50] Leucht S, Hartung B. Perazine for schizophrenia. Cochrane Database Syst Rev 2006;(2):CD002832.
[51] Leucht S, Kissling W, McGrath J, White P. Carbamazepine for schizophrenia. Cochrane Database Syst Rev 2007;(3):CD001258.
[52] Leucht S, Kissling W, McGrath J. Lithium for schizophrenia. Cochrane Database Syst Rev 2007;(3):CD003834.
[53] Lewis R, Bagnall AM, Leitner M. Sertindole for schizophrenia. Cochrane Database Syst Rev 2005;(3):CD001715.
[54] Macritchie KA, Geddes JR, Scott J, Haslam DR, Goodwin GM. Valproic acid, valproate and divalproex in the maintenance treatment of bipolar disorder. Cochrane Database Syst Rev 2001;(3):CD003196.
[55] Macritchie K, Geddes JR, Scott J, Haslam D, de Lima M, Goodwin G. Valproate for acute mood episodes in bipolar disorder. Cochrane Database Syst Rev 2003;(1):CD004052.
[56] Marques LO, Lima MS, Soares BG. Trifluoperazine for schizophrenia. Cochrane Database Syst Rev 2004;(1):CD003545.
[57] Marriott RG, Neil W, Waddingham S. Anti-psychotic medication for elderly people with schizophrenia. Cochrane Database Syst Rev 2006;(1):CD005580.
[58] Marshall M, Rathbone J. Early intervention for psychosis. Cochrane Database Syst Rev 2006;(4):CD004718.
[59] Matar HE, Almerie MQ. Oral fluphenazine versus placebo for schizophrenia. Cochrane Database Syst Rev 2007;(1):CD006352.
[60] Mota NE, Lima MS, Soares BG. Amisulpride for schizophrenia. Cochrane Database Syst Rev 2002;(2):CD001357.

[61] Nolte S, Wong D, Lachford G. Amphetamines for schizophrenia. Cochrane Database Syst Rev 2004;(4):CD004964.
[62] Pekkala E, Merinder L. Psychoeducation for schizophrenia. Cochrane Database Syst Rev 2002;(2):CD002831.
[63] Premkumar TS, Pick J. Lamotrigine for schizophrenia. Cochrane Database Syst Rev 2006;(4):CD005962.
[64] Punnoose S, Belgamwar MR. Nicotine for schizophrenia. Cochrane Database Syst Rev 2006;(1):CD004838.
[65] Quraishi S, David A. Depot flupenthixol decanoate for schizophrenia or other similar psychotic disorders. Cochrane Database Syst Rev 2000;(2):CD001470.
[66] Quraishi S, David A. Depot haloperidol decanoate for schizophrenia. Cochrane Database Syst Rev 2000;(2):CD001361.
[67] Rathbone J, McMonagle T. Pimozide for schizophrenia or related psychoses. Cochrane Database Syst Rev 2007;(3):CD001949.
[68] Rendell JM, Gijsman HJ, Keck P, Goodwin GM, Geddes JR. Olanzapine alone or in combination for acute mania. Cochrane Database Syst Rev 2003;(3):CD004040.
[69] Rendell JM, Gijsman HJ, Bauer MS, Goodwin GM, Geddes GR. Risperidone alone or in combination for acute mania. Cochrane Database Syst Rev 2006;(1):CD004043.
[70] Rendell JM, Geddes JR. Risperidone in long-term treatment for bipolar disorder. Cochrane Database Syst Rev 2006;(4):CD004999.
[71] Rummel C, Hamann J, Kissling W, Leucht S. New generation anti-psychotics for first episode schizophrenia. Cochrane Database Syst Rev 2003;(4):CD004410.
[72] Rummel C, Kissling W, Leucht S. Antidepressants for the negative symptoms of schizophrenia. Cochrane Database Syst Rev 2006;3:CD005581.
[73] Soares BG, Fenton M, Chue P. Sulpiride for schizophrenia. Cochrane Database Syst Rev 2000;(2):CD001162.
[74] Soares BG, Lima MS. Penfluridol for schizophrenia. Cochrane Database Syst Rev 2006;(2):CD002923.
[75] Srisurapanont M, Kittiratanapaiboon P, Jarusuraisin N. Treatment for amphetamine psychosis. Cochrane Database Syst Rev 2001;(4):CD003026.
[76] Srisurapanont M, Maneeton B, Maneeton N. Quetiapine for schizophrenia. Cochrane Database Syst Rev 2004;(2):CD000967.
[77] Tharyan P, Adams CE. Electroconvulsive therapy for schizophrenia. Cochrane Database Syst Rev 2005;(2):CD000076.
[78] Trevisani VF, Castro AA, Neves Neto JF, Atallah AN. Cyclophosphamide versus methylprednisolone for treating neuropsychiatric involvement in systemic lupus erythematosus. Cochrane Database Syst Rev 2006;(2):CD002265.
[79] Tuominen HJ, Tiihonen J, Wahlbeck K. Glutamatergic drugs for schizophrenia. Cochrane Database Syst Rev 2006;(2):CD003730.
[80] Tuunainen A, Wahlbeck K, Gilbody SM. Newer atypical anti-psychotic medication versus clozapine for schizophrenia. Cochrane Database Syst Rev 2000;(2):CD000966.
[81] Volz A, Khorsand V, Gillies D, Leucht S. Benzodiazepines for schizophrenia. Cochrane Database Syst Rev 2007;(1):CD006391.
[82] Wahlbeck K, Cheine M, Essali MA. Clozapine versus typical neuroleptic medication for schizophrenia. Cochrane Database Syst Rev 2000;(2):CD000059.
[83] Waraich PS, Adams CE, Roque M, Hamill KM, Marti J. Haloperidol dose for the acute phase of schizophrenia. Cochrane Database Syst Rev 2002;(3):CD001951.
[84] Webb RT, Howard L, Abel KM. Anti-psychotic drugs for non-affective psychosis during pregnancy and postpartum. Cochrane Database Syst Rev 2004;(2):CD004411.
[85] Whitehead C, Moss S, Cardno A, Lewis G. Antidepressants for people with both schizophrenia and depression. Cochrane Database Syst Rev 2002;(2):CD002305.
[86] Wijkstra J, Lijmer J, Balk F, Geddes J, Nolen WA. Pharmacological treatment for psychotic depression. Cochrane Database Syst Rev 2005;(4):CD004044.

[87] Wong D, Adams CE, David A, Quraishi SN. Depot bromperidol decanoate for schizophrenia. Cochrane Database Syst Rev 2004;(3):CD001719.

[88] Young AH, Geddes JR, Macritchie K, Rao SN, Vasudev A. Tiagabine in the maintenance treatment of bipolar disorders. Cochrane Database Syst Rev 2006;3:CD005173.

[89] van Tulder M, Furlan A, Bombardier C, Bouter L; Editorial Board of the CochraneCollaboration Back Review Group. Updated method guidelines for systematic reviews in the Cochrane Collaboration back review group. Spine 2003;28(12):1290-9.

[90] Higgins J, Green S. Cochrane handbook for systematic reviews of interventions version 5.0.0. edn. Oxford: The Cochrane Collaboration, 2008.

[91] Moher D, Cook DJ, Eastwood S, Olkin I, Rennie D, Stroup DF. Improving the quality of reports of meta-analyses of randomized controlled trials: the QUOROM statement. Quality of Reporting of Meta-analyses. Lancet 1999;354:1896-900.

[92] Sampaio C, Ferreira J, Costa J.[Numbers needed for treatment and their respective confidence intervals: useful tools to assess clinical significance and uncertainty associated with medical interventions] Rev Port Cardiol 2000;19(12):1303-8.[Portuguese]

[93] Ebrahim S. The use of numbers needed to treat derived from systematic reviews and meta-analysis. Caveats and pitfalls. Eval Health Prof 2001;24(2):152-64.

[94] Moncrieff J, Wessely S, Hardy R. Active placebos versus antidepressants for depression. Cochrane Database Syst Rev. 2004;(1):CD003012.

[95] Boutron I, Estellat C, Guittet L, Dechartres A, Sackett DL, Hróbjartsson A, Ravaud P. Methods of blinding in reports of randomized controlled trials assessing pharmacologic treatments: a systematic review. PLoS Med 2006;3(10):e425.

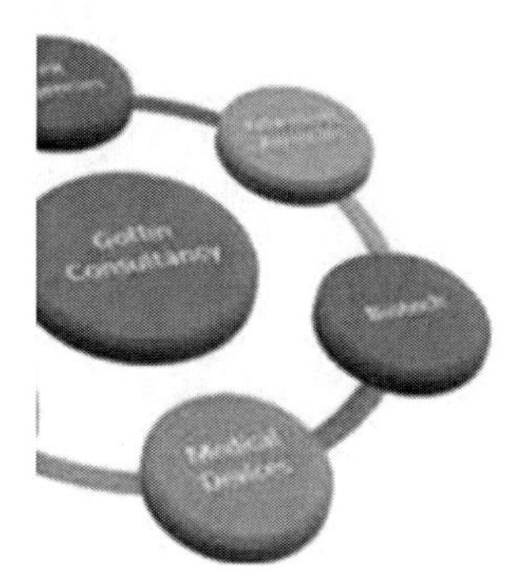



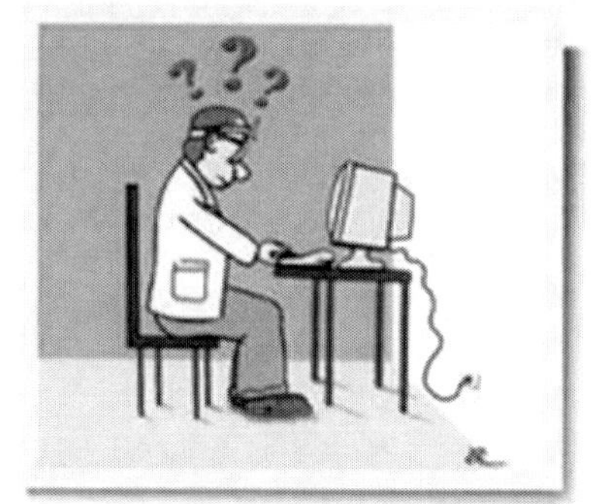

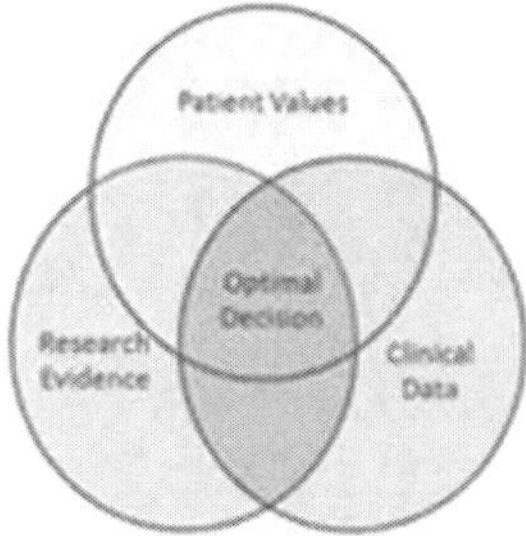



Evidence Based Medicine: when best evidence from research meets clinical information and patient values, optimal decisions are possible ©MedPie.com

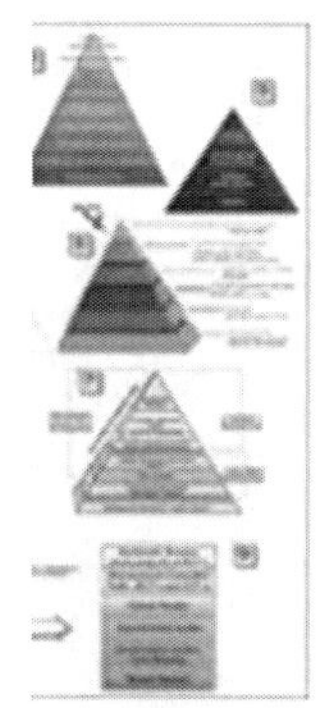

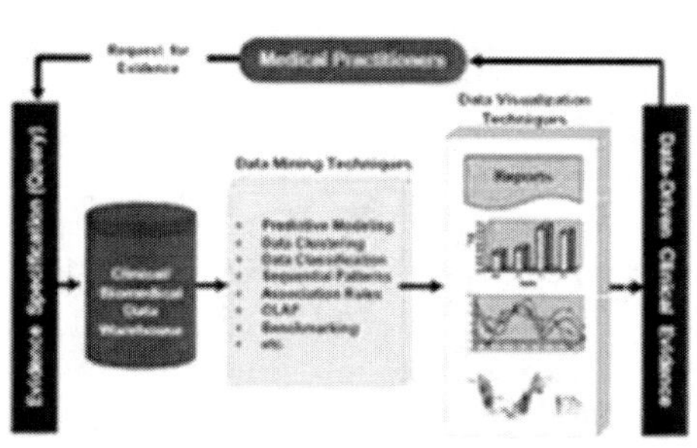



The Proposed Data Mining Info-Structure

| Level of Evidence | Grading Criteria | Grade of Recommendati |
|---|---|---|
| 1a | Systematic review of RCTs including meta-analysis | A |
| 1b | Individual RCT with narrow confidence interval | A |
| 1c | All and none studies | B |
| 2a | Systematic review of cohort studies | B |
| 2b | Individual cohort study and low quality RCT | B |
| 2c | Outcome research study | C |
| 3a | Systematic review of case-control studies | C |
| 3b | Individual case-control study | C |
| 4 | Case-series, poor quality cohort and case-control studies | C |
| 5 | Expert opinion | D |

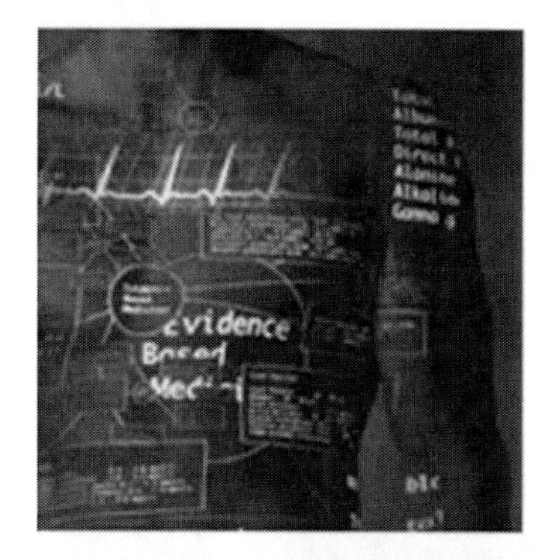

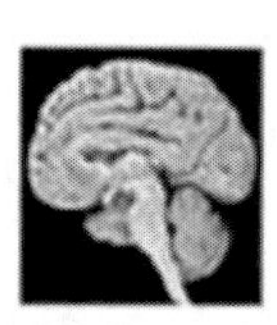

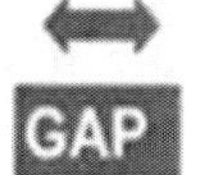



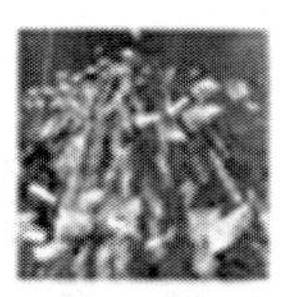

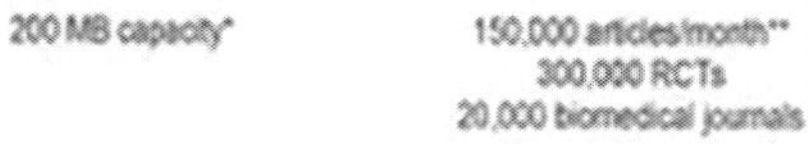



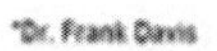



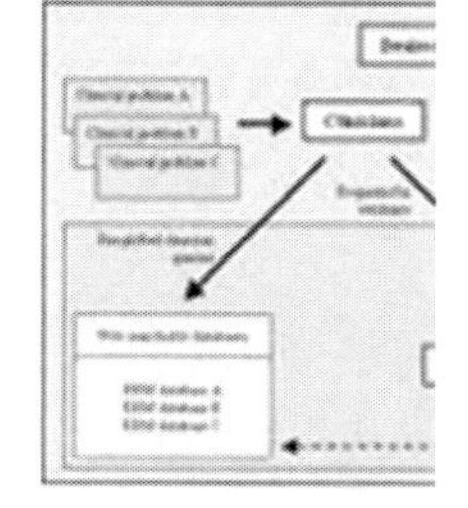

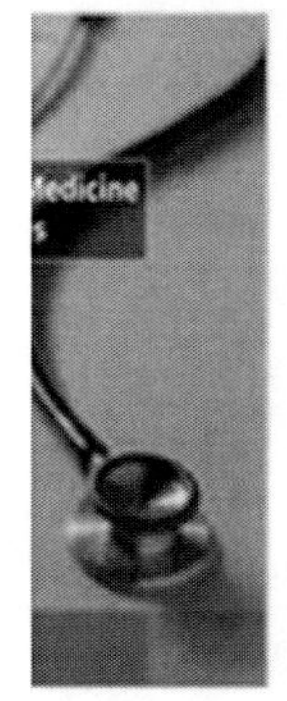



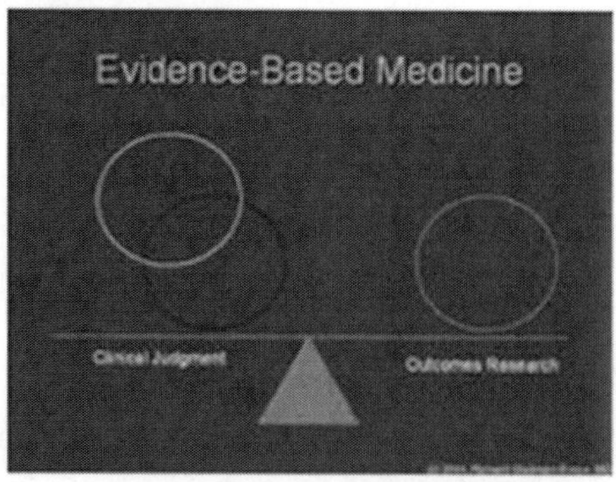



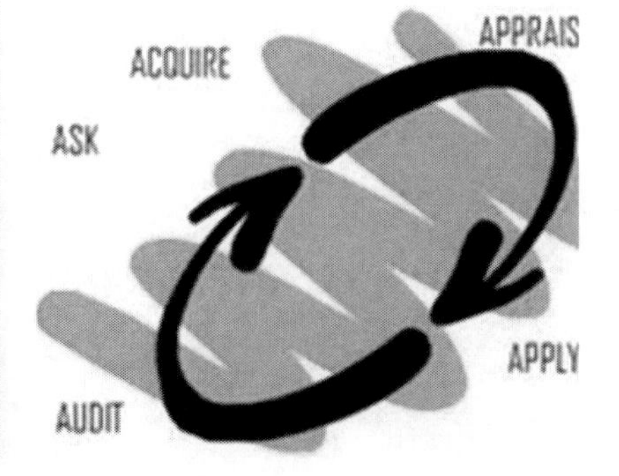

*Chapter XVI*

# Is the biochemical hypothesis for the etiology of the mental diseases substantiated?

We review the understanding of the etiology of the mental diseases, which has changed considerably during the last three decades. We consider the results from psycho-neuro-pharmacology and the derived historical, biochemical hypotheses for the mental diseases, and find that they have not been substantiated.

We analyse the popular, biochemical hypothesis of the diseases depression and schizophrenia and find that the standard biochemical hypotheses are not substantiated. We suggest a mechanism for the pacifying effect of the antipsychotic drugs. When it comes to the etiology of the two most common mental diseases both of these seem to be caused by disturbed psychosexual development, causing a degenerated intent, in accordance with Bleuler's classical description and understanding of schizophrenia. We present a psychobiological and more holistic models of the mental diseases and their etiology, which we find more plausible than the historical, biochemical and genetic models.

## Introduction

All transmitter systems known so far are present in both rats and humans; they must therefore be considered to be very stable in an evolutionary perspective (1). But here are significant differences also in the vertebrate brains; it looks as if man to a much higher degree than animals is in control of his fundamental mental functions such as attention, sleep, and motor activity. In man all these functions are under control of the will and are assumed to be ruled from the cerebral cortex. This is in accordance with the known development of the cerebral neocortex and above all the fronto-orbital lobes. Because mental diseases such as depression and schizophrenia are hardly found in animals, it seems reasonable to believe that mental diseases are caused by regulation from the cerebral cortex rather than deregulation in one or several of the ascending systems. The rational-mechanical interpretation of reality favors the hypothesis of a defect in the ascending systems, while the energetic-informational interpretation of reality favors a complex cerebral deregulation. Research has concentrated on the ascending systems, partly because of the documented effect of the antidepressants and the neuroleptics. However little is known about the descending, neural systems.

Seen from a rational interpretation of reality we think it is natural to assume, that mental diseases are caused by an inherited, mechanical defect in the brain such as a defect in an enzyme or a receptor. When psychopharmacological drugs were invented, they were seemingly able to reduce many of the symptoms of mental illnesses, i.e. the hallucinatory behaviour of schizophrenic patients. The mentally ill patients became much more calm and easier to care for, and members of the patient's family often appreciated the results of the treatment, in spite of the rate of cure was rarely found to be significantly improved compared to the traditional methods of psychotherapy and holistic therapy. Especially the obedience of the patients was often radically improved, and the lack of resistance and the cooperation was seen as important signs of improvement.

This led to a number of hypotheses, as it was assumed that the effect of the drugs was a simple compensation for specific defects behind the mental diseases. This interpretation has, however, in spite of many years of research and thousands of published papers not lead to the expected full understanding of the aetiology of mental diseases; quite on the contrary mental illness and human brain function seems more mysterious and hard to understand from a chemical perspective than ever.

This chapter provides arguments to reject the hitherto proposed simple hypotheses about a link between biochemical, molecular defects and mental disease. For instance, in spite of a great scientific effort neither schizophrenia nor depression has been linked to such defect genes or other specific biochemical defects; and this fact was clear to researchers already in 1989 (2).

## Psychoneurophamacology

Almost every drug that affects the brain does so in terms of influences on synaptic transmissions (3). Antidepressants and neuroleptics as well as several other types of psychotropic drugs often work on one or more ascending mono-aminergic transmitter system (with serotonine (5HT), norepinephrine (NE) or dopamine (DA) as transmitter), whose nuclei are present in the brain stem or the diencephalon. Pharmacological interaction with systems with acetylcholine (Ach) or gamma-aminobutyrate (GABA) can, however, also give a similar effect. Reserpin was the first antipsychotic drug that were shown to empty the monoamines from their storage vesicles, making them accessible to degradation by mitochondria-tied monoamine oxidase. The discovery of such compounds lead to the formation of the hypothesis of genetically specified dysfunction in these systems as a possible cause of schizophrenia, and serotonine and norepinephrine of depression.

The monoamine systems (5HT, NE, DA) are supposed to be the primary site of action of many psychotropic drugs and have therefore been the subject of intensive research activity. But in spite of this the precise nature of the exact relation between the monoamine systems, the mental effect of the drugs, physiology, and behaviour is still not understood in details. Because of their great diversity the monoaminergic systems can be assumed to attend to general regulatory functions. The function of the serotonergic systems is the least understood.

They seem to function through a neural inhibiting tonus especially to the limbic system, correlated to muscle tonus. Dopaminergic systems possibly regulate motor activity and the activity of thoughts. Regulation of outwardly directed attention is possibly connected to the noradrenergic systems.

# Model examples of mental disorders

Depression and schizophrenia can be seen as examples of mental illness, which is the heavy workload in any psychiatric center or practice. Depression is characterized by constantly bad mood, self-disapproval, a low self-confidence, and a negative self-image (4). Schizophrenia most frequently occurs at the age 15-35 years and is characterized by lack of zest for life and disorganization of logical thought most often together with auditory hallucinations and paranoid delusions (5), together with emotional flattening and social withdrawal (comp. Bleuler 1911). Depressed and schizophrenic patients constitute far the greatest part of the mentally ill patients. These two mental diseases will be the subjects of the further discussion in this chapter, because they represent the best known and investigated mental disorders existing today.

# Depression

Studies of monozygote twins showed that if twins grow up together, the concordance as regards depression is higher for monozygote twins (33-79%) than for dizygote twins (54%) (6). A concordance of 79% in the heaviest cases showed that even in these cases monozygotic twins have a considerable freedom to develop in their own way despite having the same genes and living in the same environment.

## Studies of adaptation

A study of 29 adopted bipolar depressive patients showed that 31% of the patients had adoptive parents who suffered from affective diseases, in contrast to only 9% of the biological parents. In the case of non-depressive adopted children 2% of their adoptive parents suffered from affective diseases. These data, reviewed by (7) suggested that the environmental factors dominate in the ratio 2:1 against the "early factors", at least in this case. A simple Mendelian inheritance seems unlikely. We hypothesize that intrauterine information transmitting interactions between the mother and child are responsible for the remaining cases not explained by genetics and environment.

Most affective diseases have a cyclic nature, most notably bipolar depression that hardly tallies with a genetic defect or a descending cerebral dysfunction. In the well-known "winter-depression" the light factor seems to play a key role.

It seems that environmental factors as well as genetic factors and other early factors, of which we favor intrauterine information transmitting interactions, play a role in the development of depressive diseases. As there is a very close contact between mother and child in utero, and adopted children of course spend their foetal lives in their mother's womb, twin studies are not able to distinguish between the two kinds of factors.

## The effectiveness of antidepressants compared to placebo

For many years it was thought that antidepressants were more active than placebo, but around year 2000 the understanding of the active placebo effect led to re-investigation and comparison of the most efficient antidepressants (the tricyclic antidepressant) with active placebo, and quite chocking it was found that these drugs, being the most potent antidepressant drugs know, was not at all better that placebo (8). Before that it was generally believed that app. 65% of non-psychotic depressive patients respond to imipramine, while app. 30% responds to placebo; all heterocyclic antidepressants had the response figures of 65-75% after one month treatment compared to 20-40% response to placebo. Generally speaking, the worse a depression is, the better the antidepressant fares compared to the passive placebo (7), but this difference is obviously annihilated when it comes to active placebo.

The above-mentioned old studies were conducted in a way that opened up to criticism. Even a 50% reduction in the Hamilton rating score (9) were clinically called a response, but in fact this was only a mild relief of symptoms. More importantly most researchers only included patients that completed the experiment, but did not inform about how many patients that did not complete the experiment – and they did not count these as non-responders, what most of them perhaps were. Moreover it was rarely told how many patients the subjects are chosen from, and there were serious problems with the criteria for election for the experiment. Only patients that do respond positively to the drugs were included in most of the studies, creating a tremendous bias: "Most of the controlled clinical studies exclude patients who have not responded to antidepressants in the past" (10). In most cases the studies report no results of the duration of the recovery or of the frequency of relapse, and long-term follow-ups are extremely rare. So it is easy to see today how the inefficient, antidepressive drugs were artificially turned into active and valuable drugs by the research that was almost always paid for by the pharmaceutical industry.

## The hypothesis of depression

Around 1990 research of the effect of antidepressants led to a fundamental revision of the earlier hypotheses. Most researchers seem to agree that the simple hypothesis of depression as caused by lack of monoamines was not verified. This hypothesis was partly based on the assumption that the drugs worked through an increased supply of transmitter substances (NE and 5HT) in the synapses in a clinical time variance of the effect of between 7- 45 days (7), a much longer time than the quickly induced biochemical effect. Moreover drugs e.g. iprindol and mianserin, which are not reuptake- or MAO-inhibitors, in a significant way were found to be as efficient as the classical drugs. In addition amphetamine, which is a reuptake-inhibitor, cannot effectively be used in the treatment of depressions.

Studies of monoamine-turnover in laboratory animals, long term treated with antidepressants or electroshock, showed no significant deviation from normal. The influence of the reuptake-blocking seems to be submitted to a feedback-regulated mechanism exerting its effect through auto-receptors. None of these findings are sufficient in themselves in order to reject the hypothesis, "but together they provide a powerful argument for its re-examination and suggest that antidepressants act in a more complex manner than that envisaged by the monoamine deficiency hypothesis of depression" concluded Elliot and Stephenson in 1989 (4).

### Psychotherapy, holistic therapy and depression

Since 1975 great methodological and technical improvements have been made, including improvement of methods of evaluating 1) the condition of the patient, 2) the qualifications of the therapist, 3) the contents of the therapy and 4) the improved situation of the patient. Central coordination of therapist training and evaluation programs has apparently resulted in a minor revolution in this area. The results are mixed, but some researchers have concluded that there are large differences in effectiveness between the different therapies (9).

Recent research has documented that depressed patients were helped better by psychotherapy than by psychiatric standard treatment (11-13). One of the best predictors for response to interpersonal therapy is a pathological picture indicating endogen depression! It seems reasonable to conclude, that mental factors are of tremendous importance concerning affective diseases (14,15). We interpret the existing data in the following way: Mental illnesses are caused primarily by psychological factors, not by genes, as genes cannot be changed by psychotherapy. More efficient that psychotherapy alone is the combination of psychotherapy and bodywork, and holistic therapy like clinical holistic medicine, also including work with philosophy of life and sexuality (16-25).

## Schizophrenia

Evidently schizophrenia is not randomly distributed within a population, but is more frequent within exposed families than in the population as a whole ($p<0.001$) (26). In recent twin studies the concordance between pairs of twins growing up together is larger between monozygotic (31-78%) than between dizygotic twins (6- 28%). These studies also show that 22-69% of monozygotic twins growing up together do not both develop schizophrenia (ibid.). This point towards a dominant influence of environmental factors. Since several investigations have shown that monozygotic twins to a far higher degree than dizygotic twins share the same environment, friends, and attitudes of their parents and teachers (ibid.), the greater concordance might as well be attributed to these environmental likenesses.

Studies have found a significantly higher occurrence of schizophrenia among children adopted by schizophrenic parents and among adopted children, whose biological parents were schizophrenic, compared to the average population. In some studies no significant difference was found, however. Studies of monozygotic twins not growing up together were of much greater value than studies of monozygotic twins growing up together. The adopted children have, however, often spent a smaller or larger time together with the mother, and in all circumstances they had had the opportunity to adapt to the mother within the womb. The information transmitting interactions have had the time to work.

What is transferred from one generation to the next is not a simple tendency towards the development of schizophrenia, not even a non-specific tendency towards the development of psychiatric diseases, but a tendency towards bad psychosocial functioning, "These findings provide an increasingly complex, but informative, picture of the nature of transmitted liability to schizophrenia" (26).

Since 1916 it has been known, that schizophrenia does not follow a classic Mendelian inheritance pattern, thus, it is obvious to imply a polygenic inheritance. Models for polygenic inheritance, however, are flexible, because they are very difficult to falsify.

From all this, it seems that the studies of adopted monozygotic children could suggest the importance of" early factors", but it is not known, whether these are of a genetic or an intrauterine nature. In addition, it is evident, that environmental factors play a great role.

## Hypotheses for schizophrenia

Several hypotheses for schizophrenia have been proposed, but the dopamine hypothesis seemed for many years to be the only transmitter hypothesis, that could not be definitively falsified (see historical review in (5)). The dopamine hypothesis was founded in the effect on dopaminergic systems of many of the original neuroleptics. The hypothesis says that schizophrenia is caused by a(genetically inherited) hyper-activity of the dopaminergic system.

The hypothesis came in different versions each considering one of several possibilities with regard to the function of DA in the psychotic brain. Either there was too fast a DA-metabolism, or a too large a receptor sensitivity (5). Unfortunately for the believer in the dopamine hypothesis, post mortem studies or other studies did not provide evidence for an increased DA-turnover in the brain of people with schizophrenia. An up regulation of D2-receptors as a consequence of the administration of neuroleptics in the brain of schizophrenics was not found. There is still no positive evidence for occurrence of changed D2-frequency in untreated schizophrenics. Thus there is no evidence for any molecular hypothesis for schizophrenia, not even for the dopamine hypothesis. This is in agreement with the fact that schizophrenia occurs in episodes - a fact that is very difficult to explain in terms of a defect in a transmitter system. The earlier mentioned simple hypotheses about schizophrenia as caused by simple biochemical defects or disturbances were around 1990 abandoned in favor of more complex explanations of the brain function.

From 1990 to 2008 came a large series of Cochrane metaanalysis analysing the effect of all kinds and types of antipsychotic drugs on a number of different illnesses and mental states (27-103). Quite surprisingly it was found that every time an antipsychotic drug was tested against placebo, the patients' mental state was not found to be significantly improved. Behaviour was still found to be modified, but the effect of the behaviour was just pacification, not an improvement. Hallucinations and other symptoms of mental illness was not at all relieved by the drugs, which does not deserve its name "antipsychotic medicine" anymore, as the drugs are not at all antipsychotic, only tranquillizing the patients. It was also documented in these studies that the adverse effects of the drugs were very severe; they basically took the patient's energy and autonomy away, thus giving the obedient and more socially acceptable picture of an improved patient, which from an existential perspective was actually losing his quality of life as a sad consequence of the treatment. The Cochrane analyses finally made it impossible to believe in the biochemical hypothesis of schizophrenia and the other psychotic mental illness; they were simply not substantiated.

### Negative and positive symptomatology

The subdivision of schizophrenics into a positive and a negative symptomatology has a long history and seems to be supported by morphological studies (104). The positive symptoms are hallucinations, delusions and some types of thought disturbances as derailment, neologisms and incoherency. The negative symptoms are lack of function in a number of areas, such as social withdrawal, weakened affect, reduced motivation, psycho motor retardation, and poverty of speech.

It was around 1990 commonly understood, that the negative symptoms are not disappearing by use of neuroleptics, but only with the Cochrane studies systematic exploration of the effects of the drugs on the positive effects was it documented that the positive symptoms were not improved either.

There is clinical evidence showing that negative symptoms may be connected with too low a dopamine activity. It is known that Parkinson disease is often associated with social withdrawal and deflated affect. Large doses of neuroleptics may trigger the negative symptoms, besides motor inhibition, while chronic l-dopa administration, which counteracts neuroleptics, sometimes is able to alleviate deflated affect, withdrawn emotions, and apathy.

This means that schizophrenic patients can be divided into a "hyper-dopaminergic" group with positive symptoms, and a "hypo-dopaminergic" group with negative symptoms. The words "hyper" and "hypo" refer to the pharmaceutical compensation that seems to remove the symptoms, and not necessarily to the DA-activity of the patients. The variance in neuropsychological state cannot in itself support a biochemical hypothesis for schizophrenia. Taken all together it is clear today that the biochemical hypothesis for schizophrenia is in no way substantiated.

## Discussion

The passive placebo effect seems to be the same for anti-schizophrenic (antipsychotic drugs) as for antidepressants (5); the active placebo effect is only known for the antidepressant drugs, as nobody yet has investigated this with the antipsychotic drugs. The psychological and sexual factors seem to be dominant in schizophrenia as well as in depression. In studies of neuroleptics, the fact that 2 of three or more were non-responders showed that the brain has a great adaptive capacity to compensate the sedating influences of the neuroleptics.

It has been known for a long time that the side effects of neuroleptics closely resemble Parkinson's disease, which is known to be associated by the decay of dopaminergic neurons; the strongest evidence for the dopaminergic effect is the fact that the clinical efficiency of many neuroleptics is closely correlated to their displacement of 3H-spiroperidol and 3H-haloperidol from D2-receptors (5,104). When it was shown, that there was a good correlation between the clinical efficiency of neuroleptics and D2-binding, it seemed reasonable to assume that neuroleptics worked through the D2-receptor. Today a whole new generation of neuroleptics with quite different affinity profiles (27-103,105) has been created. Among the newly identified neuroleptics are compounds that by thorough clinical testing has been shown to be as effective as the old ones, while they on the whole have no affinity to DA-receptors (e.g. clozapin; less tested is flulerlapin, and BW 234 U). These compounds are all found to be "effective" in animal models. It has been shown, that they in general are clinically effective, since it is no longer possible to associate neuroleptic activity with D2-binding. Hence there is no pharmacological evidence, that psychosis is associated with the DA-systems (5). Webster and Jordan concluded in 1989: "The controversy over neuroleptic treatment and the state of D2-receptors remain unsolved." Today this is finally solved: The illness called schizophrenia is not at all connected to the D2-receptors.

The considerable time-elapse, before the effect of the neuroleptics occurs, points to a complex interaction between drug and brain. As the discontinuation of the drug rarely leads to an immediate aggravation of symptoms, it is evident, that the effects of the drugs cannot be explained by a simple interaction between a drug and a transmitter system.

Neuroleptics have not improved during the past 50 years (28) and while patients' mental health according to the many new Cochrane metaanalysis stays totally unaffected their bodies suffers. A vast fraction of the patients get serious side effects, such as tardive dyskinesia and tardive psychosis, the consequences of which are still uncertain. In spite of intensive studies the patients that selectively respond to these drugs have not been characterized (106).

Finally there is no clinical evidence that neuroleptics should be more active against schizophrenic psychoses than against any other kind of psychosis (107). Therefore there is no reason to limit the DA-hypothesis to schizophrenia; it should comprise all kinds of psychoses. Discontinuation of neuroleptics rarely seems to result in acute aggravation of the schizophrenic symptoms. The schizophrenic symptoms seem to arrive in episodes, a detail that proposes a very complex mechanism.

One of the strangest arguments of the 80'ies, interesting for its historical value, is that the pharmacological effect is due to adaptation to the drug. This hypothesis is of cause not plausible, because adaptation should lower the effect of the neuroleptics, not increase them, but in the 80'ies researches in antipsychotic drugs often suspended all reason to prove what they believed was be true. But this is not so rare in science.

## A suggestion of the mechanism of psychopharmacological drugs

The key problem in understanding the mechanism of antidepressants and neuroleptics seems to be the great time delay of their effect. The pharmacological effect takes a few hours, the central nervous system adaptation to this effect presumably takes a few days, but the clinical effect often takes a month or more. The hypothesis of adaptation at receptor level as a mechanism behind the clinical effect does not seem plausible given the time discrepancy. The pharmacological effect of antidepressants generally seems to be an argumentation of synaptic activity, where neuroleptics (e.g. reserpine) may induce depression.

About 1990 it seemed reasonable to assume, that antidepressants respectively neuroleptics compensated a hypo-activity respectively a hyper-activity in the brain as a whole, not at any specific site of action for a specific drug. This compensation could give the complete neural system a "push" in the right direction towards normal function and normal interpretation of reality. According to this interpretation the time delay of the clinical effect was seen as inertia in the adaptation at the higher (mental) levels of the brain.

We suggest that the cognitive content of mental disease corresponds to a large number of considerations and decisions that take a long time to accumulate in one's model of reality in the brain. This inertia in the change of perception of reality leads to the time delay in any treatment of depression and schizophrenia, whether it is done by pharmacological means or by electro chock (ECT), psychotherapy and holistic therapy.

But the most obvious hypothesis for the function of the drugs is much simpler: Poisoning. As time goes by, and the patients loose energy due to severe poisoning, the behaviour becomes more and more obedient, passive and without the initiative and rebellion that characterizes autonomous beings. The psychopharmacological drugs are simple socializing the patients by depraving them of their life energy. This interpretation seems to be in almost perfect accordance with the findings of the Cochrane studies of antipsychotic drugs.

## The etiology of depression and schizophrenia

In 1990 it was found that depression could be counteracted through interaction with many different transmitter systems. This pointed towards a complex mechanism and not a simple one tied to a single transmitter system. Reuptake in itself could also be excluded as a mechanism, because cocaine and amphetamine did not act as antidepressants. Compensatory up regulation of beta-receptors was often seen, but not always (107), thus this could not be the general regulation mechanism. Adaptation to a drug, including receptor adaptation through increased sensitivity, was suggested as a mechanism. This did not seem likely, because such an adaptation should eliminate the disturbance and thus decrease rather than increase. In this way reduce instead of increase the effect of the antidepressants. It seems absurd to suppose that such an adaptation should give a whole new effect as for example to alleviate a depression. An adaptation to a psychotropic drug normally takes about four days (108), whereas the effect of antidepressants often does not assert its effect before about six weeks (7).

The long interval before the effect shows up indicated a very complex mechanism instead of a simple molecular mechanism. The same conclusion was indicated by the fact that about one third of the patients did not respond to antidepressants at all. The placebo effect – known today to account for the full effect (8) of the antidepressant drugs – caused by the expectations to a treatment, indicated an important mental factor. Inheritance studies suggested that a certain amount of genetic transmission could not be excluded. Spontaneous remission was well known in patients with depression, but would not be likely in the case of a genetic programmed biochemical error. The periodical nature of manic depression (bipolar depression) was also difficult to connect to a genetic deficiency.

Today we know that psychotherapy is superior to drugs, and we know that the psychopharmacological drugs themselves are only giving positive effects through psychological mechanisms – the placebo effect.

The conclusion therefore is, that environmental factors are more important for the etiology of mental illness than genetic defects. As defect genes causing mental illness has never been found, the "early factor" seemingly important in the etiology of schizophrenia is more likely to be information-transmitting interactions between mother and child in and outside the womb. Inheritance studies showed that environmental factors played a decisive role in the etiology of schizophrenia. Early factors, such as genetic and/or intrauterine factors, were of minor importance. We hypothesize that information-transmitting interactions in utero and in early childhood were more important than genetic factors.

Studies of neuroleptics have shown a considerable placebo effect and a substantial group of non-responders, as is also the case in antidepressants. New generations of neuroleptics forced researchers around 1990 to reject the earlier assumption of schizophrenia was tied to the dopaminergic transmitter system. The long lapse of time before the effect manifest itself (7-30 days) corresponded badly with the time for the chemical effect (2 hours) or the time of adaptation at receptor level (a few days). Moreover, the episodic occurrence of schizophrenia makes it hard to maintain simple, molecular hypotheses for schizophrenia.

The positive and negative symptomatology seems to show, that schizophrenia covers a broad spectrum from "hypo" to "hyper" dopaminergic activity. Finally, neuroleptics assert their effect non-specifically against all psychoses, not only against schizophrenia. All in all no evidence for any molecular hypothesis seems to have been found. On the contrary, there is clear evidence for the importance of environmental and psychological factors.

# References

[1] McGeer PL, Eccles JC, McGeer EG. Molecular neurobiology of the mammalian brain. New York: Plenum Press, 1987.
[2] Meltzer HY. Psychopharmacology. The third generation of progress. New York: Raven, 1987.
[3] Snyder SH. Molecular strategies in neuropsychopharmacologic research. In: Meltzer HY, ed. Psychopharmacology. The third generation of progress. New York: Raven, 1987.
[4] Elliot JM, Stephenson JD. Depression. In: Webster RA, Jordan CC, eds. Neurotransmitters, drugs and disease. Oxford: Blackwell, 1989.
[5] Webster RA, Jordan CC. Neurotransmitters, drugs and disease. Oxford: Blackwell, 1989.
[6] Gershon ES, Berrettini W, Nurnberger J, Goldin LR. Genetics and affective illness. In: Meltzer HY, ed. Psychopharmacology. The third generation of progress. New York: Raven, 1987.
[7] Brotman AW, Falk WE, Gelenberg AJ. Pharmacologic treatment of depressive subtypes. Psychiatr Med 1988;6(3):92-113.
[8] Moncrieff J, Wessely S, Hardy R. Active placebos versus antidepressants for depression. Cochrane Database Syst Rev. 2004;(1):CD003012.
[9] Williams JBW. A structured interview guide for the Hamilton Depression Rating Scale. Arch Gen Psychiatry 1988;45(8):742-7.
[10] Weissman MM, Jarrett RB, Rush AJ. Psychotherapy and its relevance to the pharmacotherapy of major depression: a decade later (1976-1985). In: Meltzer HY, ed. Psychopharmacology. The third generation of progress. New York: Raven, 1987.
[11] Leichsenring F, Rabung S, Leibing E. The efficacy of short-term psychodynamic psychotherapy in specific psychiatric disorders: a meta-analysis. Arch Gen Psychiatry 2004;61(12):1208-16.
[12] Leichsenring F. Are psychodynamic and psychoanalytic therapies effective? A review of empirical data. Int J Psychoanal 2005;86(Pt 3):841-68.
[13] Leichsenring F, Leibing E. Psychodynamic psychotherapy: a systematic review of techniques, indications and empirical evidence. Psychol Psychother 2007;80(Pt 2):217-28.
[14] Beck A. Cognitive therapy and the emotional disorders. New York: Int Univ Press, 1976.
[15] Beck A. Cognitive therapy of depression. London: Guildford, 1979.

[16] Ventegodt S, Kandel I, Merrick J. Clinical holistic medicine (mindful short-term psychodynamic psychotherapy complimented with bodywork) in the treatment of schizophrenia (ICD10-F20/DSM-IV Code 295) and other psychotic mental diseases. ScientificWorldJournal 2007;7:1987-2008.
[17] Ventegodt S, Kandel I, Merrick J. Clinical holistic medicine: how to recover memory without "implanting" memories in your patient. ScientificWorldJournal 2007;7:1579-89.
[18] Ventegodt S, Clausen B, Omar HA, Merrick J. Clinical holistic medicine: holistic sexology and acupressure through the vagina (Hippocratic pelvic massage). ScientificWorldJournal 2006;6:2066-79.
[19] Ventegodt S, Clausen B, Merrick J. Clinical holistic medicine: pilot study on the effect of vaginal acupressure (Hippocratic pelvic massage). ScientificWorldJournal 2006;6:2100-16.
[20] Ventegodt S, Clausen B, Merrick J.Clinical holistic medicine: the case story of Anna. III. Rehabilitation of philosophy of life during holistic existential therapy for childhood sexual abuse. ScientificWorldJournal 2006;6:2080-91.
[21] Ventegodt S, Thegler S, Andreasen T, Struve F, Enevoldsen L, Bassaine L, Torp M, Merrick J.Clinical holistic medicine (mindful, short-term psychodynamic psychotherapy complemented with bodywork) in the treatment of experienced impaired sexual functioning. ScientificWorldJournal 2007;7:324-9.
[22] Ventegodt S, Kandel I, Neikrug S, Merric J. Clinical holistic medicine: holistic treatment of rape and incest trauma. ScientificWorldJournal 2005;5:288-97.
[23] Ventegodt S, Morad M, Hyam E, Merrick J. Clinical holistic medicine: holistic sexology and treatment of vulvodynia through existential therapy and acceptance through touch. ScientificWorldJournal. 2004 Aug 4;4:571-80.
[24] Ventegodt S, Morad M, Kandel I, Merrick J. Clinical holistic medicine: problems in sex and living together. ScientificWorldJournal 2004;4:562-70.
[25] Ventegodt S, Morad M, Merrick J. Clinical holistic medicine: holistic pelvic examination and holistic treatment of infertility. ScientificWorldJournal 2004;4:148-58.
[26] Kendler KS. The genetics of schizophrenia: A current perspective. In: Meltzer HY, ed. Psychopharmacology. The third generation of progress. New York: Raven, 1987.
[27] Abhijnhan A, Adams CE, David A, Ozbilen M. Depot fluspirilene for schizophrenia. Cochrane Database Syst Rev 2007;(1):CD001718.
[28] Adams CE, Awad G, Rathbone J, Thornley B. Chlorpromazine versus placebo for schizophrenia. Cochrane Database Syst Rev 2007;(2):CD000284.
[29] Amato L, Minozzi S, Pani PP, Davoli M. Antipsychotic medications for cocaine dependence. Cochrane Database Syst Rev 2007;(3):CD006306.
[30] Arunpongpaisal S, Ahmed I, Aqeel N, Suchat P. Antipsychotic drug treatment for elderly people with late-onset schizophrenia. Cochrane Database Syst Rev 2003;(2):CD004162.
[31] Bagnall A, Lewis RA, Leitner ML. Ziprasidone for schizophrenia and severe mental illness. Cochrane Database Syst Rev 2000;(4):CD001945.
[32] Bagnall A, Fenton M, Kleijnen J, Lewis R. Molindone for schizophrenia and severe mental illness. Cochrane Database Syst Rev 2007;(1):CD002083.
[33] Ballard C, Waite J. The effectiveness of atypical antipsychotics for the treatment of aggression and psychosis in Alzheimer's disease. Cochrane Database Syst Rev 2006;(1):CD003476.
[34] Basan A, Leucht S. Valproate for schizophrenia. Cochrane Database Syst Rev 2004;(1):CD004028.
[35] Belgamwar RB, Fenton M. Olanzapine IM or velotab for acutely disturbed/agitated people with suspected serious mental illnesses. Cochrane Database Syst Rev 2005;(2):CD003729.
[36] Binks CA, Fenton M, McCarthy L, Lee T, Adams CE, Duggan C. Pharmacological interventions for people with borderline personality disorder. Cochrane Database Syst Rev 2006;(1):CD005653.
[37] Carpenter S, Berk M, Rathbone J. Clotiapine for acute psychotic illnesses. Cochrane Database Syst Rev 2004;(4):CD002304.
[38] Chakrabarti A, Bagnall A, Chue P, Fenton M, Palaniswamy V, Wong W, Xia J. Loxapine for schizophrenia. Cochrane Database Syst Rev 2007;(4):CD001943.
[39] Chua WL, de Izquierdo SA, Kulkarni J, Mortimer A. Estrogen for schizophrenia. Cochrane Database Syst Rev 2005;(4):CD004719.
[40] Coutinho E, Fenton M, Quraishi S. Zuclopenthixol decanoate for schizophrenia and other serious mental illnesses. Cochrane Database Syst Rev 2000;(2):CD001164.

[41] Cure S, Rathbone J, Carpenter S. Droperidol for acute psychosis. Cochrane Database Syst Rev 2004;(4):CD002830.
[42] David A, Adams CE, Eisenbruch M, Quraishi S, Rathbone J. Depot fluphenazine decanoate and enanthate for schizophrenia. Cochrane Database Syst Rev 2005;(1):CD000307.
[43] David A, Quraishi S, Rathbone J. Depot perphenazine decanoate and enanthate for schizophrenia. Cochrane Database Syst Rev 2005;(3):CD001717.
[44] DeSilva P, Fenton M, Rathbone J. Zotepine for schizophrenia. Cochrane Database Syst Rev 2006;(4):CD001948.
[45] Dinesh M, David A, Quraishi SN. Depot pipotiazine palmitate and undecylenate for schizophrenia. Cochrane Database Syst Rev 2004;(4):CD001720.
[46] Duggan L, Brylewski J. Antipsychotic medication versus placebo for people with both schizophrenia and learning disability. Cochrane Database Syst Rev 2004;(4):CD000030.
[47] Duggan L, Fenton M, Rathbone J, Dardennes R, El-Dosoky A, Indran S. Olanzapine for schizophrenia. Cochrane Database Syst Rev 2005;(2):CD001359.
[48] El-Sayeh HG, Morganti C. Aripiprazole for schizophrenia. Cochrane Database Syst Rev 2006;(2):CD004578.
[49] Elias A, Kumar A. Testosterone for schizophrenia. Cochrane Database Syst Rev 2007;(3):CD006197.
[50] Fenton M, Rathbone J, Reilly J, Sultana A. Thioridazine for schizophrenia. Cochrane Database Syst Rev 2007;(3):CD001944.
[51] Gibson RC, Fenton M, Coutinho ES, Campbell C. Zuclopenthixol acetate for acute schizophrenia and similar serious mental illnesses. Cochrane Database Syst Rev 2004;(3):CD000525.
[52] Gilbody SM, Bagnall AM, Duggan L, Tuunainen A. Risperidone versus other atypical antipsychotic medication for schizophrenia. Cochrane Database Syst Rev 2000;(3):CD002306.
[53] Gillies D, Beck A, McCloud A, Rathbone J, Gillies D. Benzodiazepines alone or in combination with antipsychotic drugs for acute psychosis. Cochrane Database Syst Rev 2005;(4):CD003079.
[54] Hartung B, Wada M, Laux G, Leucht S. Perphenazine for schizophrenia. Cochrane Database Syst Rev 2005;(1):CD003443.
[55] Hosalli P, Davis JM. Depot risperidone for schizophrenia. Cochrane Database Syst Rev 2003;(4):CD004161.
[56] Huf G, Alexander J, Allen MH. Haloperidol plus promethazine for psychosis induced aggression. Cochrane Database Syst Rev 2005;(1):CD005146.
[57] Hunter RH, Joy CB, Kennedy E, Gilbody SM, Song F. Risperidone versus typical antipsychotic medication for schizophrenia. Cochrane Database Syst Rev 2003;(2):CD000440.
[58] Jayaram MB, Hosalli P, Stroup S. Risperidone versus olanzapine for schizophrenia. Cochrane Database Syst Rev 2006;(2):CD005237.
[59] Jesner OS, Aref-Adib M, Coren E. Risperidone for autism spectrum disorder. Cochrane Database Syst Rev 2007;(1):CD005040.
[60] Joy CB, Adams CE, Rice K. Crisis intervention for people with severe mental illnesses. Cochrane Database Syst Rev 2006;(4):CD001087.
[61] Joy CB, Adams CE, Lawrie SM. Haloperidol versus placebo for schizophrenia. Cochrane Database Syst Rev 2006;(4):CD003082.
[62] Kennedy E, Kumar A, Datta SS. Antipsychotic medication for childhoodonset schizophrenia. Cochrane Database Syst Rev 2007;(3):CD004027.
[63] Kumar A, Strech D. Zuclopenthixol dihydrochloride for schizophrenia. Cochrane Database Syst Rev 2005;(4):CD005474.
[64] Leucht S, Hartung B. Benperidol for schizophrenia. Cochrane Database Syst Rev 2005;(2):CD003083.
[65] Leucht S, Hartung B. Perazine for schizophrenia. Cochrane Database Syst Rev 2006;(2):CD002832.
[66] Leucht S, Kissling W, McGrath J, White P. Carbamazepine for schizophrenia. Cochrane Database Syst Rev 2007;(3):CD001258.
[67] Leucht S, Kissling W, McGrath J. Lithium for schizophrenia. Cochrane Database Syst Rev 2007;(3):CD003834.
[68] Lewis R, Bagnall AM, Leitner M. Sertindole for schizophrenia. Cochrane Database Syst Rev 2005;(3):CD001715.

[69] Macritchie KA, Geddes JR, Scott J, Haslam DR, Goodwin GM. Valproic acid, valproate and divalproex in the maintenance treatment of bipolar disorder. Cochrane Database Syst Rev 2001;(3):CD003196.

[70] Macritchie K, Geddes JR, Scott J, Haslam D, de Lima M, Goodwin G. Valproate for acute mood episodes in bipolar disorder. Cochrane Database Syst Rev 2003;(1):CD004052.

[71] Marques LO, Lima MS, Soares BG. Trifluoperazine for schizophrenia. Cochrane Database Syst Rev 2004;(1):CD003545.

[72] Marriott RG, Neil W, Waddingham S. Antipsychotic medication for elderly people with schizophrenia. Cochrane Database Syst Rev 2006;(1):CD005580.

[73] Marshall M, Rathbone J. Early intervention for psychosis. Cochrane Database Syst Rev 2006;(4):CD004718.

[74] Matar HE, Almerie MQ. Oral fluphenazine versus placebo for schizophrenia. Cochrane Database Syst Rev 2007;(1):CD006352.

[75] Mota NE, Lima MS, Soares BG. Amisulpride for schizophrenia. Cochrane Database Syst Rev 2002;(2):CD001357.

[76] Nolte S, Wong D, Lachford G. Amphetamines for schizophrenia. Cochrane Database Syst Rev 2004;(4):CD004964.

[77] Pekkala E, Merinder L. Psychoeducation for schizophrenia. Cochrane Database Syst Rev 2002;(2):CD002831.

[78] Premkumar TS, Pick J. Lamotrigine for schizophrenia. Cochrane Database Syst Rev 2006;(4):CD005962.

[79] Punnoose S, Belgamwar MR. Nicotine for schizophrenia. Cochrane Database Syst Rev 2006;(1):CD004838.

[80] Quraishi S, David A. Depot flupenthixol decanoate for schizophrenia or other similar psychotic disorders. Cochrane Database Syst Rev 2000;(2):CD001470.

[81] Quraishi S, David A. Depot haloperidol decanoate for schizophrenia. Cochrane Database Syst Rev 2000;(2):CD001361.

[82] Rathbone J, McMonagle T. Pimozide for schizophrenia or related psychoses. Cochrane Database Syst Rev 2007;(3):CD001949.

[83] Rendell JM, Gijsman HJ, Keck P, Goodwin GM, Geddes JR. Olanzapine alone or in combination for acute mania. Cochrane Database Syst Rev 2003;(3):CD004040.

[84] Rendell JM, Gijsman HJ, Bauer MS, Goodwin GM, Geddes GR. Risperidone alone or in combination for acute mania. Cochrane Database Syst Rev 2006;(1):CD004043.

[85] Rendell JM, Geddes JR. Risperidone in long-term treatment for bipolar disorder. Cochrane Database Syst Rev 2006;(4):CD004999.

[86] Rummel C, Hamann J, Kissling W, Leucht S. New generation antipsychotics for first episode schizophrenia. Cochrane Database Syst Rev 2003;(4):CD004410.

[87] Rummel C, Kissling W, Leucht S. Antidepressants for the negative symptoms of schizophrenia. Cochrane Database Syst Rev 2006;3:CD005581.

[88] Soares BG, Fenton M, Chue P. Sulpiride for schizophrenia. Cochrane Database Syst Rev 2000;(2):CD001162.

[89] Soares BG, Lima MS. Penfluridol for schizophrenia. Cochrane Database Syst Rev 2006;(2):CD002923.

[90] Srisurapanont M, Kittiratanapaiboon P, Jarusuraisin N. Treatment for amphetamine psychosis. Cochrane Database Syst Rev 2001;(4):CD003026.

[91] Srisurapanont M, Maneeton B, Maneeton N. Quetiapine for schizophrenia. Cochrane Database Syst Rev 2004;(2):CD000967.

[92] Tharyan P, Adams CE. Electroconvulsive therapy for schizophrenia. Cochrane Database Syst Rev 2005;(2):CD000076.

[93] Trevisani VF, Castro AA, Neves Neto JF, Atallah AN. Cyclophosphamide versus methylprednisolone for treating neuropsychiatric involvement in systemic lupus erythematosus. Cochrane Database Syst Rev 2006;(2):CD002265.

[94] Tuominen HJ, Tiihonen J, Wahlbeck K. Glutamatergic drugs for schizophrenia. Cochrane Database Syst Rev 2006;(2):CD003730.

[95] Tuunainen A, Wahlbeck K, Gilbody SM. Newer atypical antipsychotic medication versus clozapine for schizophrenia. Cochrane Database Syst Rev 2000;(2):CD000966.
[96] Volz A, Khorsand V, Gillies D, Leucht S. Benzodiazepines for schizophrenia. Cochrane Database Syst Rev 2007;(1):CD006391.
[97] Wahlbeck K, Cheine M, Essali MA. Clozapine versus typical neuroleptic medication for schizophrenia. Cochrane Database Syst Rev 2000;(2):CD000059.
[98] Waraich PS, Adams CE, Roque M, Hamill KM, Marti J. Haloperidol dose for the acute phase of schizophrenia. Cochrane Database Syst Rev 2002;(3):CD001951.
[99] Webb RT, Howard L, Abel KM. Antipsychotic drugs for non-affective psychosis during pregnancy and postpartum. Cochrane Database Syst Rev 2004;(2):CD004411.
[100] Whitehead C, Moss S, Cardno A, Lewis G. Antidepressants for people with both schizophrenia and depression. Cochrane Database Syst Rev 2002;(2):CD002305.
[101] Wijkstra J, Lijmer J, Balk F, Geddes J, Nolen WA. Pharmacological treatment for psychotic depression. Cochrane Database Syst Rev 2005;(4):CD004044.
[102] Wong D, Adams CE, David A, Quraishi SN. Depot bromperidol decanoate for schizophrenia. Cochrane Database Syst Rev 2004;(3):CD001719.
[103] Young AH, Geddes JR, Macritchie K, Rao SN, Vasudev A. Tiagabine in the maintenance treatment of bipolar disorders. Cochrane Database Syst Rev 2006;3:CD005173.
[104] Losonczy MF, Davidson M, Davis KL. The dopamine hypothesis of schizophrenia. In: Meltzer HY, ed. Psychopharmacology. The third generation of progress. New York: Raven, 1987.
[105] Tamminga CA, Gerlach J. New neuroleptics and experimental antipsychotics in schizophrenia. In: Meltzer HY, ed. Psychopharmacology. The third generation of progress. New York: Raven, 1987.
[106] Hollister LE. Novel drug treatments for schizophrenia. Psychopharmacol Bull 1987;23(1):82-4.
[107] Blackwell B. Newer antidepressant drugs. In: Meltzer HY, ed. Psychopharmacology. The third generation of progress. New York: Raven,1987.
[108] Falk JL, Feingold DA. Environmental and cultural factors in the behavioural action of drugs. In: Meltzer HY, ed. Psychopharmacology. The third generation of progress. New York: Raven, 1987.

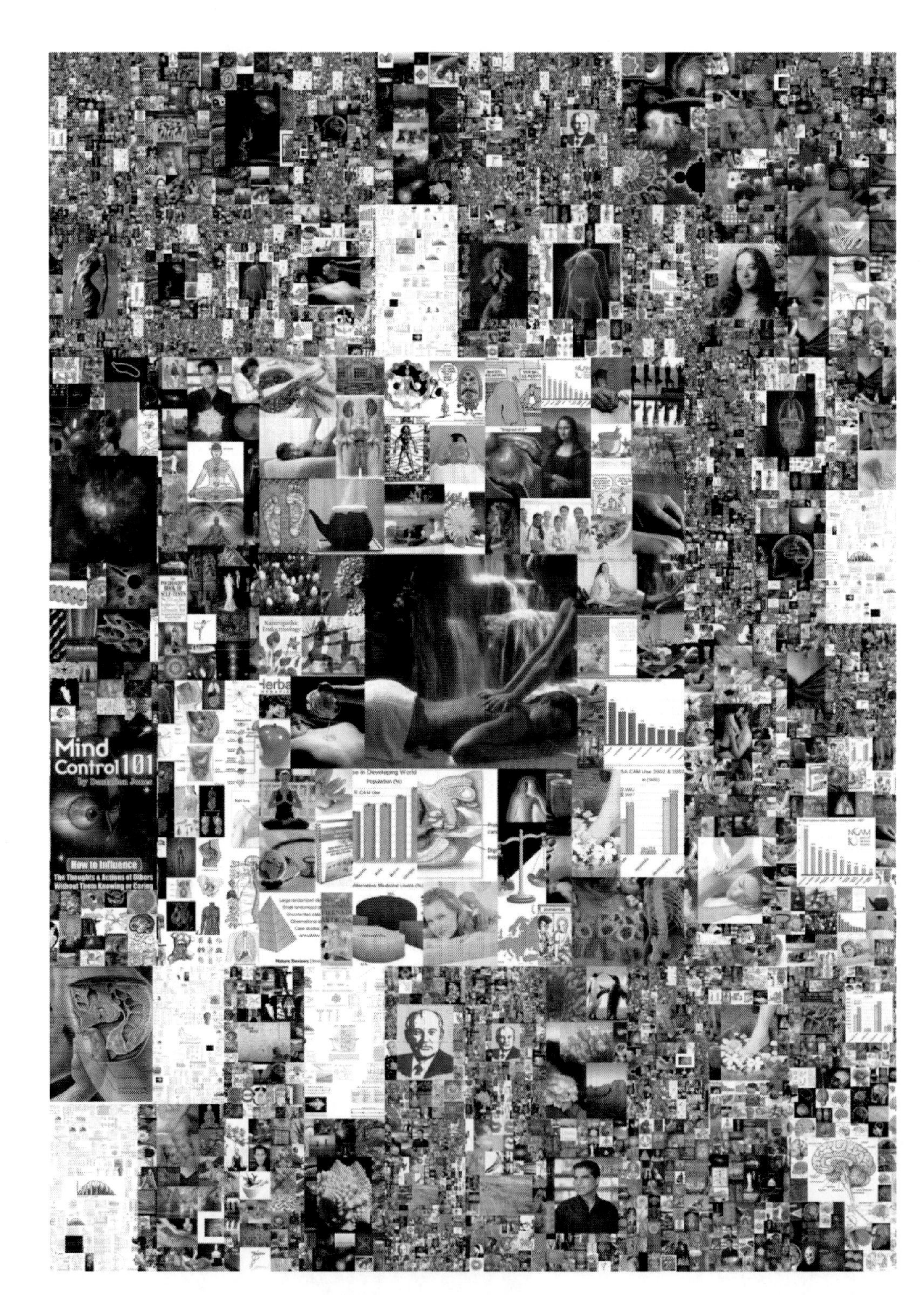
Mind
Control 101
How to Influence
The Thoughts & Actions of Others
Without Them Knowing or Caring
Naturopathic Endocrinology
Nature Reviews

*Chapter XVII*

# The therapeutic value of anti-psychotic drugs used in Denmark

The metaanalysis in the previous chapter took us six month to perform. Often you will not have this amount of time to make an analysis of the therapeutic value of drugs. Fortunately there is a simple way to get to a rough estimate of the total benefits and harms of a drug, and this is simply looking at the ratio of good and bad effects of a drug. Normally a drug will have one good effect and 10 or 100 adverse effects, each with its own likelihood to occur. The way these adverse effects are measured is that they only count when they become clinically significant. This means that all adverse effects are of similar gravity. Therefore the likelihood of getting an adverse effect can be calculating from adding up all the likelihoods for getting all the adverse effects. We call this "Total Number Needed to treat to Harm" ($NNH_{total}$). This number is normally about 3, meaning that one patient in three will get a significant adverse effect. But for many drugs this number is 2, one or even, as we saw with the antipsychotic drugs, lower than one, meaning that every single patient is likely to get an adverse effect – a harm – from the drug.

It is no secret that the pharmaceutical companies always will argue that the positive effect is so important and valuable for the patient that the side effects can never be an argument for not taking their product. The fact is that they could easily measure the total effect of a drug on the patient's quality of life and self-rated health before and after giving the drug, and in this way document a total beneficial effect of their drug. But this analysis is almost never done, obviously because the harm of most drugs are dominating the beneficial effects. This becomes very obvious when you make the calculation of the Therapeutic Value, $TV=NNH_{total}/NNT$. This shows how many patients are helped compared to how many patients are harmed. If this is above 1, the drug is as a rule beneficial; if it is about 1, it is of no value – the benefits and harms balances – and if it is below 1, it harms more than it benefits. Most patients will take the drugs also when it is about one, but if they knew that TV was below one, most rational being would stop taking it.

Of course life is not black and white, and sometimes there might be a good reason to run a great risk. But if you do, you should know that you are doing it. It might be useful to get out of strongly destructive behaviour, also if the price is a piece of your physical health. So we do not say that you should never take a risk and that all drugs are bad. But be aware. Strong commercial interest is pushing the drugs, and this mean that you need to be cautious and careful. You need to think for yourself, and you need all the information to make the right decision.

A rough estimate of the therapeutic value of a drug can be established from the ratio "Number Needed to Treat to Harm/Number Needed to Treat to Benefit" (NNH/NNT or NNtH/NNtB). The ratio illuminate the degree to which the treatment with the drug respects the ethical rule of "first do no harm"; if the ratio is >1 the drug helps more than it harms and is thus primarily beneficial. We need to compare the upper confidence limit of the NNtB with the lower confidence limit of the NNtH to assure that a drug helps and does not harm the patient. We compared NNH/NNT ratio from the Cochrane meta-analyses of the commonly used antipsychotic drugs in Denmark and found that all antipsychotic drugs used in Denmark had a NNH/NNB< 1, and often 1/5 and 1/10, meaning that the drugs are likely to harm many more patients than they help.

Antipsychotic drugs are known to have not only physical adverse effects, but also mental, existential, social and sexual side effects that are seldom included in the studies, giving a strong bias in favor of the drugs. Important factors that are often ignored in the studies were: suicides from drug-induced depression, suicide attempts and their consequences, spontaneous drug-induced death, drug-induced self-molestation, damage to learning and working ability, sexual function, social function, self-esteem and self-confidence, and cognitive factors. Antipsychotic drugs on the Danish market today have a very low therapeutic value and seems to be harmful to the patients. From an ethical perspective antipsychotic drugs can therefore not be used as a standard treatment for any mental illness. Further scientific investigation into the significance of this finding is urgently needed. Antipsychotic drugs might still be justified in the treatment of specific subgroups of patients like violent and sexually aggressive, acute psychotic, schizophrenic patients.

## Introduction

In medicine it has always been important to avoid harm to your patient: "primum non nocere" – first do no harm. To serve the patient's best interest a physician must be certain that the drugs are helping and not causing harm to the patient. Most patients will accept mild adverse effects, and serious adverse effects can be tolerated if they are rare and the drugs is useful, but it is unethical to give drugs that severely harm a substantial fraction of the patients, and it becomes a really serious ethical problem if a drug harms more patients than it helps.

In medical science today we use the concept "Number Needed to Treat to Benefit" (NNT or NNtB) about the number of patients that must be treated for one to be helped, and the Number Needed to Treat to Harm (NNtH or NNH) to tell the number of patients that must be treated for one to be harmed. NNtB and NNtH are measured with an uncertainty (CI means confidence interval at p=.05), so there are always a highest and a lowest value for each NNT measure. To be sure that a drug really helps and does not harm we need to compare the lowest empirically supported value (i.e., the upper confidence limit, or pessimistic harms assessment) with the highest empirically supported value of the Number Needed to Treat to Benefit (NNtB), i.e. a pessimist's assessment of benefits. In principle the NNtH/NNtB ratio can be calculated better, if all positive and negative effects were added up to one number; the importance of each treatment effect factor should be multiplied with its likelihood before taken into the addition, and a negative effect should be given negative value. The problem with such a "smart" strategy is that the result will be totally dependent on the number of included factors – what makes it less smart than it appears at first glance.

# Psychotropic drugs

We have compared the Cochrane meta-analyses of the commonly used antipsychotic drugs in Denmark (1-27) (see table 1). Surprisingly we found that almost all the drugs were harming more patients than they were helping, and often five or even 10 times more. We typically found NNtB to be 5-20 and NNtH 2-5. Just using a drug, which needs 10 patients treated for one to be helped, seems highly unethical, if a large fraction of the patients are harmed. Another serious problem is that the placebo effect is included in the results, making many drugs look active, when they are only slightly more effective that placebo.

A serious problem with the data is that they are provided by the industry, which has an interest in marketing their products. We found that most of the trials reviewed of the pharmaceuticals were designed to be very kind to the drugs. Only a small improvement of psychotic symptoms is often taken as help for the patient, in spite of the sad fact that these drugs rarely cure any patient for any disease. On the other hand the industry-imposed design has looked mostly at short-term physical adverse effects and often many extremely serious mental (28), social, existential, sexual, financial and other adverse effects and side effects were not included in the studies. Among some of the important factors often ignored in the studies were: suicides from drug-induced depression (28,39), suicide attempts and their consequences or spontaneous drug-induces death (4,30), drug-induced self-molestation (cutting etc), damage to learning and working ability, sexual function, social function, self-esteem, self-confidence and quality of life (4), notably including some adverse phenomena which physicians, and even psychiatric investigators, rarely have been trained to probe into. Other important biases have also been found (31). All this makes the NNtH likely to be systematically much too large and the NNtB likely to be systematically much too small, giving a very severe bias in favor of the drugs in the pharmaceutical studies, and most unfortunately also to the Cochrane meta-analyses re-using these data most often without any chance of mounting the appropriate critique. We definitely need to collect this information for the drugs being used to day.

It has been argued that the positive effects are qualitatively more important than the negative effects of the drugs, but we have analyzed this and found that both positive and negative changes were registered, when they were clinically noticeable. It therefore seems likely that NNtB and NNtH numbers build on equality noticeable phenomena, and therefore comparable. The fact that the antipsychotic drugs have highly unfavourable NNH/NNT ratios cannot be dismissed by the argument the positive effects of the drugs (i.e. the anti-hallucinating effect) are more important than the negative side effects (i.e. severe obesity). We found that there is not one single, antipsychotic, psychopharmacological drug that can be used without harming the patients more than benefiting them; NNH/NNT were always <1 (see table 1).

**Table 1. NNH/NNB ratios for the antipsychotic drugs used in Denmark (1-23) are when calculated as described below always smaller than one, often 1/5 and sometimes less than 1/10, implying that many more patients are harmed than benefited by the antipsychotic drugs, making them unethical to use. NNH/NNT is calculated here according to the principles of securing a positive effect for the patient, see text; if calculated without this principle the NNtH/NNtB ratio will still often be less than one. The list of drugs is found in (31)**

| *"Atypical" antipsychotics* |
|---|
| Sertindole (N05AE03) [1] NNtB: 'very much improved' as compared to those taking placebo NNT 7.9, CI 4.3 to 41.1<br>NNtH: almost as haloperidol. Akathisia - 8mg: 1 study, n=245, RR 0.2, CI 0.1 to 0.5, NNH 6.0, CI 4.1 to 11.2; 16mg: 1 study, n=252, RR 0.1, CI 0.0 to 0.3, NNH 5.4, CI 3.9- 9.0; 20mg: 1 study, n=253, RR 0.3, CI 0.2 to 0.7, NNH 7.3, CI 4.6 to 17.9; 24mg: 2 studies, n=524, RR 0.5, CI 0.3 to 0.7, NNH 8.6, CI 5.6 to 18.3. Tremor - 8mg: 1 study, n=245, RR 0.3, CI 0.1 to 0.7, NNH 8.5, CI 5.2 to 24.0; 16mg: 1 study, n=252, RR 0.2, CI 0.1 to 0.5, NNH 7.3, 4.8 to 15.6; 20mg: 1 study, n=253, RR 0.2, CI 0.1 to 0.6, NNH 7.8, CI 4.9 to 18.1; 24mg: 2 studies, n=524, RR 0.4, CI 0.2 to 0.6, NNH 8.2, CI 5.6 to 15.3. For Hypertonic - 24mg: 2 studies, n=524, RR 0.5, CI 0.3 to 0.8, NNH 12.4, CI 7.5 to 35.0. NNtH/NNtB=4/41.1= 0.097<br>Ziprasidone (N05AE04) [2] NNtB: As haloperidol. NNtH: Not calculated; almost as haloperidol.<br>Clozapin (N05AH02), No Cochrane study found<br>Olanzapine (N05AH03) [3] NNtB: 'no important clinical response' NNT 8 CI 5 to 27<br>NNtH: weight gain NNH 5 CI 4 to 7). Insufficient data. NNtH/NNtB=4/27= 0.15<br>Quetiapine (N05AH04) [4] NNtB 11 CI 7 to 55. NNtH: Movement disorders NNH 4 CI 4 to 5. Dry mouth NNH 17 CI 7 to 65. Sleepiness NNH 18 CI 8 to 181. NNtH/NNtB=7/55= 0.13. No summarized data of spontaneous patient death (4 of 728 died in one RCT, 2 of 618 died in an other RCT).<br>Amisulpride (N05AL05) [5] NNtB not specified: NNT 3 CI 3 to 7. NNtH: Need for antiparkinson drugs: NNH 4 CI 3 to 6. Agitation NNH 11 CI 6 to 50. NNtH/NNtB=3/7= 0.43 (Chlorpromazine used as reference´).<br>Risperidone (N05AX08)[6,7] NNtB: As Olanzapine. NNtH: sexual dysfunction abnormal ejaculation NNH 20 CI 6 to 176. Impotence RR 2.43 CI 0.24 to 24.07. One third of people given either drug experienced some extrapyramidal symptoms (n=893, 3 RCTs, RR 1.18 CI 0.75 to 1.88) but 25% of people using risperidone require medication to alleviate extrapyramidal adverse effects (n=419, 2 RCTs, RR 1.76 CI 1.25 to 2.48, NNH 8 CI 4 to 25). Weight gain: NNH 7 CI 6 to 10). NNtH/NNtB=4/27= 0.15<br>Aripiprazole (N05AX12) [8] NNtB: NNT 5 CI 4 to 8. NNtH: Need for antiparkinson drugs NNtH 4 CI 3 to 5. (Previous study included NNtH: Insomnia NNH 4 CI 3 to 9.) NNtH/NNtB=3/8= 0.37 |
| *High-dose typical antipsychotics* |
| Chlorpromazine (N05AA01) [9] NNtB: Prevents relapse, longer term data: NNT 4 CI 3 to 5. Improves symptoms and functioning NNT 6 CI 5 to 8. NNtH: Sedation: NNH 5 CI 4 to 8. Acute movement disorder NNH 32 CI 11 to 154. Need for antiparkinson drugs NNH 14 CI 9 to 28. Lowering of blood pressure with accompanying dizziness NNH 11 CI 7 to 21. Considerable weight gain NNH 2 CI 2 to 3. NNtH/NNtB=2/5= 0.15<br>Levomepromazine (N05AA02). No Cochrane study found<br>Promazine (N05AA03). No Cochrane study found<br>Thioridazine (N05AC02)[10] NNtB: "global state outcomes" NNT of 2 CI 2 to 3; NNtH: Sedation NNH 4 CI 2 to 74. Cardiac adverse effects NNH 3 CI 2 to 5. NNTH/NNTB=2/3= 0.67<br>Melperone (N05AD03), No Cochrane study found<br>Pipamperone (N05AD05) No Cochrane study found<br>Chlorprothixene (N05AF03)No Cochrane study found |
| *Middle-dose typical antipsychotics* |
| Perphenazine (N05AB03) [11]NNtB: 2 CI 1 to 20. NNtH: invalid data.<br>Depot perphenazine decanoate[12]: NNtB as clopenthixol decanoate and other antipsychotic drugs. Need for anticholinergic drugs (one RTC NNtH 4 and another NNtH 10), movement disorders (RR 1.36, CI 1.1 to 1.8 |

**Table 1. (Continued)**

| |
|---|
| NNT 5). NNtH/NNtB = 4/8 = 0.50 (Chlorpromazine used as reference).<br><br>Zuclopenthixol (N05AF05) [13] NNtB: Patient not unchanged or worse: NNT 10 CI 6 to 131. NNtH: Extraparamydal symptoms NNH 2 CI 2 to 31. Need for antiparkinson drugs NNH 3 CI 3 to 17. NNtH/NNtB=3/131= 0.023<br><br>Zuclopenthixol decanoate [14] NNtB: Prevented or postponed relapses NNT 8, CI 5-53. NNtH: Adverse effects NNH 5, CI 3-31. NNtH/NNtB=3/53= 0.057 |
| *Low-dose typical antipsychotics* |
| Fluphenazine (N05AB02) [15] NNtB: NNT= placebo (not effective). NNtH: Experiencing extrapyramidal effects such as akathisia NNH 13 CI 4 to 128. NNtH/NNtB=4/Infinite= 0.00<br>Haloperidol (N05AD01) [16] NNtB: NNT 3 CI 2 to 5/Global improvement NNT 3 CI 2.5 to 5. NNtH: Acute dystonia NNH 5 CI 3 to 9. Need for antiparkinson drugs NNH 3 CI 2 to 5. NNtH/NNtB=2/5= 0.40<br>Flupentixol (N05AF01) [17] NNtH/NNtB: as other depot antipsychotics.<br>Pimozide (N05AG02) [18] NNtB: Prevents relapse NNT 4 CI 3 to 22. NNTH: Tremor NNH 6 CI 3 to 44- Need for antiparkinson drugs NNH 3 CI 2 to 5. NNtH/NNtB=2/22= 0.091<br>Penfluridole (N05AG03) [19] NNtB: 'improvement in global state' NNT 3 CI 2 to 10 – as chlorpromazine, fluphenazine, trifluoperazine, thioridazine, or thiothixene. NNtH as chlorpromazine, fluphenazine, trifluoperazine, thioridazine, or thiothixene. NNtH/NNtB=4/10= 0.40<br>Sulpiride (N05AL01) [20] NNtH/NNtB: evidence is limited and data relating to claims for its value against negative symptoms is not trial-based.<br><br>New generation antipsychotics[21]: NNtH: Of the new generation drugs, only clozapine was associated with significantly fewer extrapyramidal side-effects (EPS) (RD=-0.15, 95% CI -0.26 to -0.4, p=0.008) and higher efficacy than low-potency conventional drugs. These findings might have been biased by the use of the high-potency antipsychotic haloperidol as a comparator in most of the trials. First episode schizophrenia[22]: NNH 3 CI 2 to 6 The results of this review are inconclusive.<br><br>Antipsychotics in treatment of childhood onset psychoses[23]: NNtH/NNtB: There are few relevant trials and, presently, there is little conclusive evidence regarding the effects of antipsychotic medication for those with early onset schizophrenia. Some benefits were identified in using the atypical antipsychotic clozapine compared with haloperidol but the benefits were offset by an increased risk of serious adverse effects. Early intervention for psychosis[24]: NNtB: Six month follow up: less likely to develop psychosis at a six month follow up NNT 4 CI 2 to 20, 12 month follow up: Not significant! NNtH: Weight gain etc., insufficient data |
| *Other drugs sometimes used against psychosis* |
| prochlorperazine (N05AB04), No antipsychotic Cochrane study found<br>periciazine (N05AC01), No Cochrane study found<br>tetrabenazine (N05AK01) No antipsychotic Cochrane study found<br>Litium (N05AN01) [25] NNTB: as placebo (not efficient). NNTH: Insufficient data.<br>NNTH/NNTB=something/infinite<<1<br><br>Benzodiazepines [26] NNTB: NNT 3 CI 2 to 17. NNTH: Maybe worse than placebo. NNTH/NNTB= 100/17? Probably >1<br><br>Valproate [27] NNTB: Insufficient data. NNTH: Insufficient data<br>acepromazine (N05AA04), No Cochrane study found |

During the last 10 years the many Cochrane units all over the world have provided us with highly valuable meta-analyses. Because of this unique source of scientifically established high-level knowledge, we now in our opinion know that the ethical treatment of many psychiatric disorders is still psychotherapy, which on one hand in many studies has been documented to help and on the other never has been documented to harm the patients (see 32-34).

To compare NNtH and NNtB will always to some extend be comparing apples and pears; this problem can only be solved by measuring one integrated endpoint of both positive and negative effect like *global quality of life* (which can be measured with a simple questionnaire like the QOL1 with one questions on self-assessed global quality of life (35)), self-assessed physical and mental health, or self-assessed ability of functioning in a number of relevant domains (work, social life, family, sexuality). We recommend the use of a wise and balanced combination of self-assessed mental and physical health, global quality of life, and ability in general as the endpoints for any medical treatment. The low ratio NNH/NNT is the likely reason that the pharmaceutical industry systematically has avoided the use of such endpoint that illuminates the effect of the drugs on the whole person.

It has also avoided long-term documentation of adverse effects, in spite of many physicians and patients have been asking for these data for years.

We suggest that we call the inverse number NNH/NNT for "the ethical treatment value of the drug". The way it is calculated is in a way "double pessimistic"; we estimate that a drug with NNH/NNT>10 has a 99% chance to be a primarily beneficial (valuable) drug, and a NNH/NNT value<1/10 signifies a 99% risk of being a primarily harmful drug. We suggest that the NNH/NNT value of "penicillin in the treatment of syphilis" (about 100) can be a benchmark for a highly valuable drug.

If effects and side effects are mechanistically related, like the better mobility after curing a femoral fracture leading to an increased future fracture rate, the above-mentioned "smart" formula must be used. The last important thing is that most symptoms and side effects are reversible, but brain damage, suicide and dead are not. Suicide is a negative effect that is much more difficult to tolerate that all other adverse effects and every study must therefore include a long-term survey of increased or diminished suicide rate.

The last thing to consider is that placebo often has a NNT=3; the difference between the antipsychotic drugs and placebo are therefore only marginal; an alternative explanation to a therapeutic effect is the fact that you can feel the drug in your brain, destroying the blindness of the study and creating an "active placebo" effect. If this is the case, we are actually only using placebo to treat, but with high risk of causing side effects and serious harm to the patients. This has never been investigated for the antipsychotic drugs neither by the pharmaceutical companies nor by neutral researchers, and this must urgently be done.

# Conclusion

In conclusion, the NNH/NNT ratio might be the needed guideline for evaluating the therapeutic effect of drugs; when this analysis is carried out on the antipsychotic drug using the upper confidence limit of NNT and the lower confidence limit of NNH for the comparison, we find that all antipsychotic drugs used in Denmark are more harmful than beneficial.

We presume that the antipsychotic drugs on the market today in Denmark are very much the same as in all other countries, as the same drugs are used almost everywhere. The analysis indicates that the antipsychotic drugs are likely not to improve health and thus to be without any net therapeutic value; they are likely to be primarily harmful to the patients. This does not mean that the drugs cannot to be used for life-saving and other compelling reasons, like on extremely aggressive, patients that urgently needs to be calmed down, or on acute psychotic sexually violent schizophrenic patients etc., but they cannot be used ethically as a standard treatment for any kind of mental illness.

On the other hand recent research comparing psychotherapy with psychiatric treatment has documented psychotherapy to be helpful to many groups of patients (32-34), and also more helpful than the psychiatric standard treatment, without having the adverse effects of the anti-psychotic drugs.

We believe that the NNH/NNT ratio is the best indicator we have today of the total therapeutic value (benefit versus harm) of a drug, but we must admit that it is a crude summary index of benefit-vs.-harm. For a better evaluation of a medical treatment we need to use a combined measure of *global quality of life* (like QOL1 and QOL5) (35), self-assesses health (36), and self-assessed ability (in a number of relevant domains) (36).

We need urgently - for the sake of all patients - to be able to estimate the total therapeutic value of a drug (or any other treatment) more accurate in the future, and recommend that all clinical trials in the future use *global QOL and self-assessed physical and mental health* as obligatory outcomes; long term studies including all relevant dimensions like *loss of working and studying ability, suicide, and spontaneous drug-induced death* are also absolutely necessary for an ethical evidence-based medicine in psychiatry.

# References

[1] Lewis R, Bagnall AM, Leitner M. Sertindole for schizophrenia. Cochrane Database Syst Rev 2005;(3):CD001715.
[2] Bagnall A, Lewis RA, Leitner ML. Ziprasidone for schizophrenia and severe mental illness. Cochrane Database Syst Rev 2000;(4):CD 001945.
[3] Duggan L, Fenton M, Rathbone J, Dardennes R, El-Dosoky A, Indran S. Olanzapine for schizophrenia. Cochrane Database Syst Rev 2005;(2):CD001359.
[4] Srisurapanont M, Maneeton B, Maneeton N. Quetiapine for schizophrenia. Cochrane Database Syst Rev 2004;(2):CD000967.
[5] Mota NE, Lima MS, Soares BG. Amisulpride for schizophrenia. Cochrane Database Syst Rev 2002;(2):CD001357.
[6] Jayaram MB, Hosalli P. Risperidone versus olanzapine for schizophrenia. Cochrane Database Syst Rev 2005;(2):CD005237.
[7] Jesner OS, Aref-Adib M, Coren E. Risperidone for autism spectrum disorder. Cochrane Database Syst Rev 2007;(1):CD005040.
[8] El-Sayeh HG, Morganti C. Aripiprazole for schizophrenia. Cochrane Database Syst Rev 2006;(2):CD004578.
[9] Adams CE, Awad G, Rathbone J, Thornley B.Chlorpromazine versus placebo for schizophrenia. Cochrane Database Syst Rev 2007;(2):CD000284
[10] Fenton M, Rathbone J, Reilly J, Sultana A. Thioridazine for schizophrenia. Cochrane Database Syst Rev 2007;(3):CD001944.
[11] Hartung B, Wada M, Laux G, Leucht S. Perphenazine for schizophrenia.Cochrane Database Syst Rev 2005;(1):CD003443.
[12] Quraishi S, David A. Depot perphenazine decanoate and enanthate for schizophrenia. Cochrane Database Syst Rev 2000;(2):CD001717.
[13] Kumar A, Strech D. Zuclopenthixol dihydrochloride for schizophrenia. Cochrane Database Syst Rev 2005;(4):CD005474.

[14] Coutinho E, Fenton M, Quraishi S. Zuclopenthixol decanoate for schizophrenia and other serious mental illnesses. Cochrane Database Syst Rev 2000;(2):CD001164.
[15] Matar HE, Almerie MQ. Oral fluphenazine versus placebo for schizophrenia. Cochrane Database Syst Rev 2007;(1):CD006352.
[16] Joy CB, Adams CE, Lawrie SM. Haloperidol versus placebo for schizophrenia. Cochrane Database Syst Rev 2006;(4):CD003082.
[17] Quraishi S, David A. Depot flupenthixol decanoate for schizophrenia or other similar psychotic disorders. Cochrane Database Syst Rev 2000;(2):CD001470.
[18] Rathbone J, McMonagle T. Pimozide for schizophrenia or related psychoses. Cochrane Database Syst Rev 2007;(3):CD001949.
[19] Soares BG, Lima MS. Penfluridol for schizophrenia. Cochrane Database Syst Rev 2006;(2):CD002923.
[20] Soares BG, Fenton M, Chue P. Sulpiride for schizophrenia. Cochrane Database Syst Rev 2000;(2):CD001162.
[21] Leucht S, Wahlbeck K, Hamann J, Kissling W. New generation antipsychotics versus low-potency conventional antipsychotics: a systematic review and meta-analysis. Lancet 2003;361(9369):1581-9.
[22] Rummel C, Hamann J, Kissling W, Leucht S. New generation antipsychotics for first episode schizophrenia. Cochrane Database Syst Rev 2003;(4):CD004410.
[23] Kennedy E, Kumar A, Datta S.Antipsychotic medication for childhood-onset schizophrenia. Cochrane Database Syst Rev 2007;(3):CD004027.
[24] Marshall M, Rathbone J. Early intervention for psychosis. Cochrane Database Syst Rev 2006;(4):CD004718.
[25] Leucht S, Kissling W, McGrath J. Lithium for schizophrenia. Cochrane Database Syst Rev 2007;(3):CD003834.
[26] Volz A, Khorsand V, Gillies D, Leucht S. Benzodiazepines for schizophrenia. Cochrane Database Syst Rev 2007;(1):CD006391.
[27] Basan A, Leucht S.Valproate for schizophrenia. Cochrane Database Syst Rev 2004;(1):CD004028.
[28] SBU-rapport nr. 133/1 og 133/2. Treatment with neuroleptics [Behandling med neuroleptika]. Stockholm: Statens beredning för utvärdering av medicinsk metodik 1997;2:81. [Swedish]
[29] Qin P, Nordentoft M.Suicide risk in relation to psychiatric hospitalization: evidence based on longitudinal registers. Arch Gen Psychiatry 2005;62(4):427-32
[30] Lindhardt A, et al. The use of antipsychotic drugs among the 18-64year old patients with schizophrenia, mania, or bipolar affective disorder. National bord of Heath, Copenhagen[ Forbruget af antipsykotika blandt 18-64 årige patienter med skizofreni, mani eller bipolar affektiv sindslidelse". Copenhagen: Sundhedsstyrelsen, 2006 [Danish]
[31] Chaves AC, Seeman MV. Sex selection bias in schizophrenia antipsychotic trials.J Clin Psychopharmacol 2006;26(5):489-94.
[32] Leichsenring F, Rabung S, Leibing E. The efficacy of short-term psychodynamic psychotherapy in specific psychiatric disorders: a meta-analysis. Arch Gen Psychiatry 2004;61(12):1208-16.
[33] Leichsenring F. Are psychodynamic and psychoanalytic therapies effective?: A review of empirical data. Int J Psychoanal 2005;86(Pt 3):841-68.
[34] Leichsenring F, Leibing E. Psychodynamic psychotherapy: a systematic review of techniques, indications and empirical evidence. Psychol Psychother 2007;80(Pt 2):217-28.
[35] Lindholt JS, Ventegodt S, Henneberg EW. Development and validation of QoL5 for clinical databases. A short, global and generic questionnaire based on an integrated theory of the quality of life. Eur J Surg 2002;168(2):107-13.
[36] Ventegodt S, Henneberg EW, Merrick J, Lindholt JS. Validation of two global and generic quality of life questionnaires for population screening: SCREENQOL and SEQOL. ScientificWorldJournal 2003;3:412-21.

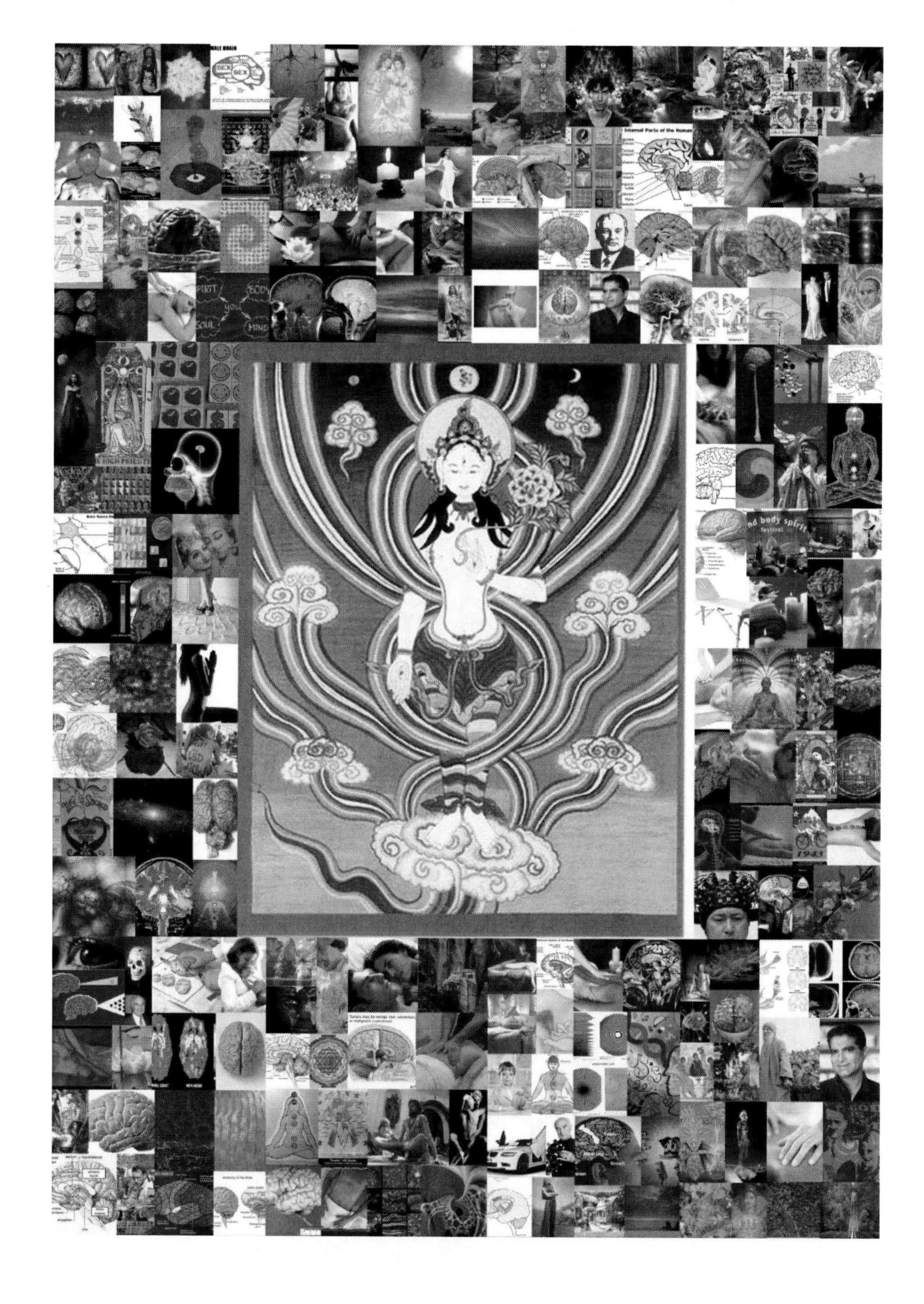

*Chapter XVIII*

# How does antipsychotic drugs and non-drug therapy effect Quality-Adjusted Life-Years (QALY) in persons with borderline and psychotic mental illness?

It is impossible for patients, physicians and health-politicians to know, which treatment to choose if the treatment outcome is not in one integrative measure. To evaluate the total outcome of the treatment of borderline and psychotic mentally ill patients with antipsychotic drugs compared to non-drug treatments, we choose the two major outcomes "quality of life" (QOL) and "survival time" integrated into one total outcome measure, the Quality-Adjusted Life Years (QALY). We estimated total outcome in QALY (Δ QALY) by multiplying the estimated difference in global QOL (Δ QOL) and the estimated difference in survival time (Δ survival time): $\Delta$ QALY= $\Sigma_{\text{all outcomes}}(\Delta QOL \times \Delta \text{ survival time})$. We included factors like suicide and spontaneous drug-induced death that is normally not included in clinical randomized trials of antipsychotic drugs. We found that the total outcome of treatments with antipsychotic drugs was about –2 QALY; the total outcome from non-drug therapies (psychodynamic psychotherapy, clinical holistic medicine) was about +8 QALY. When the total outcomes of the treatments were measured in QALY, antipsychotic drugs harmed the patients, while the patients benefited from the non-drug therapies. Antipsychotic drugs violate the medical ethics of Hippocrates, "First do no harm"; non-drug therapy is therefore the rational treatment for the borderline and psychotic mental illnesses. Treatment with antipsychotic drugs is only justified, when prolonged non-drug therapy has failed.

## Introduction

To evaluate the total outcome in medicine there are two general outcomes of primary interest: *survival* and *global quality of life*. These two measures can easily be integrated into Quality-

Adjusted Life Years (QALY) (1). A positive QALY-contribution comes from positive effects of a treatment, and a negative QALY-contribution comes from a negative effect, called the adverse or side effects, like for example the patient's death caused either by drug-induced suicide or by the toxic adverse effects. Recent studies on all mentally ill patients in Denmark revealed a high risk of suicide (2) and unexplained death associated with psychiatric treatment and antipsychotic drugs (3). NNT (number needed to treat) and NNH (number needed to harm) numbers have been calculated for the treatment with antipsychotic drugs (4) and for the non-drug treatment (5), and the NNHs have been added up to a total NNH (4,5). Only some aspects of effects and side effects were related to QOL judged from the empery from the QOL-research (6-10); the NNT and NNH related to global QOL were thus evaluated on an empirical basis to estimate the size of the impact on QOL both of the positive and negative effects, to find the total impact on QOL of the treatment. Then the treatments impact on survival was evaluated. All in all the results made it possible to estimate the total positive and negative impact of the two alternative treatments in the dimensions *QOL* and *survival time*. From this we calculated the QALY impact of the different treatments of mentally ill with antipsychotic drugs and without these drugs, to compare them and find the rational, evidence-based treatment.

The borderline and psychotic, mentally ill patients and their physicians can today choose between either a drug treatment or a non-drug therapy like psychodynamic psychotherapy (11-15) or scientific CAM (complementary and alternative medicine i.e. clinical holistic medicine) (16-18). Till this day many different outcomes and adverse effects have made the picture highly unclear to the patients, the doctor, and the political decision maker. This study aims to provide the integrated outcome data needed to make a scientific comparison of the therapeutic value of the competing treatments and thus the data needed for a rational choice.

## Our review

The QALY analyses of the effect of the non-drug treatments were rather trivial; although we had no data on survival, we had no reason to believe that any patient's life was shortened because of non-drug therapy (5). Quite on the contrary it seemed the therapy would prevent suicide and prolong life, but no accurate data could be found, so we did not include this in our calculations. We found QOL to be improved (11), or more often positive effects indicating that QOL was improved for the mentally ill patients (6-8) including patients with schizophrenia (9,10), thus giving a positive QALY outcome of non-drug therapy for mental illness.

The analysis of the QALY outcome for the treatment of mentally ill patients with antipsychotic drugs was much more complicated, so we had to build it partly on a meta-analysis on the total outcome of antipsychotic drugs (4), and partly on other studies as there were factors difficult to include in the traditional effect study due to lack of data. Factors like suicide rates and spontaneous drug-induced over-mortality were most often not included in the randomized clinical trials, so this information needed to be collected from separate studies. So we build the QALY-meta-analysis on the outcomes of antipsychotic drugs, and included the factors that were not included in the studies, to get a more complete picture of the positive and negative effects of antipsychotic drugs. Thus the present analysis contains more information and therefore is likely to give a more accurate picture than the documentation provided by the pharmaceutical industry.

We estimated the total outcome in QALY by multiplying the estimated difference in global QOL and the estimated difference in survival time: $\Delta$ QALY= $\sum_{\text{all outcomes}}(\Delta\text{QOL x } \Delta$ survival time). We made all estimations conservatively, to avoid adding a bias here. We estimated conservatively the average patient to be 25 years old at treatment start; we know that most persons with schizophrenia are diagnosed between 15 and 25 years of age. The antipsychotic treatment is normally continuing for the rest of the patient's life, which we conservatively set to last for 65 years (which is shorter than the average life span of about 75). We used the measure "global QOL" and not health-related QOL, which is not based on QOL-theory, but only on ad hoc measures (19) and preferred values confirmed with many different measures to large values only confirmed by one measure. We avoided the problems related to QALY described in an earlier paper (1).

# What did we find?

Recent Cochrane meta-analysis has shown that all antipsychotic drugs share the effect profile of chlorpromazine with a similar toxicity (20). We only found the outcome "mental state" relevant to QOL, as "relapse", "behaviour" and "global state/global impression" all related to behaviour, or to a mix of behaviour and mental state. For comparison a normal life in Denmark is 75 life-years (21) of a mean 70% QOL (12,13) equivalent to 52.5 QALY.

## Antipsychotic drugs, positive QALY-contributions

For antipsychotic drugs we found no improvement in mental state in our meta-analysis of 79 Cochrane meta-analyses of antipsychotic drugs (4). The analysis included all relevant data on subjective dimensions like fear, agitation, hallucinations, confusion etc. None of the dimensions related to global QOL showed any improvement; thus the positive contribution from improvement of mental state was 0.00 QALY.

## Antipsychotic drugs, negative QALY-contributions

We found in our meta-analysis (4) that severe adverse effects were very common with antipsychotic drugs, on average every patient had at least 1.66 adverse effects (11). We know from an earlier study that people with one or two health problems on average have a global quality of life that is 74.2% compared to people without health problems who have a global QOL of 76.1% (12); the health problems is therefore associated with a loss of global QOL of 1.9% for as long as the drugs are taken, which is normally all life if treated with antipsychotic drugs. This sums up to a QALY impact of –1.9% QOL x 40 Years= -0.76 QALY.

2.04% of the patients in the schizophrenic spectrum committed suicide in direct connection to starting the drug treatment (during psychiatric admission) and another 2.80% committed suicide immediately after admission (0-6 month) (22) giving a total of 4.84% of the patients with psychotic mental illnesses committing suicide in connection to the treatment with antipsychotic drugs, which is standard treatment in Denmark. As these patients are normally young (estimated mean of 25 years) and life expectancy of at least 65 years (conservative estimate), with at least a QOL of 41.4% (schizophrenia) (the global QOL for schizophrenic patients in Denmark (13)), this sums up to a QALY impact of –4.84% x 41.4% QOL x 40 Years= -0.80 QALY.

We know that antipsychotic drugs is associated with an 25% increased likelihood of unexplained sudden death, which normally is about 0.3% a year (23) and this continues for every year the drugs are taken; this sums up to a total of 40 years x 0.25 over-mortality/year, equal to10 times the normal mortality from spontaneous death of 0.3%; each death takes in average 20 years from the person's life. The total likelihood for spontaneous death is thus 3%. This sums up to a QALY impact of -3% x 20 years x 41.4% QOL= -0.25 QALY. The total QALY outcome of antipsychotic drugs is –1.81 QALY (see table 1).

## Non-drug therapy, positive QALY-contributions

Psychodynamic psychotherapy have in uncontrolled studies cured 1/3 to 1/8 of the schizophrenic patients (9,10) and clinical holistic medicine have cured 57% of patients who felt mentally ill (11); a conservative calculation of non-drug therapy gives us a permanent improvement of QOL of 20%; the QALY contribution is thus 40 years x 20% QOL = 8 QALY. The 20% improvement in global QOL is confirmed by measuring the global QOL before, after and one year after non-drug treatment (11,24).

**Table 1. QALY outcome from treatments with antipsychotic drugs and the non-drug treatments (PP= psychodynamic psychotherapy; CHM= clinical holistic medicine)**

| Treatment | QALY contribution |
|---|---|
| Antipsychotic drugs, positive treatment effect | + 0.00 QALY |
| Antipsychotic drugs, adverse effects | -0.76 QALY |
| Antipsychotic drugs, suicide | -0.80 QALY |
| Antipsychotic drugs, spontaneous death | -0.25 QALY |
| **Total QALY contribution, antipsychotic drugs** | **-1.81 QALY** |
| Non-drug treatment (PP, CHM), positive | +8.00 QALY |
| treatment effects | |
| Non-drug treatment (PP, CHM), adverse effects | -0.00 QALY |
| Non-drug treatment (PP, CHM), suicide | + 0.00<br>(preventive effects, size unknown) |
| Non-drug treatment (PP,CHM), spontaneous death | -0.00 QALY |
| **Total QALY contribution,** | |
| **non-drug treatment (PP, CHM)** | **+ 8.00 QALY** |

### Non-drug therapy, negative QALY-contributions

Adverse effects are generally considered not to be a problem in non-drug therapy, and suicide is very rare and actually more likely to be prevented that to be provoked (5-11,25). There is no indication of spontaneous death happening more often than usual (5). Conservatively estimated the QALY contribution from this is +0.00 QALY. The total QALY outcome from the non-drugs treatment psychodynamic psychotherapy and clinical holistic medicine is thus about 8 QALY (see table 1).

## Discussion

The method of QALY has been criticized because of the many different ways QOL can be measured (1), giving very different results depending on the QOL-measure. We find this critique to be correct when it comes to health-related QOL; we have therefore measured global QOL in 11 different ways (12-15,19) and have learned that the measure of global QOL is fairly robust, and surprisingly independent of theory and composition of questions in the questionnaire (12,13,19).

This means that global QOL can be seen as a real, measurable phenomenon, and the measure of global QOL as an expression of a person's global state of life. The multiplication of global QOL and life years have been criticized also for being too simple; a long life with poor quality of life could be worse than being dead (1) and suicide could therefore be a rational act. We do not find any of these considerations conflicting with our estimations. We conclude that the presented conservative estimates are fair and free from bias.

## Conclusion

In the treatment of the psychotic mentally ill patient, the total outcome of the treatment with antipsychotic drugs is -2 QALY, while the total outcome of non-drug therapies (psychodynamic psychotherapy and clinical holistic medicine) is +8 QALY (see table 1). The treatment with antipsychotic drugs is harming the patient, while the treatment with the non-drug therapy is beneficial judged from a QALY analysis. We must therefore strongly recommend non-drug therapy to patients with borderline and psychotic mental illnesses, whenever possible and warn against the extensive use of antipsychotic drugs.

## References

[1] Ventegodt S, Merrick J, Andersen NJ. Measurement of quality of life VI: Quality-adjusted life years (QALY) are an unfortunate use of quality of life concept. ScientificWorldJournal 2003;3:1015-9.

[2] Qin P, Nordentoft M. Suicide risk in relation to psychiatric hospitalization: evidence based on longitudinal registers. Arch Gen Psychiatry 2005;62(4):427-32.

[3] Lindhardt A, ed. The use of antipsychotic drugs among the 18-64 year old patients with schizophrenia, mania, or bipolar affective disorder. Copenhagen: National Board Health, 2006. [Danish]

[4] Ventegodt S, Flensborg-Madsen T, Andersen NJ, Samberg BØ, Struve F, Merrick J. Therapeutic value of antipsychotic drugs: A critical analysis of Cochrane meta-analyses of the therapeutic value of anti-psychotic drugs. Lancet, submitted.
[5] Ventegodt S, Kandel I, Merrick J. A metaanalysis of side effects of psychotherapy, bodywork, and clinical holistic medicine. J Complement Integr Med, submitted.
[6] Leichsenring F, Rabung S, Leibing E. The efficacy of short-term psychodynamic psychotherapy in specific psychiatric disorders: a meta-analysis. Arch Gen Psychiatry 2004;61(12):1208-16.
[7] Leichsenring F. Are psychodynamic and psychoanalytic therapies effective?: A review of empirical data. Int J Psychoanal 2005;86(Pt 3):841-68.
[8] Leichsenring F, Leibing E. Psychodynamic psychotherapy: a systematic review of techniques, indications and empirical evidence. Psychol Psychother 2007;80(Pt 2):217-28.
[9] Modestin J, Huber A, Satirli E, Malti T, Hell D. Long-term course of schizophrenic illness: Bleuler's study reconsidered. Am J Psychiatry 2003;160(12):2202-8.
[10] Searles HF. Collected papers on schizophrenia. Madison, CT: Int Univ Press, 1965:15–18.
[11] Ventegodt S, Thegler S, Andreasen T, Struve F, Enevoldsen L, Bassaine L, Torp M, Merrick J. Clinical holistic medicine (mindful, short-term psychodynamic psychotherapy complemented with bodywork) in the treatment of experienced mental illness. ScientificWorldJournal 2007;7:306-9.
[12] Ventegodt S. [Livskvalitet i Danmark]. Quality of life in Denmark. Results from a population survey.Copenhagen: Forskningscentrets Forlag, 1995. [partly in Danish]
[13] Ventegodt S. [Livskvalitet hos 4500 31-33 årige]. The Quality of Life of 4500 31-33 year-olds. Result from a study of the Prospective Pediatric Cohort of persons born at the University Hospital in Copenhagen. Copenhagen: Forskningscentrets Forlag, 1996. [partly in Danish]
[14] Ventegodt S. [Livskvalitet og omstændigheder tidligt i livet]. The quality of life and factors in pregnancy, birth and infancy. Results from a follow-up study of the Prospective Pediatric Cohort of persons born at the University Hospital in Copenhagen 1959-61. Copenhagen: Forskningscentrets Forlag, 1995. [partly in Danish]
[15] Ventegodt S. [Livskvalitet og livets store begivenheder]. The Quality of Life and Major Events in Life. Copenhagen: Forskningscentrets Forlag, 2000. [partly in Danish]
[16] Ventegodt S, Kandel I, Merrick J. Principles of holistic medicine. Philosophy behind quality of life. Victoria, BC: Trafford, 2005.
[17] Ventegodt S, Kandel I, Merrick J. Principles of holistic medicine. Quality of life and health. New York: Hippocrates Sci Publ, 2005.
[18] Ventegodt S, Kandel I, Merrick J. Principles of holistic medicine. Global quality of life. theory, research and methodology. New York: Hippocrates Science, 2005.
[19] Ventegodt S. Measuring the quality of life. From theory to practice. Copenhagen: Forskningscentrets Forlag, 1996.
[20] Adams CE, Awad G, Rathbone J, Thornley B. Chlorpromazine versus placebo for schizophrenia. Cochrane Database Syst Rev 2007;(2):CD000284.
[21] Gunnersen SJ. Statistical yearbook. Copenhagen: Statistics Denmark, 2007.
[22] Qin P, Nordentoft M.Suicide risk in relation to psychiatric hospitalization: evidence based on longitudinal registers. Arch Gen Psychiatry 2005;62(4):427-32
[23] Lindhardt A, et al. [Forbruget af antipsykotika blandt 18-64 årige patienter med skizofreni, mani eller bipolar affektiv sindslidelse]. Copenhagen: Sundhedsstyrelsen, 2006. [Danish]
[24] Ventegodt S, Thegler S, Andreasen T, Struve F, Enevoldsen L, Bassaine L, Torp M, Merrick J. Clinical holistic medicine: Psychodynamic short-time therapy complemented with bodywork. A clinical follow-up Study of 109 patients. ScientificWorldJournal 2006;6:2220-38.
[25] Polewka A, Maj JC, Warchoł K, Groszek B. [The assessment of suicidal risk in the concept of the presuicidal syndrome, and the possibilities it provides for suicide prevention and therapy--review]. Przegl Lek 2005;62:399-402. [Polish]

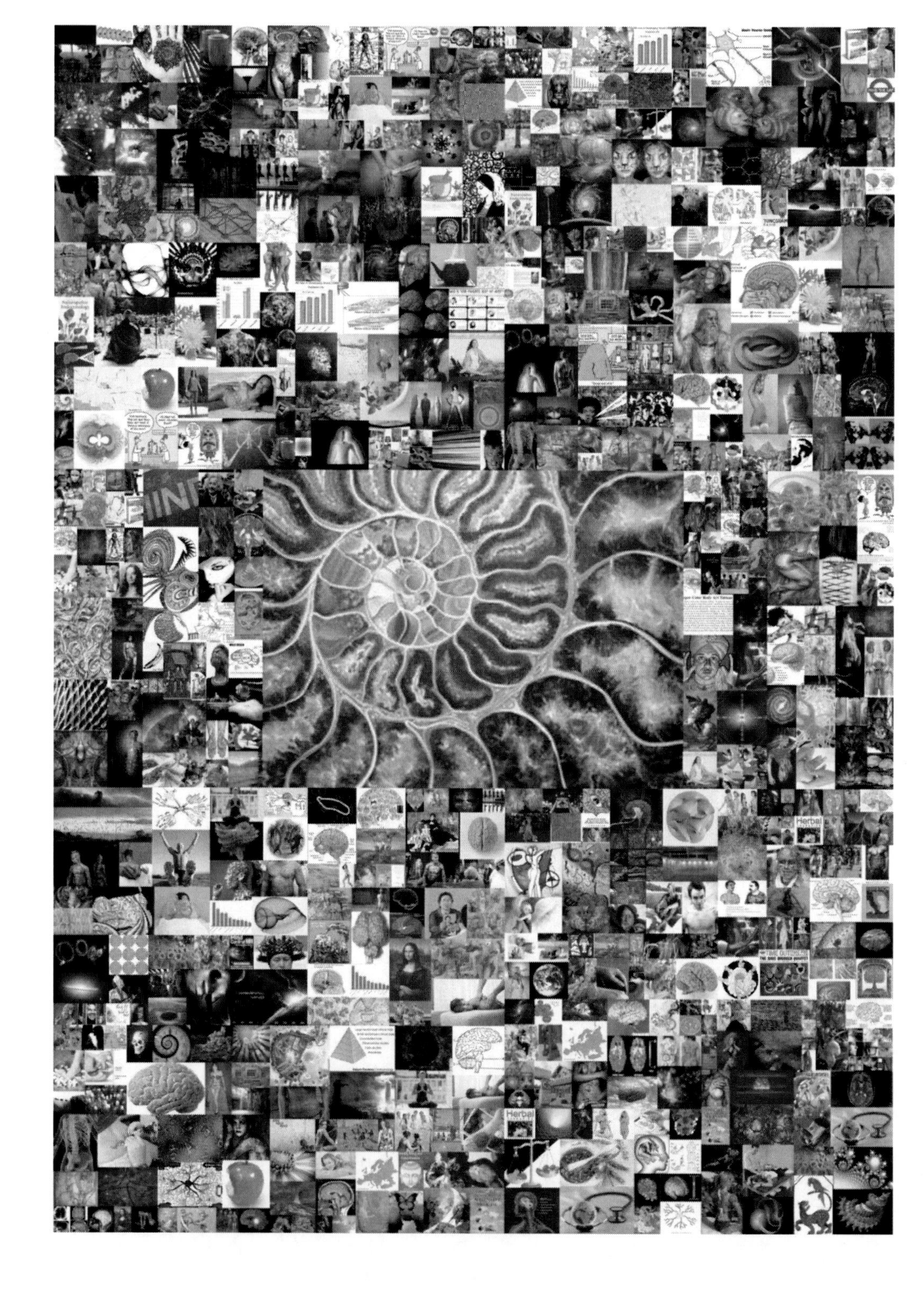

*Chapter XIX*

# When biomedicine is inadequate

The modern, biomedical physician, which is the most common type of physician at least in Northern Europe, is using pharmaceuticals as his prime tool. Unfortunately this tool is much less efficient than you might expect from the biochemical theory. The belief in drugs as the solution to the health problems of mankind, overlooking important existing knowledge on quality of life, personal development and holistic healing seems to be one good reason why around every second citizen of our modern society is chronically ill and stays ill in spite of treatment with pharmaceutical drugs.

The bio-medical paradigm and the drugs are certainly useful, where in many situations we could not do without the drugs (like antibiotics), but administering penicillin to cure infections or disease in young age is not without consequences, as the way we perceive health and medicine is influenced by such experiences. When we get a more severe disease in midlife, we also believe drugs will make us healthy again. But at this age the drugs do not work efficiently anymore, because we have turned older and lost much of the biological coherence that made us heal easily, when we were younger. Now we need to assume responsibility, take learning and improve our quality of life. We need a more holistic medicine that can help us back to life by allowing us to access our hidden resources.

The modern physician cannot rely solely on drugs, but also have holistic tools in his medical toolbox. This is the only way we can improve the general health of our populations. Whenever NNT (number needed to treat) is 3 or higher, the likelihood to cure the patient is less that 33%, which is not satisfying to any physician. In this case he must ethically try something more in order to cure his patients, which are the crossroads where both traditional manual medicine and the tools of a scientific holistic medicine are helpful.

The NNTs of pharmaceutical drugs are often 10, 20 and 50, making their use statistically almost irrelevant to most patients; as we have seen in section one the NNTs of drugs for chronic mentally illness is often 50 or higher meaning that less than 2% of the patients get better. The rest of the patients must put their hope in an alternative type of treatment.

# Introduction

About one in two persons have a chronic disease – unpleasant complaints such as arthritis, migraine, allergy, diabetes, low back pain or depression – despite numerous visits to their family physician or to specialists and generous use of advanced biomedicine (1). About half the chronic patients even seek alternative treatment (CAM) (2), which is gaining increasing trust among the population, but often to no avail – the disease usually does not go away. Holistic medicine (3-26) on the other hand is often considered obsolete by the physicians and not mastered by the complementary therapists and is therefore not used. Therefore most chronic patients stay ill for life.

In our modern society, partly due to longer life expectancy, illness has become something that people have to learn to live with. Often we see one disease followed by another and it is not uncommon for older people to have five or ten different ailments taking up to a dozen different kinds of medications. We also observe a steady decline in functional capacity of middle-aged or elderly people, who rely solely on biomedicine.

One of the most brutal tendencies of the biomedical paradigm (27) is that it often creates resignation and thus allows disease to control the individual. Symptoms can often be alleviated to some extent, but the causes of the disease are beyond the reach of acknowledgement due to the inherent philosophy of the bio-medical paradigm: the overwhelming complexity of the biochemical description of man. Therefore, biomedicine is rarely able to help people get rid of the cause of their disease, which in our understanding often is to be found in the quality of the life the patients lead, and not in their genes or metabolism. The diseases plaguing our patients are often caused by life-style.

In our opinion, modern biochemistry is generally incapable of helping people to draw on their hidden resources. Thus, the human resources that should help us overcome the disease remain hidden. That is our harshest criticism of biomedicine as holistically oriented physicians. On the pretext of being able to help, it takes responsibility for and away from patients and thereby deprives them of the opportunity to wake up and help themselves – and patients let the physician do so. The consciousness-based medicine that we are striving to develop serves the opposite purpose, namely to help people help themselves. Many people have good experiences with biomedical treatment, since we all have an infection or ailment at some time, which was cured. With all its technological perfection and scientific character, biomedicine appears extremely convincing and makes us confident that it will provide a cure the next time something goes wrong. Unfortunately, the bitter truth is that once you get seriously ill, you usually remain ill for the rest of your life. Biomedicine cannot make you well again or cure the chronic illness.

Below, we provide some examples of quite common disease and disorders for which biomedicine, in our experience as physicians, has proven inadequate. A colleague with more experience and greater insight in biomedicine might possibly be able to do a better job, so we will let readers draw their own conclusions on the numerous short and somewhat sad case histories.

# Chronic disorders

The following case reports describe chronic disorders and complaints for which biomedicine has no effective remedy or cure, as is so often the case.

> *Female, aged 21 years with chronic dizziness.*
> The patient suffers from chronic dizziness. Blood chemistry normal, except CRP (C-reactive protein), which is marginally outside the normal range. Against this background we discuss whether the patient may have another illness that would explain the dizziness, e.g. a virus affecting the acoustic nerve. The patient is told to return, if the symptoms do not go away by themselves.

Dizziness is more frequently encountered in older persons with increasing age. Most cases are benign and self-limited, but still a risk factor for falls in the older patient. Dizziness with no apparent organic cause is common and from a biomedical perspective very little can be done about it. "A virus affecting the acoustic nerve," says the biomedical doctor, which is the explanation given to the patient to excuse, why we cannot help, because there is not much we can do about a virus. Indeed, the dizziness will very often cease within six months.

However, this story might look different in a holistic perspective. Frequently, the dizziness either passes quickly, or it continues for the rest of the patient's life. In either case it is unlikely to be caused by a virus. We believe that this kind of dizziness is generally caused by a loss of vital energy due to inner conflicts and lack of confrontation with both the internal and external reality. When the patient does not have enough energy to obtain an overview of life, this kind of dizziness occurs, like motion sickness. It simply becomes difficult to orientate oneself in the world, tying down the vital energy, but when this conflict is solved, the dizziness will miraculously vanish.

> *Male, aged 25 years with chronic sore throat.*
> No fever, sore throat for four weeks. Also pricking sensation in the tongue. Oral cavity: slightly red and swollen, no coating. Glands in the sternoclavicular region swollen bilaterally. Strep A: negative. To be reassessed in two weeks. Pricking sensation in the tongue possibly due to allergy. Prescribe Zyrtec [cetirzine] for the patient to try.

There is no effective treatment against a chronic burning and pricking sensation in the tongue and throat, when there is no external cause. In our opinion, irritation of the tissue – a burning, hot and pricking sensation – is a clear sign of a blockage or hidden feelings. Symptoms can be alleviated by antihistamines, and the effect may last for a few hours, but in the long term this is not a lasting solution. The patients suffer their entire lives. Sometimes they "grow" out of it, sometimes their illness takes on a more serious nature.

> *Female, aged 42 years with tinnitus.*
> Noise in the ear, so that the patient finds it difficult to talk to other people. /Tinnitus/ Prescribe audiometry prior to assessment of the need for hearing aid with masking device. Note: Tinnitus may decrease if the patient's possible depression improves, the picture of this suspected depression is unfortunately not so clear that is justifies a treatment. Hearing test shows nearly complete loss of hearing at high frequencies (over 2000Hz). Referred to audiologist for hearing aid with masking device.

Tinnitus is a term to describe an internal noise perceived by the person. The cause can be otologic, metabolic, neurologic, pharmacologic, dental or psychological, but also due to vascular abnormalities, tympanic muscle disorders or central nervous system anomalies. A complete otolaryngeal evaluation and audiometry should be performed in order to find the potential cause. Tinnitus is a very difficult problem to treat, with a prevalence of 14.2% in Gothenburg (28), thought to be representative for the Nordic countries.

## Overweight

Childhood, adolescent and adult obesity presents one of the most challenging and frustrating problems in medical practice. Obesity is of particular concern because of the health risks associated with it. These risks include hypertension, hyperlipidaemia, hypertriglyceridemia, diabetes mellitus, coronary heart disease, pulmonary and renal problems, surgical risks, and degenerative joint disease. Obesity causes significant morbidity as well as a decreased life-expectancy. Obesity is a major public health problem. Recent data from the Third National Health and Nutrition Examination Survey (NHANES) in the United States suggested that 22% of children and adolescents are overweight, and 11% are obese. Among the general population, the survey revealed that between 1987 and 1993 overweight prevalence increased 3.3% for men and 3.6% for women. Total overweight prevalence among American males is now 33% and for females 36% (29).

*Female, aged 30 years with severe overweight.*

The patient weighs 99 kg, BMI 44.5 = severe overweight (obese class III). Headache and tingling sensation in left hand. Also many episodes of reflux. Gastroscopy should be considered if the problem persists. Patient must return for weight-loss plan.

This patient needs a life. Slight tingling sensation in her hand. Our guess is that she has more important issues to worry about. Why focus on the hand, when her entire body needs to be reviewed? And why look only at the body when her entire life has gone off track? This might seem a hard judgment, but in our opinion, a weight-loss plan or a reduction in calorie intake for that matter would be of little help to her, as she no doubt already has tried all dietary cures on the market to lose weight. To conquer her overweight she has to address the fundamental problems, of which her overweight is a result.

The real weakness of biomedicine is that it does not support the patient in taking responsibility for his or her own life; this weakness is not only a fault of biomedicine as it is shared by the majority of alternative treatments. It is often the case that the person (physician or alternative healer) giving treatment does something with the patient on the basis of the own knowledge of the physician or healer. Physicians are often highly skilled, and it is tempting to take control and know what is right. However, that is generally not the best possible help for the patient. The best result will not be achieved, until the patient plays an active part, uncovers his or her basic needs and finds out how to fulfil them.

## When pain persists

Acute pain is a normal sensation triggered in the nervous system to alert you to possible injury and the need to take care of yourself, but chronic pain is different. Chronic pain persists. Pain signals keep firing in the nervous system for weeks, months, even years. There may have been an initial mishap -- sprained back, serious infection, or there may be an on-going cause of pain -- arthritis, cancer, ear infection, but some people suffer chronic pain in the absence of any past injury or evidence of body damage. Many chronic pain conditions affect older adults. Common chronic pain complaints include headache, low back pain, cancer pain, arthritis pain, neurogenic pain (pain resulting from damage to the peripheral nerves or to the central nervous system itself), psychogenic pain (pain not due to past disease or injury or any visible sign of damage inside or outside the nervous system). One Dane in five lives a life of chronic pain in spite of the most effective biomedical treatment (3). The pain persists, despite analgesics, despite physiotherapy and massage, or despite antidepressants. The patient is in pain, regularly or more or less constantly, and life is not fun anymore.

Pain is what causes almost 30% of the patients to see their family physician (30) and often the physician does not succeed in removing the pain from the everyday life of the patient. We do not want to hand out morphine to people, who are not terminally ill – although that would be an effective pharmacological solution to both physical and existential pain. This could be one of the reasons, why we have so many drug addicts or so many young girls in existential pain, who become drug-addicted prostitutes. Let us make it clear that we do not share the restrictive attitude of our society to morphine. If it were up to us to decide, all adults would be allowed to buy it at the pharmacy. That would spare thousands of young people from humiliation, criminalization, marginalization, prostitution or HIV and society would save enormous amounts of money. The way we see it, the drug policy of our society reflects old moral codes and notions, instead of being an expression of real insight into human suffering.

*Male, aged 65 years with chronic pain, reduced vitality, libido and urge for isolation.*

Patient has had failing health with many complaints of pain over the last four years. He has gone through several assessments with X-rays of knees and hips, with only minimum findings. In recent years, he has had decreased vitality and libido, now urge for isolation – mostly stays at home and indoors. Born in Asia. Has lived in Denmark for 30 years, but with a four-year stay abroad in between. Denies any problems regarding language and culture. Examination: Knees almost normal findings, in particular no restricted movement, no looseness, no signs of arthritis, no patella effusion or other pathology. The patient reports slight tenderness on side of right knee. Hip also normal regarding movement. The patient complains of some pain in the extreme position [fully extended or flexed], but this is hardly relevant during normal use of the body. Below the note from the last radiological examination showing stable conditions in the patient's joints: X-ray of left hip joint compared with the right hip joint, shows, as previously, slight narrowing of the joint space on both sides, slightly more on the right than on the left. No deformation of femoral head/incipient osteoarthrosis of the hip bilaterally/.

This patient's situation is deteriorating. But what is actually the matter with him? The cultural problems appear to be insurmountable, but he denies them completely. This is a case of marginalization, perhaps even social exclusion. He is experiencing an existential desert, deep despair over no longer being useful.

We are convinced that this man's situation in life could be rescued if he acknowledges, however painfully, the actual nature of his problems. But that is a barrier only he himself can cross.

And as long as he keeps thinking: "If only there were something wrong with my hips. Then everything would come to an end, and my life would find its final and conclusive form," there is not much hope. Resignation is complete. His depression is real, but it cannot be treated in a conventional, medical sense. Life has gone off track, the patient refuses to help himself, and medication is unlikely to be of much help.

> *Female, aged 49 years with migrating aches.*
>
> Thyrotropin normal (not goitre). Swelling around the epiglottal cartilage, in my opinion not corresponding to thyroid gland. Receives physiotherapy, and we agree that the physiotherapist should also massage the neck. We discuss her fibromyalgia, rheumatism and Sjogren's syndrome, and the patient states that she has "migrating aches" that migrate from one area of the body to the next, like slight cramps. We discuss the nature of such "migrating aches". The patient is referred to a specialist.

Migrating aches are tensions that crawl about in the patient's body like worms. They are a very interesting example of tensions living a life of their own inside the body as a repository of unprocessed feelings. They are not localized in any particular site or organ, but may come and go anywhere in the body, with resulting disturbance of the organ they affect. In our opinion, fibromyalgia, rheumatism and Sjogren's syndrome are sequelae of such tension.

Biomedicine turn to a molecular analysis of the autoimmune disturbance and, at best, it regards the migrating aches as a rarity, while consciousness-based medicine considers the content of the migrating aches and takes them very seriously. If the patient's subjective complaints can be alleviated, there is a very good chance that the physical disturbances will also pass. Biomedicine rarely succeeds in proper healing of autoimmune diseases like diabetes type I or arthritis; it remains a semi-effective symptomatic treatment.

## Cancer kills one in three

It is believed that one Dane in three dies from cancer and biomedicine has thus no effective cure for cancer. Since we can live to become 100 years old, many of us will die from cancer around halfway through the life intended by nature.

> *Male, aged 66 years with prostatism.*
>
> Micturition slowly returning to normal, prostate surgery twice and surgery for urethral stricture twice. No pain. Examination: No tenderness corresponding to the bladder. Negative urine stick. Referral to hospital for assessment and treatment.

Prostate cancer, which is what this patient presumably has, is merciful; it grows very slowly and rarely spreads.

# Heart conditions

It is believed that one Dane in two dies from a cardiovascular disease, so biomedicine has obviously no effective cure against most heart conditions. The general practitioner will see the patient in the community, refer to the hospital, where they are diligently medicated and operated on. Survival statistics on these patients are not impressive. The average event free survival time is short, often said to be less than 10 years after bypass surgery, where three veins are grafted around the blocked coronary arteries; in the case of three-vessel coronary disease with varying severities of angina and left ventricular dysfunction, adjusted event-free survival (death, myocardial infarction, definite angina, or reoperation) after 6 years were only 23% (one vessel bypassed), 23% (two vessels bypassed), 29% (three vessels bypassed), and 31% (more than three vessels bypassed) (31).

> *Male, aged 52 years with balloon angioplasty and anxiety.*
>
> The patient suffers from anxiety following balloon angioplastic surgery twice [dilation of the coronary arteries with a balloon which is inflated inside the vessel]. We talk about getting rid of the anxiety by accepting it, dwelling on it, perhaps lying in his wife's arms, allowing yourself to be small and afraid – do it a 1,000 times over the next couple of years. His wife is kind and understanding and wants to support her husband. Can return for conversation.

People become afraid when they have heart problems. Years after the problems seem to have been solved, people still tremble with fear. Since half of us die from cardiovascular disease, this anxiety is justified.

We really are going to die. And the heart is our Achilles' heel, so to speak. It stops beating, and that is the end of it. Biomedicine has not solved the problem of weak hearts, although enormous progress has been made with for example enzymes that dissolve acute blood clots.

Dean Ornish and co-workers (32) have demonstrated that cardiac disease is very sensitive to improved quality of life. His work focused on making the patient "open up the heart physically, emotionally and spiritually". This is a marvellous project and a very successful one. Only, his colleagues do not really appreciate his work. For how can spiritual openings of the heart do away with coronary stenosis?

# Psychiatric disorders

Statistically, the incidence of severe mental diseases in the Nordic countries is about 13% [numbers from Norway] (33) and about one in five will at some point in life receive psychiatric treatment with psychotropic drugs.

Generally, people who become mentally ill do not recover completely, but people who have a reasonable life at the onset of their illness will often achieve sufficient symptom relief to resume their old lives after treatment.

The situation is different for people who become mentally ill before they have settled down, i.e. when they are young. A mentally ill and unstable person will find it difficult to attain a life. The many recovery studies indicate that only one in five patients diagnosed with schizophrenia attains a normalized existence; the rest of these patients have so many psychotic symptoms throughout their lives that a psychiatrist will still call them schizophrenic. Biomedicine removes some of their symptoms, but not the actual illness, as we have seen in Section one.

Institutionalization in psychiatric wards teaches them that they need not take responsibility for their survival. Our conclusion is that we need a new psychiatric approach that is better at making the patients well.

We need a psychiatric system that understands the actual cause of the psychiatric disorders and treats them on that basis. We will provide our view of such holistic theory below. For the moment, suffice it to say that when patients discover themselves and their purpose in life and learn to be true to themselves and live accordingly, it appears that they actually can become well or cope with life.

*Male, aged 60 years with depression:*

1. Patient scores HDS 20 (MIES24) on the Hamilton scale, corresponding to depression. Prescribe antidepressants. The patient has presumably been depressed for years, and has been advised not to expect any major improvement for weeks or months.
2. The patient suffers from chronic muscular pain, which may be a manifestation of the depression.

Quite frankly, the psychiatric biomedical program against depression and psychosis is not working well. Depression and psychoses may be temporarily alleviated by means of psychotropic drugs, and patients may return more or less to who they used to be, albeit perhaps a little more timid and inhibited. But surely life does not intend us to remain the way we are as people at our current stage of development, and then deteriorate physically and mentally over our adult lives? Is it not the meaning of life that we should develop, become better and more alive, and get to know ourselves better?

An episode of depression is an opportunity to take a close look at ourselves and learn lessons through questions such as: why are my shoes not comfortable to wear? What is it I feel about myself, the people around me and life in general that gives me this unsatisfactory life? Any patient who patiently and laboriously takes on the task of sorting out his own philosophy of life will, in our experience, be richly rewarded for the effort.

## Difficult medical conditions

Sometimes patients suffer from something rare and strange. The body is a highly complex structure and any disturbances may take on quite strange, special and unexpected forms of expression. The poorer the understanding of a patient's disease or condition, the more difficult it is to treat. Where should you begin and where end? Patients with rare diseases are usually referred to specialized units at the hospital, where they are transferred from one unit to another, until somebody feels competent enough to treat them. Having a rare disease may be life threatening. Patients with well-known but incurable diseases often end up in hospitals, which take care of their symptoms and give them general life support, but the normal pattern is a slow deterioration towards dead. With holistic medicine both situations may be within the physician's therapeutic reach, if only the patient is willing to work on himself.

*Male, aged 44 years with purpura.*

Patient has breathing difficulties, dizziness with headache, swelling around the eyes, sometimes feels very ill, very tired for a long period, partially far-away sensation in the head. Examination: BP 135/85. Weighs 92.5 kg – usually weighs between 55 and 59 kg. Small red patches that do not disappear on pressure! /Purpura [a dangerous rash]/ /suspected immunological disorder. New appointment when we have the results of various blood tests.

Blood test results together with the clinical purpura indicated systemic [involving the entire body] disease, which should be assessed by specialists at the hospital. Referral.

This is a very dangerous situation for him. Purpura – the image formed by thousands of micro haemorrhages in the skin – is not to be taken lightly. If he also has micro haemorrhages (small bleedings) everywhere in his internal organs, his life is at risk. The condition is difficult to treat pharmacologically, and the outcome of such 'immunological collapse' may be death in spite of the greatest expertise. We are not quite as good at adjusting imbalances of that kind, as is generally assumed.

## Stagnant existence or burnout

Stagnation is an odd phenomenon. People lose the spark of life or they have no purpose, their entire existence and all their human relations decay. In the end, they have absolutely nothing of value, and although their bodies are strong and healthy, they display numerous symptoms, reflecting repression to the body of their emotionally painful lives.

*Female, aged 37 years with typical "stagnant" picture.*

Presents with distal phalanx of the right second finger, which feels sore and "inflamed" on one side. Examination: Slight redness and tenderness corresponding to the phalanx, but unlikely to be rheumatoid arthritis or other well-defined arthropathy. Additionally: All phalanges of the digits bilaterally "rigid", cough, tenderness corresponding to the trigger points in arms and legs, severe tension in the neck, back problems – but the knee problems claimed by the patient are unlikely. The cause of the patient's complaints appears to be tension rather than inflammation. We discuss it: "I have never been able to relax", "I don't like just sitting, then I start feeling agitated," the patient says. EXERCISE in relaxation: "Sit down for 10 minutes with an egg-timer and just sit there without doing anything at all, sense how you feel. Preferably combined with massaging of the many sore muscles. Should return if the problem persists, possibly physiotherapy.

People who do not work on themselves at all or who are totally unwilling to confront their problems in life easily become stagnant. The stagnant picture includes the following aspects: "trouble" in the joints, sore muscles, dizziness and mental clouding, mixed-up human relations and a distinct lack of initiative and direction in life in general. They somehow appear "clumsy", "untidy" and poorly presented, as if they basically refuse to present themselves as people with goals in life and a meaning to their existence. The clay that should be moulded remains un-moulded. It is as if they totally lack creative and constructive spirit. Neither medication nor physiotherapy can do much about that. They need to talk about it.

*Female, aged 46 years with possible burnout.*

Constantly tired, dizzy, impaired concentration, perhaps a slight temperature, throat complaints for about 45 days. BP 130/70. Auscultation of the lungs: slight basal crackles. Throat: still slightly red, no coating. Socially: no longer happy about work. Strict boss who "forbids anything good", is not allowed to do anything, works too slowly, "the other bookkeeper is much better." /Suspected atypical pneumonia/ /suspected burnout/ Prescribe Abboticin [erythromycin]. If no marked improvement within 2 weeks, the patient should return to the clinic.

In this case, the approach was simply to prescribe the best drug that we could find for her. Then we wait to see whether the problem might disappear by itself. We hope so, but do not believe it will, although the suspected pneumonia could make the difference. It will probably take a lot more than antibiotics to get her back on her own two feet considering her complaints. We believe that she has a burnout and in need of comprehensive rehabilitation. But sometimes we are tricked. If she does, in fact, have pneumonia, she and her negative attitude might recover completely with the medicine.

## Old age

Old age is one of the strangest phenomena, because there is often a substantial difference between chronological age and physiological age. Young people may appear very old and tired – worn out and incoherent – while old people may appear extremely energetic and fit. Physiological age is determined by our personal energy level. In turn, this is determined by how much of our vital energy is free and how much of it tied to blockage and traumas. At the cellular level, the cells are forever young – they have eternal life – after all, they are 3,800,000,000 years old by now: the cells have always existed almost back to the beginning of the planet Earth, they renew themselves by division, so in principle they never become old. Therefore, it is extremely difficult to perceive age as anything but an energy problem. There is another factor, however, the life purpose (5), which may be fulfilled so that the person feels genuinely full of days. Unfortunately, hardly anybody has succeeded with that project in our time. Physiological old age is therefore to a great extent a result of accumulated inner conflicts and susceptible to holistic treatment – people may actually "become five or ten years younger" following six months of holistic therapy. By contrast, biomedical pharmaceuticals bind further vital energy by disturbing the body in all sorts of ways, so that although the symptom addressed by the treatment may become milder, the general health and well-being can in fact deteriorate. For that reason, elderly people should preferably not receive medication; nevertheless many elderly people have ten different kinds of pills in their medicine cabinet instead of three kinds at the most, which their bodies can tolerate.

*Female, aged 56 years growing old much too soon:*

1. Has slept on her side, pain corresponding to outside of left arm for last three weeks. Loss of strength assessed as being of "protection – fixation type." No sensory deficit, no affliction of feet or lower legs /to be followed up/.
2. Oedema around the ankles. Prescribe Furix [furosemide].
3. Patient requests a blood sample for gout, but there is no physical signs, so there is no immediate indication for it. "If she doesn't get it, her husband will tear the

whole clinic apart." She is informed in detail of the risk of prescribing too much medicine, if blood tests are not clinically justified and show false-positive results.
4. Productive morning cough for many months. Auscultation of the lungs: nothing abnormal discovered. No fever. May have slight bronchitis in spite of the normal examination.
5. We talk about her everyday life, which is difficult; she becomes increasingly insecure. We talk about anxiety and menopause.
6. Headache almost daily. BP 130/90.

This patient has grown old 20 years too soon. She desperately wants to be examined, since there must be a disease, which the physicians have overlooked and for which she can be treated. But no, there is no disease. A good physician knows often intuitively whether or not people are seriously ill.

To the best of our knowledge, this patient is not ill. We do not want to examine her for something, which we are certain she does not have – with the risk that the blood samples show a slight imbalance. Blood samples often shows false-positive results, some say one in twenty, but sometimes it is much more: compare i.e. the high rate of false positives in blood donor screening for antibodies to hepatitis C virus (34). So a fine rule is only to test when you suspect a specific disease. All the biomedicine in the world cannot save her. She has to save herself. Otherwise it will not happen.

*Male, aged 79 year and aged:*
1. Vision and hearing no longer good. Should have an appointment with ophthalmologist and audiometry.
2. Dandruff and dry facial skin. Should use a rich skin cream daily on the face and anti-dandruff shampoo.
3. Very dizzy. BP 160/115. Probably drinks far too little, which may also be a predisposing factor of urinary tract infection that he sometimes suffer from. The home care should make sure that he drinks at least 2 litters daily. In addition, slightly confused, possibly also slightly demented. Cannot place the hours on the face of a clock.
4. Still pain in the locomotor system. Nobligan [opioid analgesic], 50 mg capsules, as required, maximum four times daily in addition to regular medication twice daily.
5. Urinary tract infection. The urine sample today negative, excluding 2+ for blood.

Dementia affects a great many elderly people – and especially people around them. Several alternative treatments have been developed to work toward the prevention of dementia by psychosocial measures. The idea is to use empathic communication in order to make the patient feel useful again.

By contrast, biomedicine currently has no remedies for dementia. Alzheimer disease (AD) was first described by professor Alois Alzheimer, Germany, in 1906, when he reported the case of Auguste D, a 51-year old female patient, he had followed at a Frankfurt hospital since 1901 up until her death on April 8th, 1906.

Even after her death he went on to study the neuropathological features of her illness. Shortly after her death he presented her case at the 37th Conference of German Psychiatrist in Tubingen on November 4th, 1906 in which he described her symptoms: Progressive connective impairment, focal symptoms, hallucinations, delusions, psychosocial incompetence and neurobiological changes found at autopsy: plaques, neurofibrillary tangles and atherosclerotic changes.

These symptoms are still the characteristics of AD today, which is the most common cause of dementia in western countries. Clinically AD most often presents with a subtle onset of memory loss followed by a slowly progressive dementia that has a

## Discussion

The fine art of medicine is to give the patient what he or she needs to get well and healthy. For lots of reasons the drugs do not always help, and it is therefore important for modern medicine to understand, which patients will benefit and also where it will be a waste to give drugs. Many modern drugs have a NNT (Number Needed to Treat) of 2 or more (36,37), and this situation is interesting, because it means that only some of the patients will be helped. Therefore the task of the modern physician will be to know which one to treat with a drug and which patient not to treat bio-medically, but with manual medicine or consciousness-oriented holistic medicine instead.

When a drug has a NNT of 2 or more, and you have no specific reason to believe that the drug will help a specific patient, it means that the patient has a likelihood of only 50% to be helped by the drug; if the NNT is 5, the likelihood is only 20%. But any physician worth his salt wants to cure the majority of his patients. So just using a drug with an NNT of 2 is not good enough and he is forced to use another toolbox. In general, treatment with a drug of NNT higher that 2 can never stand alone, and if the NNT is 5 or higher, an alternative toolbox must desperately be sought. Interestingly consciousness-based medicine seems to be able to help most of the patients, who understand the path of personal development, if the physician masters the art of "holding" and processing, and have the love for his patients necessary to gain the trust needed for the patient to receive the holding.

Another important aspect is that the pharmaceutical industry could be much better to let us know the NNT number for various drugs, which should be placed on every package, for the physician and his patient to know. And the pharmaceutical industry could and should do much more research to determine, which groups of patients are likely to be helped by the drug (38). Most drugs work better, when a person is otherwise healthy, young, understands to cooperate with the treatment and motivated to take the drugs. It is also important that the patient believes in biomedicine, has an orderly personality to keep a high compliance, has good personal networks, employed, etc. So it is very important to include different kind of patients in a drug study and to let us know the NNT in every case. We believe that this should be regulated by law, as the companies have an obvious interest in widening the group receiving the drug, while the physician and his patients have the complete opposite interest. We need to know and find out, when to give and take the drug, and when to use alternative medical toolboxes. So understanding, where the biomedicine is likely to work and not to work is the most important issue in today's medical practice. Administering drugs with high NNT numbers blindly to our patients is not going to help much.

# Conclusion

The bio-medical paradigm is dominating our medical education in most western countries. The modern physician is using pharmaceuticals as his prime tool. Unfortunately this tool is much less efficient than you might expect from the biochemical theory. The naïve believe in drugs as the solution to health problems of mankind, overlooking important existing knowledge on quality of life, personal development and holistic healing, seems to be the main reason, why around every second citizen of our modern societies are chronically ill.

The bio-medical paradigm and the drugs are certainly useful and in many situations we could not do without the drugs, i.e. the antibiotics curing syphilis and pneumonia. But curing infections in young age is not without consequences as the way we perceive health and medicine is influenced by such experiences. When we get a more severe disease in midlife we also often believe that a drug exists that can make us healthy again. But now the drugs does not work anymore, because we have turned older and have lost much of the surplus and personal energy that made us heal easily, when we were younger. Now we need to assume responsibility, take learning, and improve our quality of life. We need a more holistic medicine that can help us back to life by allowing us to access our hidden resources.

Whenever NNT is 3 or higher, the likelihood to cure the patient is less that 33%, which is not satisfying to any physician. In this case he must for ethical reasons try something more, to cure his patients; this is where the tools of both traditional manual medicine and the tools of a scientific holistic medicine are helpful. The modern physician cannot rely solely on drugs; he must also have holistic tools in his medical toolbox. With every patient he must ask himself what he truly believes will help this patient, and this is the line of treatment he must follow. This is the only way we as physicians can improve the general health of our populations. Drugs alone will not do the job.

# References


[1] Ventegodt S. [Quality of life in Denmark. Results from a population survey.] Copenhagen: Forskningscentrets Forlag, 1995. [Danish]

[2] Danish Parliament. Rapport from the Technology Council on alternative treatment in Denmark. Christiansburg, Copenhagen: Danish Parliament, 2002. [Danish]

[3] Ventegodt S, Andersen NJ, Merrick J. Editorial: Five theories of human existence. ScientificWorldJournal 2003;3:1272-6.

[4] Ventegodt S. The life mission theory: A theory for a consciousness-based medicine. Int J Adolesc Med Health 2003;15(1):89-91.

[5] Ventegodt S, Andersen NJ, Merrick J. The life mission theory II: The structure of the life purpose and the ego. ScientificWorldJournal 2003;3:1277-85.

[6] Ventegodt S, Andersen NJ, Merrick J. The life mission theory III: Theory of talent. ScientificWorldJournal 2003;3:1286-93.

[7] Ventegodt S, Merrick J. The life mission theory IV. A theory of child development. ScientificWorldJournal 2003;3:1294-1301.

[8] Ventegodt S, Andersen NJ, Merrick J. The life mission theory V. A theory of the anti-self and explaining the evil side of man. ScientificWorldJournal 2003;3:1302-13.

[9] Ventegodt S, Andersen NJ, Merrick J. Holistic medicine: Scientific challenges. ScientificWorldJournal 2003;3:1108-16.

[10] Ventegodt S, Andersen NJ, Merrick J. Holistic Medicine II: The square-curve paradigm for research in alternative, complementary and holistic medicine: A cost-effective, easy and scientifically valid design for evidence based medicine. ScientificWorldJournal 2003;3:1117-27.
[11] Ventegodt S, Andersen NJ, Merrick J. Holistic Medicine III: The holistic process theory of healing. ScientificWorldJournal 2003;3: 1138-46.
[12] Ventegodt S, Andersen NJ, Merrick J. Holistic Medicine IV: The principles of the holistic process of healing in a group setting. ScientificWorldJournal 2003;3:1294-1301.
[13] Ventegodt S, Andersen NJ, Merrick J. Quality of life theory I. The IQOL theory:An integrative theory of the global quality of life concept. ScientificWorldJournal 2003;3:1030-40.
[14] Ventegodt S, Merrick J, Andersen NJ. Quality of life theory II. Quality of life as the realization of life potential: A biological theory of human being. ScientificWorldJournal 2003;3:1041-9.
[15] Ventegodt S, Merrick J, Andersen NJ. Quality of life theory III. Maslow revisited. ScientificWorldJournal 2003;3:1050-7.
[16] Ventegodt S, Andersen NJ, Merrick J. Quality of life philosophy: when life sparkles or can we make wisdom a science? ScientificWorldJournal 2003;3:1160-3.
[17] Ventegodt S, Andersen NJ, Merrick J. QOL philosophy I: Quality of life, happiness, and meaning of life. ScientificWorldJournal 2003;3: 1164-75.
[18] Ventegodt S, Andersen NJ, Kromann M, Merrick J. QOL philosophy II: What is a human being? ScientificWorldJournal 2003;3:1176-85.
[19] Ventegodt S, Merrick J, Andersen NJ. QOL philosophy III: Towards a new biology. ScientificWorldJournal 2003;3:1186-98.
[20] Ventegodt S, Andersen NJ, Merrick J. QOL philosophy IV: The brain and consciousness. ScientificWorldJournal 2003;3:1199-1209.
[21] Ventegodt S, Andersen NJ, Merrick J. QOL philosophy V: Seizing the meaning of life and getting well again. ScientificWorldJournal 2003;3:1210-29.
[22] Ventegodt S, Andersen NJ, Merrick J. QOL philosophy VI: The concepts. ScientificWorldJournal 2003;3:1230-40.
[23] Merrick J, Ventegodt S. What is a good death? To use death as a mirror and find the quality in life. BMJ Rapid Response 2003 Oct 31.
[24] Ventegodt S, Merrick J, Andersen NJ. Quality of life as medicine. A pilot study of patients with chronic illness and pain. ScientificWorld Journal 2003;3:520-32.
[25] Ventegodt S, Merrick J, Andersen NJ. Quality of life as medicine II. A pilot study of a five day "Quality of Life and Health" cure for patients with alcoholism. ScientificWorld Journal 2003;3:842-52.
[26] Ventegodt S, Morad M, Hyam E, Merrick J. Clinical holistic medicine: Use and limitations of the biomedical paradigm. ScientificWorldJournal 2004;4:295-306.
[27] Ventegodt S, Clausen B, Langhorn M, Kromann M, Andersen NJ, Merrick J. Quality of life as medicine III. A qualitative analysis of the effect of a five days intervention with existential holistic group therapy: a quality of life course as a modern rite of passage. ScientificWorld Journal 2004;4:124-33.
[28] Axelsson A, Ringdahl A. Tinnitus--a study of its prevalence and characteristics. Br J Audiol 1989;23(1):53-62.
[29] Bjorntorp P, ed. International textbook of obesity. Chichester: John Wiley, 2001.
[30] Hasselstrom J, Liu-Palmgren J, Rasjo-Wraak G. Prevalence of pain in general practice. Eur J Pain 2002;6(5):375-85.
[31] Bell MR, Gersh BJ, Schaff HV, Holmes DR Jr, Fisher LD, Alderman EL, et al. Effect of completeness of revascularization on long-term outcome of patients with three-vessel disease undergoing coronary artery bypass surgery. A report from the Coronary Artery Surgery Study (CASS) Registry. Circulation 1992;86(2):446-57.
[32] Ornish D, Brown SE, Scherwitz LW, Billings JH, Armstrong WT, Ports TA, et al. Can lifestyle changes reverse coronary heart disease? Lancet 1990;336(8708):129-33.
[33] Sandanger I, Nygard JF, Ingebrigtsen G, Sorensen T, Dalgard OS. Prevalence, incidence and age at onset of psychiatric disorders in Norway. Soc Psychiatry Psychiatr Epidemiol 1999;34(11):570-9.

[34] Prohaska W, Wolff C, Lechler E, Kleesiek K. High rate of false positives in blood donor screening for antibodies to hepatitis C virus. Cause of underestimation of virus transmission rate? Klin Wochenschr 1991;69(7):294-6. [German]
[35] Merrick J, Kandel I, Morad M. Health needs of adults with intellectual disability relevant for the family physician. ScientificWorldJournal 2003;3:937-45.
[36] Smith R. The drugs don't work. BMJ 2003;327(7428):0-h.
[37] Dyer O. City reacts negatively as GlaxoSmithKline announces for a new drugs. BMJ 2003;327:1366.
[38] Gøtzsches P. Bias in double-blind trials. Dan Med Bull 1990;37:329-36.

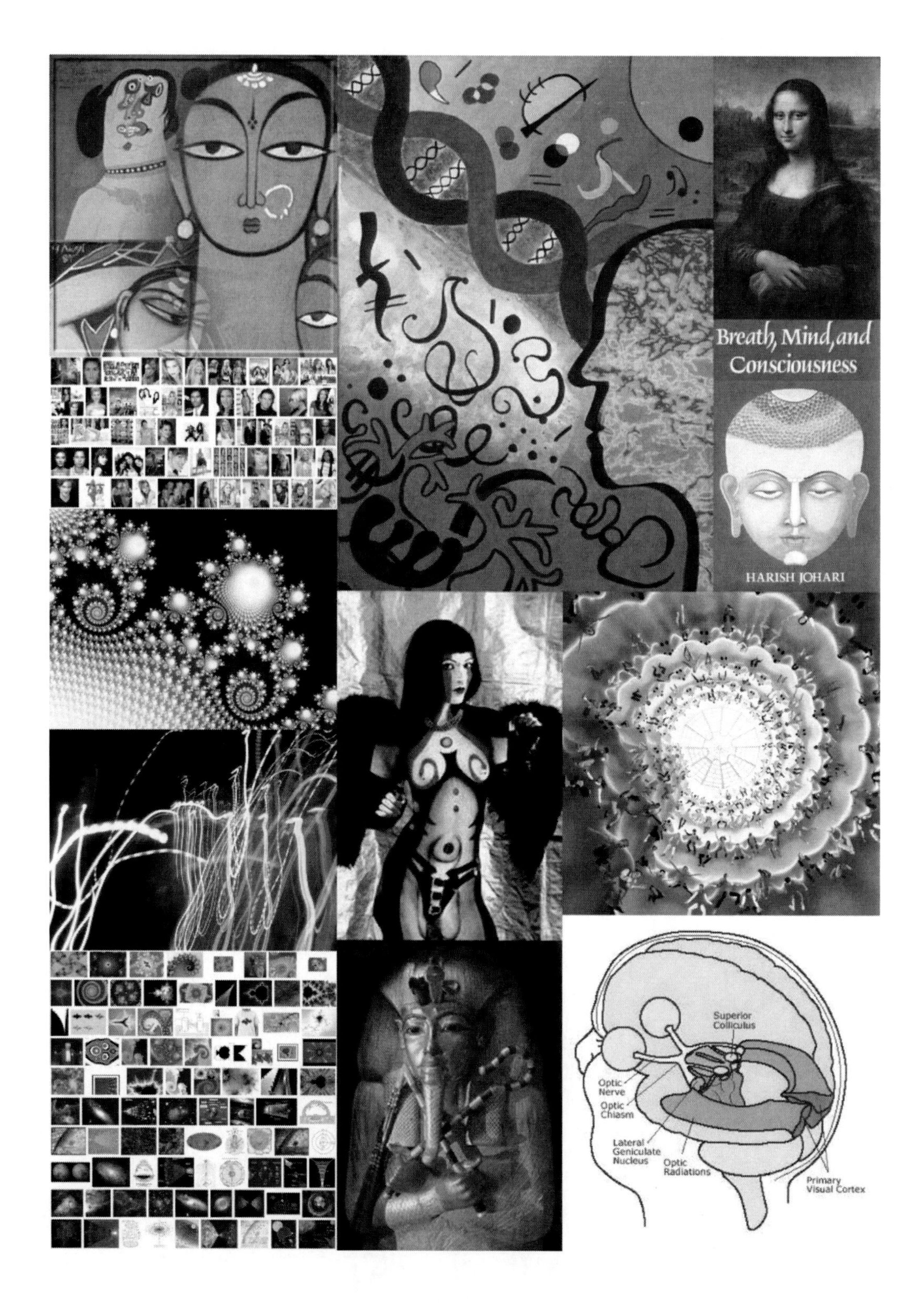
Breath, Mind, and Consciousness
HARISH JOHARI
Superior Colliculus
Optic Nerve
Optic Chiasm
Lateral Geniculate Nucleus
Optic Radiations
Primary Visual Cortex

*Chapter XX*

# Holistic healing in religion, medicine and psychology

The abstract aim of the human endeavours in the field of religion, medicine and psychology is basically the same: healing of human existence. Most interestingly, the process of holistic healing seems to be the same in all cultures, at all times and in all human endeavours. We try in this chapter to document the common nature of holistic healing and to describe how healing is related to personal development, especially development of the human consciousness enabling it to embrace and comprehend both the depth of self and the depth of the surrounding world. This development is necessary for the mentally ill patient to heal and recover.

We argue that only by deepening the worldview, i.e. making our personal cosmology more complex, will we be able to reach the threshold for holistic healing. When we heal, not only our spirit and heart are healed, but also our body and mind, explaining why holistic healing has been such an important concept in all the religious and medical system of the world's premodern cultures.

Holistic healing thus seems to be the core concept of the Hippocratic Greek medicine, the origin of modern medicine. We compare this to modern holistic healing in the holistic medical clinic that uses the concept of applied salutogenesis to induce healing not only of existential and sexual disorders, but also of serious illness, such as cancer and schizophrenia.

We argue that only if the patient is willing to abandon his simplistic worldview, he can have the fruit of holistic, existential healing and salutogenesis. In this chapter the religious experience is defined as the personal meeting with the totality of the universe; this can be a meeting with the universe as a person, i.e. God, or it can be the meeting with the fundamental source, the emptiness, sunya(ta) that creates the world, or it can be a unification with the universal energy lowing though everybody and everything. The universal quality of holistic healing is the development of sense of coherence (salutogenesis).

# Introduction

Holistic healing is about the human healing his totality, i.e. healing of existence, or healing on an existential level (1,2). In all religions the purpose is the direct experience of the universe in its totality; in some religions like Judaism, Christianity, and Islam, the universe appears, according to the famous Jewish philosopher Martin Buber (1878-1965) (3) to be a person, a You, a God; in other religions like Hinduism, Buddhism, Islamic, Jewish and Christian mystic, and the native American, African and Australian cultures, the universe appears as the void, sunya(ta), the great emptiness, the common, creative source of everything, the universal energy penetrating everything. Independent of the universe being a person or not, the goal of the religion is to help the person back to the experience of being a part of the universe, a person welcome in the world, a person in the deepest harmony with the universe.

Most interestingly this striving for sense of coherence in religion seems to be identical with the striving for existential healing in the many different medical systems of the world's premodern cultures: The ancient Greek Hippocratic character medicine (4), the medicine wheel and peyote medicine of the native Americans (5), the tradition of the about one million African Sangomas, the medical tradition of the Australian aboriginals (6), the tradition of the shaman healers of Northern Europe's (i.e. the Sames), the tradition of druids and witches using the power of nature for healing. In modern holistic sexology we find the same intend of transcending the ego, to allow the patient to get full orgasm using the tool of surrendering to love, oneness, and sense of coherence (7-16).

The striving for sense of coherence, and the merging of own consciousness with the collective conscious is also quite remarkably the goal of depth psychology as it started with Carl Gustav Jung (1875-1961) and of one of the more recent trends in psychology called "positive psychology". Several philosophers and researchers have reflected on the fact that holistic, existential healing, sense of coherence, and oneness with the world seems to be a fundamental objective of all human endeavour. This has led to the successful concepts of perennial philosophy (18) and, as mentioned above, salutogenesis (1,2).

Taken to one single, abstract concept, all human striving seems to be about love – about loving and about being loved. Thus love being the essence of our human nature, the purpose of life (19-25) and the most fundamental motivation of our soul. Freud and the school of psychodynamic psychotherapy follow the fundamental motivations of man back to sexuality. In sexuality there is also this peculiar striving for unification, for the experience of oneness and transcendence; the full orgasm has been known to transcend ego and mind and everything else (comp. the French calling orgasm "le petit mort", i.e. the small death) and modern sexologists like Reich and Osho (Bhagwan Shree Rajneesh) believed that only the full orgasm had the power to heal man in his present, highly neurotic condition (27,28).

So it seems that holistic healing, in the most abstract sense of helping man back to being a perfect and happy, healthy, meaningful, coherent part of the universe, is the basic goal of religion, medicine and psychology. If we look at religion, medicine and psychology most of the practices have through history been holistic practices and the intent seem to always be the same: healing of human existence, holistic healing or in other words salutogenesis.

# The nature of holistic healing

The different cultures are primarily characterized by their world-view (29). To understand the structure and nature of the world-view one must go to cosmology. Most interestingly, the depth of its cosmology determines the complexity of the culture including its religion, medicine and psychology. The more complex the cosmology, the more spiritually conscious, deeper reflected philosophically, and mystical is the culture. The cosmology thus seems to determine the quality of the culture and its religion and science. The complexity of the cosmology can be analyzed in a simple way using the concept of rays; the more rays or constitutional aspects a cosmology has, the more complex is it (25,26,28). Interestingly the number of rays determines, if a culture is very spiritual or very materialistic; in a cosmology with only one ray everything is the same, and often this is taken to be matter.

Modern biomedicine is thus based on the basic idea that the world is only chemistry and atoms, i.e. matter, allowing for a most practical and operational experience of the world, inviting the use of drugs and surgery for treatment. Jewish mysticism (the Kabbalah and Tarot build on this) is a cosmology seemingly with about 10 rays, or fundamental aspects of existence, allowing for a deep mystical experience of the world, deep existential reflection and healing, and even the personal meeting with God. Most psychological systems are in between, based on dualism with mind and matter allowing for some psychological and existential depth in the analyses without going all the way to mysticism.

Using the concept of poly-ray cosmology as a fundamental frame for interpretation, it seems that the condition for holistic healing is high cosmological complexity. In Hippocratic medicine the ray-number were four corresponding to the four elements (4); in Chinese medicine the ray number was five corresponding to five Chinese elements; in Hinduism the ray number was often seven, and in native American cosmology (the medicine wheel) the ray number was often eight (the eight directions of the wheel) (28). Mystics like George Ivanovitch Gurdjieff (1877–1949) made highly ingenious analysis of the structure of the human soul, which is still very popular with business leaders worldwide (29). This becomes quite practical in the end, allowing us to conclude that to meet God and heal existentially you need to develop your consciousness into a more complex understanding of self and the world. The concept of personal development (30-37) has been crystallized out of this cultural striving for a deeper understanding.

Tools for personal development can be found in religion (prayer, meditation), medicine (healing, development of character, consciousness and self-insight into the purpose of life and talents) and psychology (psychotherapy, exercises).

# Discussion

Holistic healing, which is needed for the mentally ill patients to recover, thus basically is about the person developing a consciousness of sufficient depth and complexity to truly grasp both the world and the self, and in this understanding integrating the two into one, or creating the bridge from existence to the world.

The religious experience is often that you become one with everything, that God is within you and outside you; that you are just one string of energy arising out of the subtle, divine energies of the universe, materializing a being that again a just a dancing particle in the divine unity of everything. It has been described many times in medicine and psychology that patients even with metastatic cancer and other mortal diseases have become completely happy (38) and even spontaneously well again (39). Of course we all know stories of religious miracles, a little harder to believe for the sceptically, scientifically oriented mind. But basically, the message is the same: When you become once again one with the universe, improve your quality of life, and experience the magical sense of coherence, you will heal, not only your spirit, but also you mind and your body (40,41). The healing of the heart have often been an issue, as has sexual healing, reviving the person from the most fundamental and basic level of existence.

We have analyzed the nature of holistic healing from an existence-philosophical perspective, and found that we are born with a purpose of life, a gift of love to the world, and early in life we are forced to abandon this gift, and thus abandon the most valuable and divine aspect of our human nature. Holistic healing is basically about allowing ourselves to rediscover this hidden gem and become a unique and valuable person, not only to ourselves, but also to the surrounding world.

We have used this theory of a personal life-mission (18-25) to help patients heal, when biomedicine could not help them and have found that holistic medicine in this way could heal every second patient with physical illnesses and chronic pains, mental illnesses, existential and sexual problems (9,15,42-46). We have also found the effect of holistic healing to be lasting (47).

In practice, clinical holistic medicine has used the tools of conversational therapy, bodywork, and philosophical exercises to obtain the holistic healing and during the past 10 years cures have been developed for a number of illnesses and diseases (48-69). Very often the patients have had religious experiences and deep, spontaneous insights in self in relation to healing (7,70-72). Several patients even with mental illness, even schizophrenia and severe physical illness like cancer can seemingly be healed or helped this way (73-79).

# Conclusion

So holistic healing, as we know it from religion, medicine and (depth) psychology, might have substantial values to offer modern man. A solution for many physical, mental, existential and sexual problems of modern man comes from the holistic healing that happens, when we develop our consciousness from being one-rayed – having a simple, materialistic worldview - into a much more complex, loving and appreciative understanding of both our inner and our outer world.

The abstract aim of the human endeavours in the field of religion, medicine and psychology is basically the same: healing of human existence. Most interestingly, the process of holistic healing seems to be the same in all cultures and we have tried in this chapter to document the common nature of holistic healing and to describe how healing is related to personal development, especially development of the human consciousness making it able to embrace and comprehend both the depth of self and the depth of the surrounding world. We argue that only by deepening the worldview, i.e. making our personal cosmology more complex, will be able to reach the threshold for holistic healing. When we heal, we heal our spirit, heart, body and mind, which explain why holistic healing has been such an important concept in premodern cultures. Holistic healing thus seems to be the core concept of the Hippocratic Greek medicine, the origin of modern medicine.

We compared this to modern holistic healing in the holistic medical clinic using the concept of applied salutogenesis to induce healing not only of existential and sexual disorders, but also of serious illness like cancer and schizophrenia. We argue that only if the patient is willing to abandon his simplistic worldview, he can have the fruit of holistic, existential healing and salutogenesis. In this chapter the religious experience is defined as the personal meeting with the totality of the universe; this can be a meeting with the universe as a person, i.e. God, or it can be the meeting with the fundamental source, the emptiness, sunya(ta) that creates the world, or it can be a unification with the universal energy lowing though everybody and everything. The universal quality of holistic healing is the development of sense of coherence (salutogenesis) (80-82). Only by looking for what is common in man's fundamental endeavours of religion, medicine and psychology, can we find the abstract core of the meaning of life, and only by finding this meaning can we live a happy, healthy, able life, which we were meant to live. Development and perfection of experience seems to be the fundamental intent of the universe. Only when we surrender and start experiencing this directly can we understand existence and truly be.

# References


[1] Antonovsky A. Health, stress and coping. London: Jossey-Bass,1985.

[2] Antonovsky A. Unravelling the mystery of health. How people manage stress and stay well. San Franscisco: Jossey-Bass, 1987.

[3] Buber M. I and thou. New York: Charles Scribner, 1970.

[4] Jones WHS. Hippocrates. Vol. I–IV. London: William Heinemann, 1923-1931.

[5] Anderson EF. Peyote. The divine cactus. Tucson, AZ: Univ Arizona Press, 1996.

[6] Morgan M. Mutant message from forever: A novel of Aboriginal wisdom. London: Harper Collins, 1990.

[7] Ventegodt S, Clausen B, Merrick J.Clinical holistic medicine: the case story of Anna. III. Rehabilitation of philosophy of life during holistic existential therapy for childhood sexual abuse. ScientificWorldJournal 2006;6:2080-91.

[8] Ventegodt S, Kandel I, Merrick J.Clinical holistic medicine: how to recover memory without "implanting" memories in your patient. ScientificWorldJournal 2007;7:1579-89.

[9] Ventegodt S, Thegler S, Andreasen T, Struve F, Enevoldsen L, Bassaine L, et al.Clinical holistic medicine (mindful, short-term psychodynamic psychotherapy complemented with bodywork) in the treatment of experienced impaired sexual functioning. ScientificWorldJournal 2007;7:324-9.

[10] Ventegodt S, Kandel I, Neikrug S, Merric J. Clinical holistic medicine: holistic treatment of rape and incest trauma. ScientificWorldJournal 2005;5:288-97.

[11] Ventegodt S, Morad M, Hyam E, Merrick J. Clinical holistic medicine: holistic sexology and treatment of vulvodynia through existential therapy and acceptance through touch. ScientificWorldJournal 2004;4:571-80.

[12] Ventegodt S, Morad M, Kandel I, Merrick J. Clinical holistic medicine: problems in sex and living together. ScientificWorldJournal 2004;4:562-70.

[13] Ventegodt S, Morad M, Merrick J. Clinical holistic medicine: holistic pelvic examination and holistic treatment of infertility. ScientificWorldJournal 2004;4:148-58.

[14] Ventegodt S, Clausen B, Omar HA, Merrick J. Clinical holistic medicine: holistic sexology and acupressure through the vagina (Hippocratic pelvic massage). ScientificWorldJournal 2006;6:2066-79.

[15] Ventegodt S, Clausen B, Merrick J. Clinical holistic medicine: pilot study on the effect of vaginal acupressure (Hippocratic pelvic massage). ScientificWorldJournal 2006;6:2100-16.
[16] Ventegodt S, Struck P. Five tools for manual sexological examination: Efficient treatment of genital and pelvic pains and sexual dysfunction without side effects. J Altern Med Res 2009;1(3):247-56.
[17] Huxley A. The perennial philosophy. New York: Harper Collins, 1972.
[18] Ventegodt S, Andersen NJ, Merrick J. Editorial: Five theories of human existence. ScientificWorldJournal 2003;3:1272-6.
[19] Ventegodt S. The life mission theory: A theory for a consciousness-based medicine. Int J Adolesc Med Health 2003;15(1):89-91.
[20] Ventegodt S, Andersen NJ, Merrick J. The life mission theory II. The structure of the life purpose and the ego. ScientificWorldJournal 2003;3:1277-85.
[21] Ventegodt S, Andersen NJ, Merrick J. The life mission theory III. Theory of talent. ScientificWorldJournal 2003;3:1286-93.
[22] Ventegodt S, Andersen NJ, Merrick J. The life mission theory IV. Theory on child development. ScientificWorldJournal 2003;3:1294-1301.
[23] Ventegodt S, Andersen NJ, Merrick J. The life mission theory V. Theory of the anti-self (the shadow) or the evil side of man. ScientificWorldJournal 2003;3:1302-13.
[24] Ventegodt S, Kromann M, Andersen NJ, Merrick J. The life mission theory VI. A theory for the human character: Healing with holistic medicine through recovery of character and purpose of life. ScientificWorldJournal 2004;4:859-80.
[25] Ventegodt S, Flensborg-Madsen T, Andersen NJ, Merrick J. The life mission theory VII. Theory of existential (Antonovsky) coherence: A theory of quality of life, health and ability for use in holistic medicine. ScientificWorldJournal 2005;5:377-89.
[26] Reich W. [Die Function des Orgasmus]. Köln: Kiepenheuer Witsch, 1969. [German]
[27] Osho B. Tao. The pathless path. New York: Renaissance Books, 2002.
[28] Ventegodt S, Thegler S, Andreasen T, Struve F, Jacobsen S, Torp M, Aegedius H, Enevoldsen L, Merrick J. A review and integrative analysis of ancient holistic character medicine systems. ScientificWorldJournal 2007;12;7:1821-31.
[29] Maitri S. The spiritual dimension of the enneagram. New York: Penguin Putnam, 2001.
[30] Ventegodt S, Andersen NJ, Merrick J. Quality of life philosophy: when life sparkles or can we make wisdom a science? ScientificWorldJournal 2003;3:1160-3.
[31] Ventegodt S, Andersen NJ, Merrick J. Quality of life philosophy I. Quality of life, happiness and meaning in life. ScientificWorldJournal 2003;3:1164-75.
[32] Ventegodt S, Andersen NJ, Merrick J. Quality of life philosophy II. What is a human being ? ScientificWorldJournal 2003;3:1176-85.
[33] Ventegodt S, Andersen NJ, Merrick J. Quality of life philosophy III. Towards a new biology: Understanding the biological connection between quality of life, disease and healing. ScientificWorldJournal 2003;3:1186-98.
[34] Ventegodt S, Andersen NJ, Merrick J. Quality of life philosophy IV. The brain and consciousness. ScientificWorldJournal 2003;3:1199-1209.
[35] Ventegodt S, Andersen NJ, Merrick J. Quality of life philosophy V. Seizing the meaning of life and becoming well again. ScientificWorldJournal 2003;3:1210-29.
[36] Ventegodt S, Andersen NJ, Merrick J. Quality of life philosophy VI. The concepts. ScientificWorldJournal 2003;3:1230-40.
[37] Ventegodt S, Merrick J. Philosophy of science: How to identify the potential research for the day after tomorrow? ScientificWorldJournal 2004;4:483-9.
[38] Grof S. LSD psychotherapy: Exploring the frontiers of the hidden mind. Alameda, CA: Hunter House, 1980.
[39] Dige U. Cancer miracles. Copenhagen: Hovedland, 2000. (Danish)
[40] Spiegel D, Bloom JR, Kraemer HC, Gottheil E. Effect of psychosocial treatment on survival of patients with metastatic breast cancer. Lancet 1989;2(8668):888-91.
[41] Ornish D, Brown SE, Scherwitz LW, Billings JH, Armstrong WT, Ports TA, et al. Can lifestyle changes reverse coronary heart disease? The lifestyle heart trial. Lancet 1990;336(8708):129-33.

[42] Ventegodt S, Thegler S, Andreasen T, Struve F, Enevoldsen L, Bassaine L, et al. Self-reported low self-esteem. Intervention and follow-up in a clinical setting. ScientificWorldJournal 2007;7:299-305.
[43] Ventegodt S, Thegler S, Andreasen T, Struve F, Enevoldsen L, Bassaine L, et al. Clinical holistic medicine (mindful, short-term psychodynamic psychotherapy complemented with bodywork) in the treatment of experienced mental illness. ScientificWorldJournal 2007;7:306-9.
[44] Ventegodt S, Thegler S, Andreasen T, Struve F, Enevoldsen L, Bassaine L, et al. Clinical holistic medicine (mindful, short-term psychodynamic psychotherapy complemented with bodywork) in the treatment of experienced physical illness and chronic pain. ScientificWorldJournal 2007;7:310-16.
[45] Ventegodt S, Thegler S, Andreasen T, Struve F, Enevoldsen L, Bassaine L, et al. Clinical holistic medicine (mindful, short-term psychodynamic psychotherapy complemented with bodywork) improves quality of life, health and ability by induction of Antonovsky-Salutogenesis. ScientificWorldJournal 2007;7:317-23.
[46] Ventegodt S, Kandel I, Merrick J. A short history of clinical holistic medicine. ScientificWorldJournal 2007;7:1622-30.
[47] Ventegodt S, Thegler S, Andreasen T, Struve F, Enevoldsen L, Bassaine L, et al. Clinical holistic medicine: Psychodynamic short-time therapy complemented with bodywork. A clinical follow-up study of 109 patients. ScientificWorldJournal 2006;6:2220-38.
[48] Ventegodt S, Merrick J. Clinical holistic medicine: Applied consciousness-based medicine. ScientificWorldJournal 2004;4:96-9.
[49] Ventegodt S, Morad M, Merrick J. Clinical holistic medicine: Classic art of healing or the therapeutic touch. ScientificWorldJournal 2004;4:134-47.
[50] Ventegodt S, Morad M, Merrick J. Clinical holistic medicine: The "new medicine". The multiparadigmatic physician and the medical record. ScientificWorldJournal 2004;4:273-85.
[51] Ventegodt S, Morad M, Hyam E, Merrick J. Clinical holistic medicine: Use and limitations of the biomedical paradigm. ScientificWorldJournal 2004;4:295-306.
[52] Ventegodt S, Morad M, Kandel I, Merrick J. Clinical holistic medicine: Social problems disguised as illness. ScientificWorldJournal 2004;4:286-94.
[53] Ventegodt S, Morad M, Andersen NJ, Merrick J. Clinical holistic medicine: Tools for a medical science based on consciousness. ScientificWorldJournal 2004;4:347-61.
[54] Ventegodt S, Morad M, Hyam E, Merrick J. Clinical holistic medicine: When biomedicine is inadequate. ScientificWorldJournal 2004;4:333-46.
[55] Ventegodt S, Morad M, Merrick J. Clinical holistic medicine: Prevention through healthy lifestyle and quality of life. Oral Health Prev Dent 2004;2(Suppl 1):239-45.
[56] Ventegodt S, Morad M, Vardi G, Merrick J. Clinical holistic medicine: Holistic treatment of children. ScientificWorldJournal 2004;4:581-8.
[57] Ventegodt S, Morad M, Kandel I, Merrick J. Clinical holistic medicine: A psychological theory of dependency to improve quality of life. ScientificWorldJournal 2004;4:638-48.
[58] Ventegodt S, Morad, M, Kandel I, Merrick J. Clinical holistic medicine: Treatment of physical health problems without a known cause, examplified by hypertention and tinnitus. ScientificWorldJournal 2004;4:716-24.
[59] Ventegodt S, Morad M, Merrick J. Clinical holistic medicine: Developing from asthma, allergy and eczema. ScientificWorldJournal 2004;4:936-42.
[60] Ventegodt S, Merrick J. Clinical holistic medicine: Chronic infections and autoimmune diseases. ScientificWorldJournal 2005;5:155-64.
[61] Ventegodt S, Flensborg-Madsen T, Andersen NJ, Morad M, Merrick J. Clinical holistic medicine: A pilot study on HIV and quality of life and a suggested cure for HIV and AIDS. ScientificWorldJournal 2004;4:264-72.
[62] Ventegodt S, Merrick J. Clinical holistic medicine: Chronic pain in the locomotor system. ScientificWorldJournal 2005;5:165-72.
[63] Ventegodt S, Gringols M, Merrick J. Clinical holistic medicine: Whiplash, fibromyalgia and chronic fatigue. ScientificWorldJournal 2005;5:340-54.
[64] Ventegodt S, Merrick J. Clinical holistic medicine: Chronic pain in internal organs. ScientificWorldJournal 2005;5:205-10.

[65] Ventegodt S, Kandel I, Neikrug S, Merrick J. Clinical holistic medicine: The existential crisis – life crisis, stress and burnout. ScientificWorldJournal 2005;5:300-12.
[66] Ventegodt S, Gringols M, Merrick J. Clinical holistic medicine: Holistic rehabilitation. ScientificWorldJournal 2005;5:280-7.
[67] Ventegodt S, Morad M, Press J, Merrick J, Shek DTL. Clinical holistic medicine: Holistic adolescent medicine. ScientificWorldJournal 2004;4:551-61.
[68] Ventegodt S, Merrick J. Clinical holistic medicine: The patient with multiple diseases. ScientificWorldJournal 2005;5:324-39.
[69] Ventegodt S, Clausen B, Nielsen ML, Merrick J. Clinical holistic medicine: Advanced tools for holistic medicine. ScientificWorldJournal 2006;6:2048-65.
[70] Ventegodt S, Clausen B, Merrick J. Clinical holistic medicine: The case story of Anna. I. Long-term effect of childhood sexual abuse and incest with a treatment approach. ScientificWorldJournal 2006;6:1965-76.
[71] Ventegodt S, Clausen B, Merrick J. Clinical holistic medicine: The case story of Anna. II. Patient diary as a tool in treatment. ScientificWorldJournal 2006;6:2006-34.
[72] Clinical holistic medicine: factors influencing the therapeutic decision-making. From academic knowledge to emotional intelligence and spiritual "crazy" wisdom. ScientificWorldJournal 2007;7:1932-49.
[73] First do no harm: an analysis of the risk aspects and side effects of clinical holistic medicine compared with standard psychiatric biomedical treatment. ScientificWorldJournal 2007;7:1810-20.
[74] Biomedicine or holistic medicine for treating mentally ill patients? A philosophical and economical analysis. ScientificWorldJournal 2007;7:1978-86.
[75] Ventegodt S, Andersen NJ, Neikrug S, Kandel I, Merrick J. Clinical holistic medicine: Mental disorders in a holistic perspective. ScientificWorldJournal 2005;5:313-23.
[76] Ventegodt S, Andersen NJ, Neikrug S, Kandel I, Merrick J. Clinical holistic medicine: Holistic treatment of mental disorders. ScientificWorldJournal 2005;5:427-45.
[77] Clinical holistic medicine (mindful short-term psychodynamic psychotherapy complimented with bodywork) in the treatment of schizophrenia (ICD10-F20/DSM-IV Code 295) and other psychotic mental diseases. ScientificWorldJournal. 2007;7:1987-2008.
[78] Ventegodt S, Morad M, Hyam E, Merrick J. Clinical holistic medicine: Induction of spontaneous remission of cancer by recovery of the human character and the purpose of life (the life mission). ScientificWorldJournal 2004;4:362-77.
[79] Ventegodt S, Solheim E, Saunte ME, Morad M, Kandel I, Merrick J. Clinic holistic medicine: Metastatic cancer. ScientificWorldJournal 2004;4:913-35. Sense of coherence and physical health. Testing Antonovsky's theory. ScientificWorldJournal 2006;6:2212-9.
[80] Flensborg-Madsen T, Ventegodt S, Merrick J. Sense of coherence and physical health. A cross-sectional study using a new scale (SOC II). ScientificWorldJournal 2006;6:2200-11.
[81] Flensborg-Madsen T, Ventegodt S, Merrick J. Sense of coherence and physical health. The emotional sense of coherence (SOC-E) was found to be the best-known predictor of physical health. ScientificWorldJournal 2006;6:2147-57.
[82] Flensborg-Madsen T, Ventegodt S, Merrick J. Sense of coherence and health. The construction of an amendment to Antonovsky's sense of coherence scale (SOC II). ScientificWorldJournal 2006;6: 2133-9.

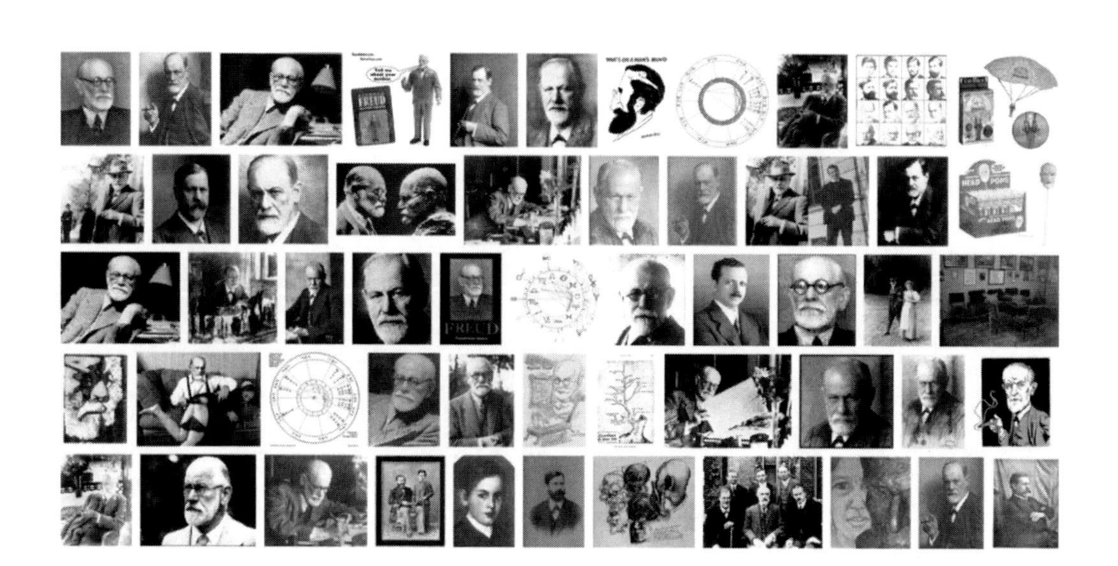
FREUD

*Chapter XXI*

# Etiology of mental diseases and the role of adult human metamorphosis in spontaneous recovery

Mentally ill patients can enter the state of adult human metamorphosis, to re-do the juvenile metamorphosis into non-human forms that was necessary for their survival in childhood. The adult human metamorphosis looks at first glance like a normal psychotic crisis of a schizophrenic patient, but when you study it closer it becomes obvious that it is actually a healing crisis, an unusual state of accelerated healing process of the type "Antonovsky-salutogenesis".

The healing crisis and the process of adult human metamorphosis seems to be the pathogenesis reversed: an inverted event of a juvenile metamorphosis, where the patient originally turned him- or herself into a non-human (often quite alien) form to survive a hostile and unfriendly environment. This often leads to severe developmental disturbances and thus to physical or mental health problems later in life.

We have observed several cases of spontaneous remission of a number of different mental diseases induced by holistic existential therapy: schizophrenia, borderline, anxiety, and bulimia. We propose that the general etiology of mental diseases is juvenile metamorphosis intended for survival, not defect genes disturbing the patient's brain chemistry. This understanding empowers us to induce salutogenesis and spontaneous recovery in also the most ill, mental patients with clinical holistic medicine.

The healing crisis could be wrongly diagnosed as a brief reactive psychosis, if the psychiatrist is without practical knowledge of the phenomenon of Antonovsky-salutogenesis; this could explain why intensive psychotherapy has been considered dangerous by some psychiatrists.

## Introduction

As we have discussed in our papers on "human development", shape and function is closely related to the organism's consciousness. Intent seems to be able to change and modify shape and function. The modifying force of intent is active though life from its very beginning, and the individual seems to be able to read what is going on in its world though the exchange of information on many levels in the individual and collective informational systems.

This opens up for radical self-modifications early in life. We suggest that the individual is actually able to transform itself into a being more fit for survival and the family it is going to soon be a part of. These transformations can be caused by dramatic events in the family, or by the environment being so rough that a normal child could not survive in it. Many dysfunctional families could qualify for this description. The most dramatic change we know of is the metamorphosis; the radical and complete transformation of an individual through an interaction between the level of intent and consciousness to the level of form and function.

We suggest that early adaptation to severely dysfunctional parents, in the womb or in early childhood, will render the individual so changed that it can present itself almost non-human; both consciousness and functions will be severely disturbed, and the person can even sometimes look not only ugly, but "alien" in bodily appearance and energy.

## Adult human metamorphosis

We have examined and treated a number of severely mentally ill patients and have observed that they often appear very unappealing physically and very alien mentally, as if they have turned themselves into some kind of "monsters" early in life. In surprisingly many cases they have adapted to extreme environments dominated by violent or sexual abuse, or severe neglect and fail. Spontaneously in the holistic existential therapy (1-6) they have entered the state of what we call adult human metamorphosis and they have spent weeks to reconnect to the human collective consciousness, as if they have lived in a system of their own non-connection to the human universe but to some strange parallel reality. It is like they are coming back from a monstrous world into the world of human beings.

Often they have felt alien; felt that they were like aliens waling the earth. So we suggest that they have metamorphosed themselves into beings with non-human intent (3,4,6-10) in some cases even using biological information from alien life forms, in fantasy or for real, if biological information can ride even the energy of the galaxies. Changing intent and the patterns of thought and perception early in life away from the typical human patterns into something else, giving the individual severe problems with relating to other people and the human world at large, is from this perspective what causes mental diseases of the schizotypical types. Presumably this also goes for the affective disorders, as the root of affective aberration likewise seem to be cognitive disturbances. So we suggest that mental diseases are caused by the individual entering metamorphosis early in life to transform into a being with non-human consciousness better able to survive an inhuman and severely dysfunctional environment. This gives some meaning to the extremely scary effects of aliens in movies: that they are here already, walking amongst us, disguised as humans. And we think they are.

All aspects of a human being except its fundamental purpose of life can be changed by human juvenile metamorphosis; the purpose of life cannot be changed, but repressed and forgotten. The person going through the process of metamorphosis seems to change functioning purpose of life and fundamental intent, and both mind and body seem to follow.

Love, consciousness and sexuality is often severely affected, and the ability to love, understand and enjoy is often damaged. The gender is often annulated or even inverted energetically; the feelings are often completely withdrawn, and mental and intellectual capacity is changed into focusing on non-living issues, very much like the loss of a "I-thou" relationship described by Martin Buber (1878-1965) (11).

# Re-metamorphosis

The metamorphosis of the human mind during the psychotic crises seems to be the most radical and drastic of the processes of healing. It happens spontaneously, when development has been radically arrested early in life, normally because of a trauma forcing the patient to let go of his or her purpose of life and substitute it with another purpose. The patients have seemingly had a psychotic episode in connection to this, often in early childhood. Often many aspects of psychosexual development has been arrested, and the people likely to go into human metamorphosis are in many ways like the butterfly's larvae, which grow and grow in size but not in any other way, until the day of metamorphosis, where the information linked to being an adult is finally accessed at once, giving a complete transformation of character, personality and consciousness.

Entering the metamorphosis is helped by intense holistic existential therapy combined with intense holding and combined with the patient's extreme intent to heal here and now and today! Healing existence must be more important than anything else, and the process of metamorphosis is taking the patient to a place of continuous healing for days. Recreation for a week or two after the introvert, psychotic crises seems mandatory, and the patient cannot work or look after kids or have other normal obligations in this period, and sometimes for an extended period of time.

Once the process of personal transformation has started it must run to its natural end. If the metamorphosis is disturbed, when the patient is in the most vulnerable state, severe harm can be done. It is very important that spouses and other family members are informed about the natural course of this kind of spontaneous healing, and they must be carefully informed about the urgent needs for tranquillity and loving care and support for days or weeks. The danger of poor living for months or years if the healing process is disrupted and the patient is sedated or drugged must be severely stressed.

An important ethical problem is if the physician or the relatives should judge what is in the best interest of the patient, when the patient enters the introvert, "psychotic" state similar to the butterfly's pupae. Often the spouse of family members not completely trusting the natures ways will react with fear and want the patient back in the old condition, while the patient him- or herself is doing everything possible to transform into a new and better version of self. Coming from fear and anger the family can cause severe damage to the patient, by interrupting the metamorphosis and arresting it at a transformational state where the patients mind is not very functional. Another dangerous aspect of this is that the person needing the transformation is often victimized early in life, and therefore of a week character allowing other people to exploit them, when they evolve into a more responsible and whole version of themselves they will often rebel against the dominance and "ownership", to become free and autonomous. It is important that the physician notice patterns of abuse in the relationship and helps the patient to understand the consequences of submitting to dominance and being owned by i.e. a spouse. If the behaviour of relatives is obviously threatening the patient's health, the physician should inform the social authorities and other relevant authorities for them to take the appropriate action.

Most interestingly human metamorphosis seems to be able to explain many religious experiences, like the 40 days in the desert where Jesus meets his creator, or Gautama Buddha's famous enlightenment, where he reaches Nirvana, the cosmic emptiness creating the world. A simple way of understanding human metamorphosis is as re-establishing the coherence with the world, getting direct access to the "web", "the nest of the world" (in prep. for publication), or the deep level of the universe we call "the matrix of energy and information"(in prep. for publication), feeding all organisms with qualities like intent and talent.

## Case stories

At many occasions during our 14 years of research in quality of life and holistic medicine at the Quality of Life Research Clinic in Copenhagen we have seen patients with the diagnoses of schizophrenia or borderline enter an extremely intense, accelerated process of healing we have called "adult human metamorphosis", because of its remarkable resemblance of a butterfly's larva entering the pupae and metamorphosing into the butterfly. The patients even sometimes look like larvae, with plump poorly demarcated body contours, immature, clumsy movement patterns, and they are characterized by having poor reality testing, as if they lived in their own world, in a parallel universe. Sometimes they have been students of remarkable intelligence, studying medicine or psychology at the university, sometimes they have been very intelligent, but not able to study, sometimes they have chosen to study nursing or occupational therapy. The patients that have come to our research clinic for holistic medicine come to our private clinic by own choice to enter our research protocol on healing the mentally ill (12,13); they normally get a grant from the Quality of Life Research Center so they are able to participate; they typically pay 25% of the therapy themselves.

> *Female university student of medicine, 24 years, borderline.*
>
> At the beginning of the treatment she was 30 kg overweight, a poor reality testing, no close friends; she was still a virgin with no interest in men, and a strange non-human uni-sex appearance. All body movements was impaired, she was slow, clumsy, and seemingly depressed, but with no emotional problems, except feeling like an alien. She was not able to look into other people's eyes. In holistic existential therapy she confronted that her 10-year-older big brother had raped her when she was five years old. The energy was that of war-rape: she was raped in the intent of repressing her. Strangely her parents wanted her eliminated and her brother was in alliance with the parents against her and he was not punished. She entered a psychotic crisis that lasted for 14 days during which she was hospitalized at the clinic. She experienced that she melted down and re-entered the human stream of consciousness – the collective human consciousness. She entered a visionary state of mind and for days she received thousands of pictures of human life from an inner source of wisdom and knowledge. When she re-appeared to the surface she was completely transformed into a wise young human remembering her true human nature. She changes her life completely, started dating boys, doing exercise,

changing diet and losing weight. In art-therapy she painted hundreds of paintings of the scenarios she has visualized during the metamorphosis.

*Female university student of psychology, 22 years, bulimia.*

Severe problems with self-esteem, looks, sexuality – not able to enjoy sex or intercourse – self-confidence, presenting severely disturbed eating patterns of overeating and vomiting. She believed she must weigh 50.00 kg. If not, she found her body disgusting. Sometimes she dressed extremely feminine in skirt and appears as a beautiful young woman, this interchanging with a much more male appearance where she varies men's pants. She also suffers from anxiety, and her sexual borders are 2 meters from her body; if men get closer she often feels intimidated. In holistic existential therapy the therapist (SV) could not get close to her for many sessions. When trust was won she finally allowed the therapist to get close emotionally and she melted down in psychotic crises, where all her problems of sexuality of low bodily self-esteem exploded. She entered a mental state of feeling totally unreal and stayed like this for days. She was hospitalized at our clinic for four days, before she can integrate the painful childhood events of failure and neglect that she has confronted; obviously she has then as a child metamorphosed into a person living in her own world not needing any contact to her parents, to avoid the pain of feeling not loved and not cared for. After the psychotic crises her condition slowly normalized and she was able to function again as a human being.

We have earlier described this kind of spontaneous healing of two schizophrenic patients (14), and we have often seen holistic sexological therapy and holistic gynecology lead to accelerated existential healing (Antonovsky salutogenesis) (15-24).

## Discussion

In a number of cases in our clinical work we have observed a radical process of spontaneous healing that seems to be adult human metamorphosis, parallel to the metamorphosis of many insects and some vertebrates. In its most radical version the person's mind is melting down and all behavioural and mental patterns are disintegrated for up to 10 days. The function of the human metamorphosis is to allow a person to catch up after many years of arrested psychosexual development. It happens spontaneously or provoked by holistic existential therapy, and is most likely to happen with people who have been violently or sexually abused in early childhood. The process is often initiated by a catharsis and a break through into old trauma of extremely intense emotional pain; rape in early childhood seems to be the paradigm. Other traumas of sufficient intensity to cause the developmental arrest which is set free by the metamorphosis is: surgery, social isolation, violence, and other events giving the child a near-death or psychic death experience. During the metamorphosis the person will re-live the extreme neural arousal and temporary psychosis of the traumatic childhood event.

It is most important to stress that the metamorphosis is not a mental disease - but a state of spontaneous healing - and it should not be treated as such. In this spontaneous healing event the patient needs loving care and tranquillity, while being "in the pupae": introvert, mentally disintegrated, seemingly psychotic and not in present time, sinking into the sea of biological information of being human, to finally reappear the way nature originally meant this person to be.

We suggest that human metamorphosis is really a biological process, and we believe that there is a complete set of genes and chemical mediators (hormones, neurotransmitters, or neuropeptides) to handle the biological side of the human metamorphosis. We believe that human metamorphosis is the most efficient healing process known to this day, and that a successful metamorphosis can save the patient from many years of therapy and sufferings. Human metamorphosis cannot only change the mind. We believe that spontaneous healing of cancer and other diseases is also often caused by human metamorphosis.

## Conclusion

Interestingly, mentally ill patients can enter the state of adult human metamorphosis, to re-do the juvenile metamorphosis into non-human forms that was beneficial for their childhood survival. The adult human metamorphosis looks at first glance like a normal psychotic crisis of a schizophrenic patient, but when you study it closer it becomes obvious that it is an unusual state of accelerated healing, a healing crisis. It is important to understand that the adult human metamorphosis is the inverted event of a juvenile metamorphosis where the patient turned him- or herself into some non-human alien form to survive; the self-transportation of human existence into a parallel dimension of existence often gives severe developmental problems and both physical and mental problems to the person later in life but was necessary for survival from an emotional point of view.

We have now carefully observed several cases of spontaneous remission of a number of different mental diseases: schizophrenia, borderline, anxiety, and bulimia. We understand the adult human metamorphosis as a confirmation of our hypothesis of aetiology of mental diseases: that they are in general caused by juvenile metamorphosis (12,13), not by defective genes and disturbed brain chemistry.

We believe that we in cracking this "secret code" have found a general way to understand and heal mental diseases, by taking them into adult human metamorphosis with clinical holistic medicine.

## References

[1] Ventegodt S, Andersen NJ, Merrick J. Holistic medicine III: The holistic process theory of healing. ScientificWorldJournal 2003;3:1138-46.
[2] Ventegodt S, Andersen NJ, Merrick J. Holistic medicine IV: Principles of existential holistic group therapy and the holistic process of healing in a group setting. ScientificWorldJournal 2003;3:1388-1400.
[3] Ventegodt S, Andersen NJ, Merrick J. The life mission theory V. A theory of the anti-self and explaining the evil side of man. ScientificWorldJournal 2003;3:1302-13.
[4] Ventegodt S, Andersen NJ, Merrick J. The life mission theory VI: A theory for the human character. ScientificWorldJournal 2004:4:859-80.
[5] Ventegodt S, Morad M, Andersen NJ, Merrick J. Clinical holistic medicine Tools for a medical science based on consciousness. ScientificWorldJournal 2004;4:347-61.
[6] Ventegodt S, Flensborg-Madsen T, Andersen NJ, Merrick J. Life mission theory VII: Theory of existential (Antonovsky) coherence: a theory of quality of life, health and ability for use in holistic medicine. ScientificWorldJournal 2005;5:377-89.

[7] Ventegodt S. The life mission theory: A theory for a consciousness-based medicine. Int J Adolesc Med Health 2003;15(1):89-91.

[8] Ventegodt S, Andersen NJ, Merrick J. The life mission theory II: The structure of the life purpose and the ego. ScientificWorldJournal 2003;3:1277-85.

[9] Ventegodt S, Andersen NJ, Merrick J. The life mission theory III: Theory of talent. ScientificWorldJournal 2003;3:1286-93.

[10] Ventegodt S, Merrick J. The life mission theory IV. A theory of child development. ScientificWorldJournal 2003;3:1294-1301.

[11] Buber M. I and thou. London: Free Press, 1971.

[12] Ventegodt S, Andersen NJ, Neikrug S, Kandel I, Merrick J. Clinical Holistic medicine: Holistic treatment of mental disorders. ScientificWorldJournal 2005;5:427-45.

[13] Ventegodt S, Andersen NJ, Neikrug S, Kandel I, Merrick J. Clinical holistic medicine: Mental disorders in a holistic perspective. ScientificWorldJournal 2005;5:313-23.

[14] Ventegodt S, Kandel I, Merrick J. Clinical holistic medicine (mindful short-term psychodynamic psychotherapy complimented with bodywork) in the treatment of schizophrenia (ICD10-F20/DSM-IV Code 295) and other psychotic mental diseases. ScientificWorldJournal 2007;7:1987-2008.

[15] Ventegodt S, Kandel I, Merrick J.Clinical holistic medicine: how to recover memory without "implanting" memories in your patient. ScientificWorldJournal 2007;7:1579-89.

[16] Flensborg-Madsen T, Ventegodt S, Merrick J. Sense of coherence and physical health. The emotional sense of coherence (SOC-E) was found to be the best-known predictor of physical health. ScientificWorldJournal 2006;6:2147-57.

[17] Ventegodt S, Clausen B, Omar HA, Merrick J. Clinical holistic medicine: holistic sexology and acupressure through the vagina (Hippocratic pelvic massage). ScientificWorldJournal 2006;6:2066-79.

[18] Ventegodt S, Clausen B, Merrick J. Clinical holistic medicine: pilot study on the effect of vaginal acupressure (Hippocratic pelvic massage). ScientificWorldJournal 2006;6:2100-16.

[19] Ventegodt S, Clausen B, Merrick J.Clinical holistic medicine: the case story of Anna. III. Rehabilitation of philosophy of life during holistic existential therapy for childhood sexual abuse. ScientificWorldJournal 2006;6:2080-91.

[20] Ventegodt S, Thegler S, Andreasen T, Struve F, Enevoldsen L, Bassaine L, Torp M, Merrick J.Clinical holistic medicine (mindful, short-term psychodynamic psychotherapy complemented with bodywork) in the treatment of experienced impaired sexual functioning. ScientificWorldJournal 2007;7:324-9.

[21] Ventegodt S, Kandel I, Neikrug S, Merric J. Clinical holistic medicine: holistic treatment of rape and incest trauma. ScientificWorldJournal 2005;5:288-97.

[22] Ventegodt S, Morad M, Hyam E, Merrick J. Clinical holistic medicine: holistic sexology and treatment of vulvodynia through existential therapy and acceptance through touch. ScientificWorldJournal 2004;4:571-80.

[23] Ventegodt S, Morad M, Kandel I, Merrick J. Clinical holistic medicine: problems in sex and living together. ScientificWorldJournal 2004;4:562-70.

[24] Ventegodt S, Morad M, Merrick J. Clinical holistic medicine: holistic pelvic examination and holistic treatment of infertility. ScientificWorldJournal 2004;4:148-58.

# Section 2. Acknowledgments

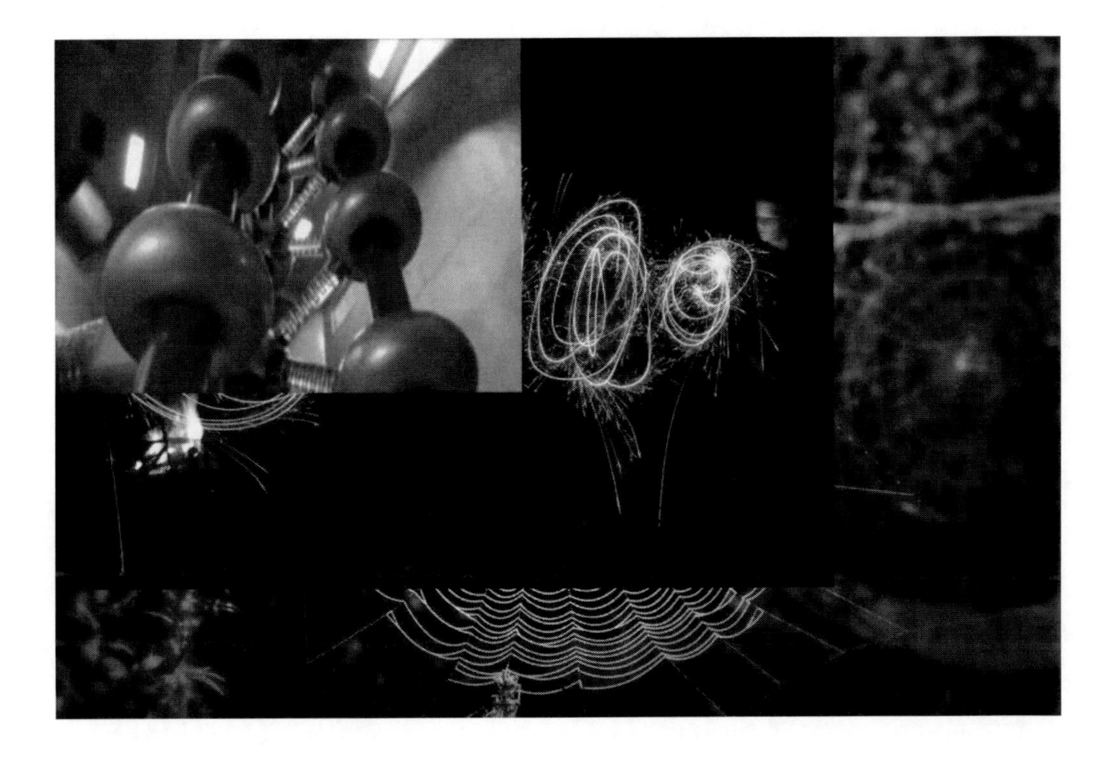

*Chapter XXII*

# About the authors

***Søren Ventegodt***, MD, MMedSci, EU-MSc-CAM is the director of the Nordic School of Holistic Medicine and the Quality of Life Research Center in Copenhagen, Denmark and an editor of several scientific journals in alternative and holistic medicine. He is responsible for a Research Clinic for Holistic Medicine and Sexology in Copenhagen and used as a popular speaker throughout Scandinavia. He has published numerous scientific or popular articles and a number of books on holistic medicine, quality of life, and quality of working life. Recently he has written textbooks on holistic psychiatry and holistic sexology. His most important scientific contributions are the comprehensive SEQOL questionnaire, the very short QOL5 questionnaire, the integrated QOL theory, the holistic process theory, the life mission theory, and the on-going Danish Quality of Life Research Survey, 1991-94 in connection with follow-up studies of the Copenhagen Perinatal Birth Cohort 1959-61 initiated at the University Hospital of Copenhagen by the late professor of pediatrics, Bengt Zachau-Christiansen, MD, PhD. 2006-2008 he was director and lecturer, Inter-University College, International Campus, Denmark in collaboration with Inter-University Consortium for Integrative Health Promotion, Inter-University College Graz, Austria and the Austrian Ministry of Education, Science and Culture. He is the author of 15 books and about 200 scientific papers on quality of life and holistic medicine. E-Mail: ventegodt@livskvalitet.org. Website: www.livskvalitet.org

***Joav Merrick,*** MD, MMedSci, DMSc, is professor of pediatrics, child health and human development affiliated with Kentucky Children's Hospital, University of Kentucky, Lexington, United States and the Division of Pediatrics, Hadassah Hebrew University Medical Center, Mt Scopus Campus, Jerusalem, Israel, the medical director of the Health Services, Division for Intellectual and Developmental Disabilities, Ministry of Social Affairs and Social Services, Jerusalem, the founder and director of the National Institute of Child Health and Human Development in Israel. Numerous publications in the field of pediatrics, child health and human development, rehabilitation, intellectual disability, disability, health, welfare, abuse, advocacy, quality of life and prevention. Received the Peter Sabroe Child Award for outstanding work on behalf of Danish Children in 1985 and the International LEGO-Prize ("The Children's Nobel Prize") for an extraordinary contribution towards improvement in child welfare and well-being in 1987. E-mail: jmerrick@zahav.net.il; Home-page: http://jmerrick50.googlepages.com/home.

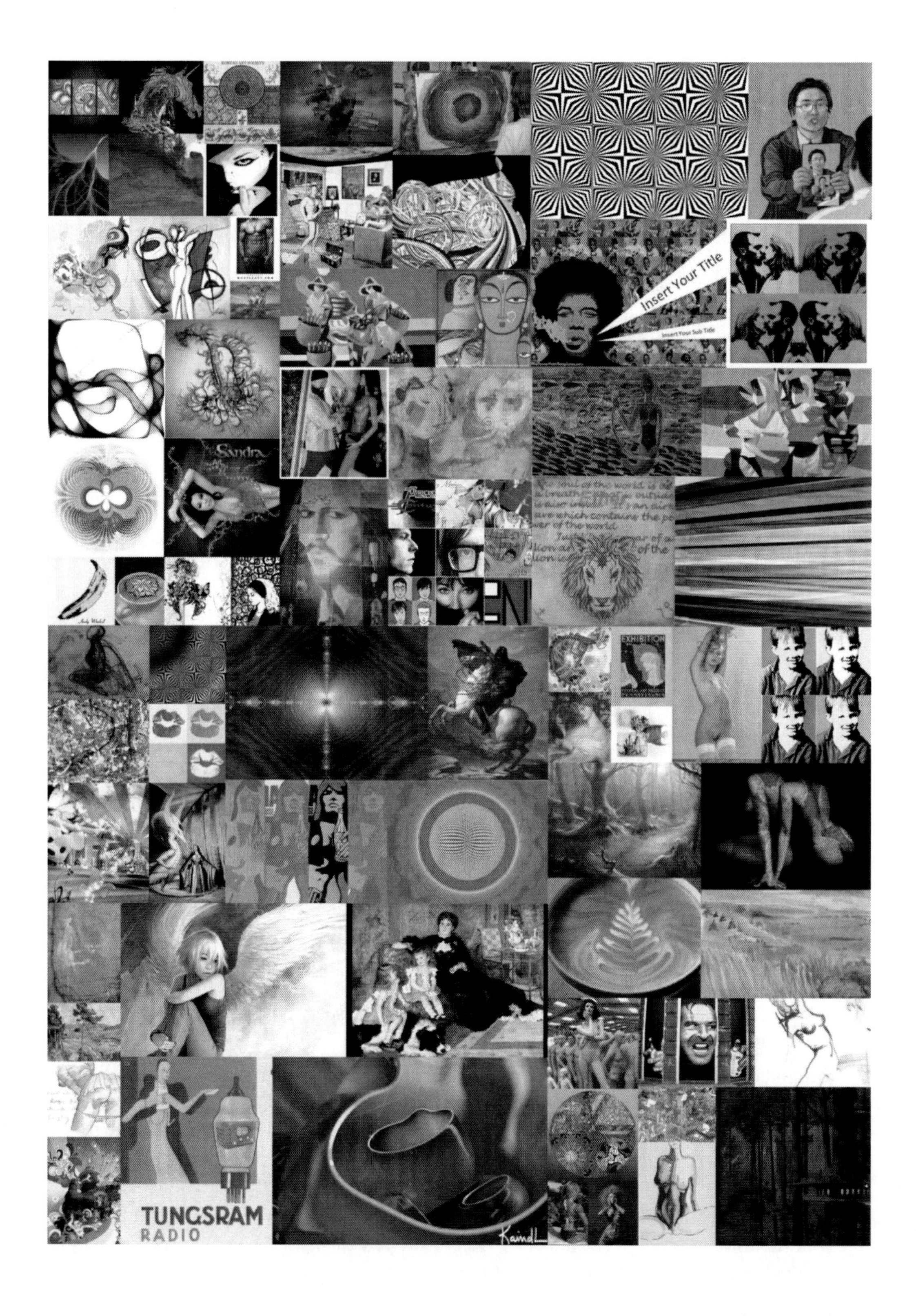
Insert Your Title
Insert Your Sub Title
Sandra
EXHIBITION
TUNGSRAM
RADIO
Kaindl

*Chapter XXIII*

# International review board

This book is written by Søren Ventegodt and Joav Merrick and the result of more than ten years of work together, but also an international collaboration with a group of very special people that we have published many papers with. This book project (a total of six books on mind-body medicine) has been a tremendous effort and we have been guided, helped and supported by a group of international collaborators and colleagues. These busy academics and clinicians have given of their time and expertise to advise us, so we wish to acknowledge their incredible support and friendship in this endeavour.

Andersen, Niels Jørgen
Andreasen, Tove
Anyanwu, Ebere C (deseased)
Bassaine, Laila
Brom, Bernard
Clausen, Birgitte
Enevoldsen, Lars
Ehiri, John E
Flensborg-Madsen, Trine
Gringols, Mark
Greydanus, Donald E
Hemmo-Lotem, Michal
Hermansen, Tyge Dahl
Hyam, Eytan
Henneberg, Eskild W
Kandel, Isack
Kromann, Maximilian
Kanu, Ijeoma
Lindholt, Jes S
Merrick-Kenig, Efrat
Morad, Mohammed
Nielsen, Maj Lyck
Neikrug, Shimshon
Omar, Hatim A
Orr, Gary
Rald, Erik
Struve, Flemming
Shek, Daniel T L
Torp, Margrethe
Thegler, Suzette

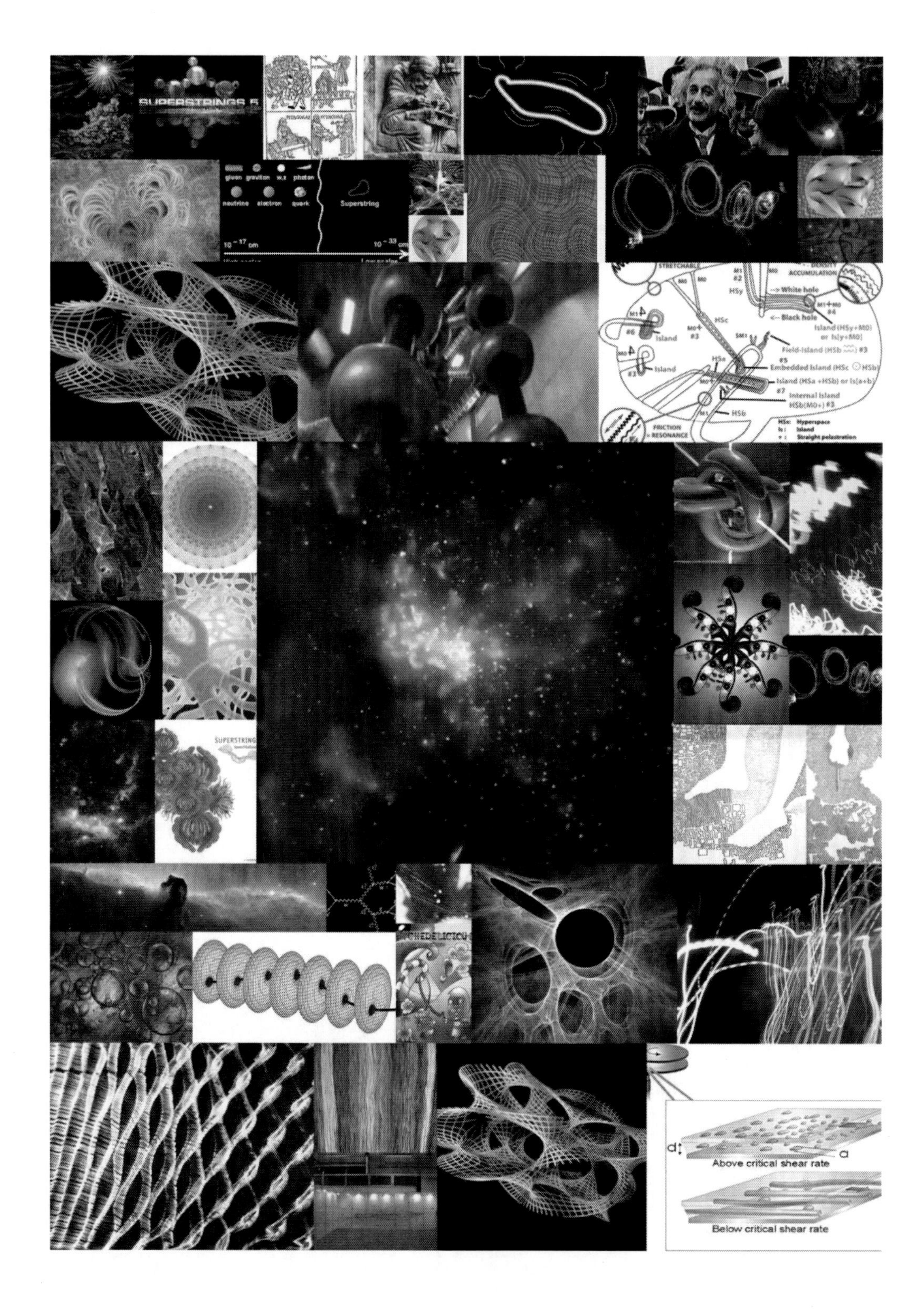

given
graviton
photon
neutrino
electron
quark
Superstring
STRETCHABLE
DENSITY ACCUMULATION
--> White hole
<-- Black hole
Island
Embedded Island
FRICTION = RESONANCE
HSa: Hyperspace
Is : Island
Above critical shear rate
Below critical shear rate

*Chapter XXIV*

# About the Quality of Life Research Center in Copenhagen, Denmark

The Quality of Life Research Center in Copenhagen was established in 1989, when the physician Søren Ventegodt succeeded in getting collaboration started with the Department of Social Medicine at the University of Copenhagen in response to the project "Quality of life and causes of disease". An interdisciplinary "Working group for the quality of life in Copenhagen" was established and when funds were raised in 1991 the University Hospital of Copenhagen (Rigshospitalet) opened its doors for the project.

The main task was a comprehensive follow-up of 9,006 pregnancies and the children delivered during 1959-61. This Copenhagen Perinatal Birth Cohort was established by the a gynaecologist and a pediatrician, the late Aage Villumsen, MD, PhD and the late Bengt Zachau-Christiansen, MD, PhD, who had made intensive studies during pregnancy, early childhood and young adulthood. The cohort was during 1980-1989 directed by the pediatrician Joav Merrick, MD, DMSc, who established the Prospective Pediatric Research Unit at the University Hospital of Copenhagen and managed to update the cohort for further follow-up register research, until he moved to Israel. The focus was to study quality of life related to socio-economic status and health in order to compare with the data collected during pregnancy, delivery and early childhood.

The project continued to grow and later in 1993, the work was organized into a statistics group, a software group that developed the computer programs for use in the data entry and a group responsible for analysis of the data.

## Quality of Life Research Center at the university medical center

The Quality of Life Center at the University Hospital generated grants, publicity with research and discussions among the professionals leading to the claim that quality of life was significant for health and disease. It is obvious that a single person cannot do much about his/her own disease, if it is caused by chemical defects in the body or outside chemical-physical influences. However, if a substantial part of diseases are caused by a low quality of life, we can all prevent a lot of disease and operate as our own physicians, if we make a personal effort and work to improve our quality of life. A series of investigations showed that this was indeed possible. This view of the role of personal responsibility for illness and health would naturally lead to a radical re-consideration of the role of the physician and also influence our society.

## Independent Quality Of Life Research Center

In 1994, The Quality of Life Research Center became an independent institution located in the center of the old Copenhagen. Today, the number of full-time employees has grown. The Research Center is still expanding and several companies and numerous institutions make use of the resources, such as lectures, courses, consulting or contract research. The companies, which have used the competence of the research center and its tools on quality of life and quality of working life, include IBM, Lego, several banks, a number of counties, municipalities, several ministries, The National Defense Center for Leadership and many other management training institutions, along with more than 300 public and private companies. It started in Denmark, but has expanded to involve the whole Scandinavian area.

The centre's research on the quality of life have been through several phases from measurement of quality of life, from theory to practice over several projects on the quality of life in Denmark, which have been published and received extended public coverage and public impact in Denmark and Scandinavia. The data is now also an important part of Veenhoven's Database on Happiness at Rotterdam University in the Netherlands.

## New research

Since The Quality-of-Life Research Center became independent a number of new research projects were launched. One was a project that aimed to prevent illness and social problems among the elderly in one of the municipalities by inspiring the elderly to improve their quality of life themselves. Another project about quality of life after apoplectic attacks at one of the major hospitals in Copenhagen and the Danish Agency for Industry granted funds for a project about the quality of work life.

## Quality of life of 10,000 Danes

There is a general consensus that many of the diseases that plague the Western world (which are not the result of external factors such as starvation, micro-organisms, infection or genetic defects) are lifestyle related and as such, preventable through lifestyle changes. Thus increasing time and effort is spent on developing public health strategies to promote "healthy" lifestyles. However, it is not a simple task to identify and dispel the negative and unhealthy parts of our modern lifestyle even with numerous behavioural factors that can be readily highlighted harmful, like the use of alcohol, use of tobacco, the lack of regular exercise and a high fat, low fibre diet.

However there is more to Western culture and lifestyle than these factors and if we only focus on them we can risk overlooking others. We refer to other large parts of our life, for instance the way we think about and perceive life (our life attitudes, our perception of reality and our quality of life) and the degree of happiness we experience through the different dimensions of our existence. These factors or dimensions can now, to some degree, be isolated and examined. The medical sociologist Aaron Antonovsky (1923-1994) from the Faculty of Health Sciences at Ben Gurion University in Beer-Sheva, who developed the salutogenic model of health and illness, discussed the dimension, "sense of coherence", that is closely related to the dimension of "life meaning", as perhaps the deepest and most important dimension of quality of life. Typically, the clinician or researcher, when attempting to reveal a connection between health and a certain factor, sides with only one of the possible dimensions stated above. A simple, one-dimensional hypothesis is then postulated, like for instance that cholesterol is harmful to circulation. Cholesterol levels are then measured, manipulated and ensuing changes to circulatory function monitored. The subsequent result may show a significant, though small connection, which supports the initial hypothesis and in turn becomes the basis for implementing preventive measures, like a change of diet. The multi-factorial dimension is therefore often overlooked.

In order to investigate this multifactorial dimension a cross-sectional survey examining close to 10,000 Danes was undertaken in order to investigate the connection between lifestyle, quality of life and health status by way of a questionnaire based survey. The questionnaire was mailed in February 1993 to 2,460 persons aged between 18-88, randomly selected from the CPR (Danish Central Register) and 7,222 persons from the Copenhagen Perinatal Birth Cohort 1959-61.

A total of 1,501 persons between the ages 18-88 years and 4,626 persons between the ages 31-33 years returned the questionnaire (response rates 61.0% and 64,1% respectively). The results showed that health had a stronger correlation to quality of life ($r= 0.5$, $p<0.0001$), than it had to lifestyle ($r=0.2$, $p< 0.0001$).

It was concluded that preventable diseases could be more effectively handled through a concentrated effort to improve quality of life rather than through an approach that focus solely on the factors that are traditionally seen to reflect an unhealthy life style.

## Collaborations across borders

The project has been developed during several phases. The first phase, 1980-1990, was about mapping the medical systems of the pre-modern cultures of the world, understanding their philosophies and practices and merging this knowledge with western biomedicine. A huge task seemingly successfully accomplished in the Quality of Life (QOL) theories, and the QOL philosophy, and the most recent theories of existence, explaining the human nature, and especially the hidden resources of man, their nature, their location in human existence and the way to approach them through human consciousness.

Søren Ventegodt visited several countries around the globe in the late 1980s and analyzed about 10 pre-modern medical systems and a dozen of shamans, Sangomas and spiritual leaders noticing most surprisingly similarities, allowing him together with about 20 colleagues at the QOL Study Group at the University of Copenhagen, to model the connection between QOL and health. This model was later further developed and represented in the integrative QOL theories and a number of publications. Based on this philosophical breakthrough the Quality of Life Research Center was established at the University hospital. Here a brood cooperation took place with many interested physicians and nurses from the hospital.

A QOL conference in 1993 with more than 100 scientific participants discussed the connection between QOL and the development of disease and its prevention. Four physicians collaborated on the QOL population survey 1993. For the next 10 years the difficult task of integrating bio-medicine and the traditional medicine went on and Søren Ventegodt again visited several centers and scientists at the Universities of New York, Berkeley, Stanford and other institutions. He also met people like David Spiegel, Dean Ornish, Louise Hay, Dalai Lama and many other leading persons in the field of holistic medicine and spirituality.

Around the year 2000 an international scientific network started to take form with an intense collaboration with the National Institute of Child Health and Human Development (NICHD) in Israel, which has now developed the concept of "Holistic Medicine". We believe that the trained physician today has three medical toolboxes: the manual medicine (traditional), the bio-medicine (with drugs and pharmacology) and the consciousness-based medicine (scientific, holistic medicine). What is extremely interesting is that most diseases can be alleviated with all three sets of medical tools, but only the bio-medical toolset is highly expensive. The physician, using his hands and his consciousness to improve the health of the patient by mobilizing hidden resources in the patient can use his skills in any cultural setting, rich or poor.

## Contact person

Director Søren Ventegodt, MD, MMedSci, MSc
Quality of Life Research Center
Frederiksberg Allé 13A, 2tv
DK-1820 Copenhagen V
Denmark
E-mail: ventegodt@livskvalitet.org
Website: www.livskvalitet.org

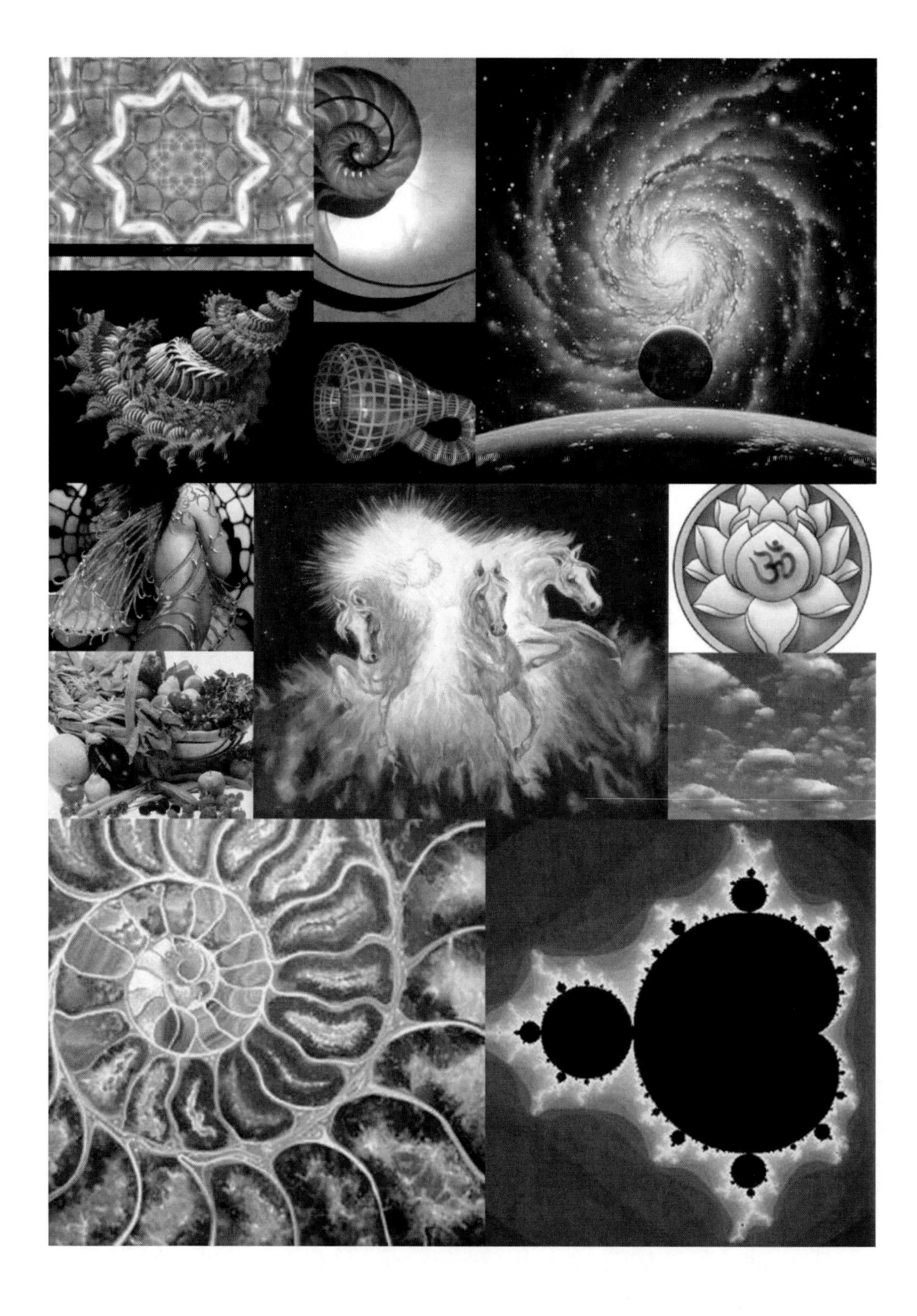

# Chapter XXV

# About the National Institute of Child Health and Human Development in Israel

The National Institute of Child Health and Human Development (NICHD) in Israel was established in 1998 as a virtual institute under the auspices of the Medical Director, Ministry of Social Affairs and Social Services in order to function as the research arm for the Office of the Medical Director. In 1998 the National Council for Child Health and Pediatrics, Ministry of Health and in 1999 the Director General and Deputy Director General of the Ministry of Health endorsed the establishment of the NICHD. In 2011 the NICHD became affiliated with the Division of Pediatrics, Hadassah Hebrew University Medical Center, Mt Scopus Campus in Jerusalem.

## Mission

The mission of a National Institute for Child Health and Human Development in Israel is to provide an academic focal point for the scholarly interdisciplinary study of child life, health, public health, welfare, disability, rehabilitation, intellectual disability and related aspects of human development. This mission includes research, teaching, clinical work, information and public service activities in the field of child health and human development.

## Service and academic activities

Over the years many activities became focused in the south of Israel due to collaboration with various professionals at the Faculty of Health Sciences (FOHS) at the Ben Gurion University of the Negev (BGU). Since 2000 an affiliation with the Zusman Child Development Center at the Pediatric Division of Soroka University Medical Center has resulted in collaboration around the establishment of the Down Syndrome Clinic at that center. In 2002 a full course on "Disability" was established at the Recanati School for Allied Professions in the Community, FOHS, BGU and in 2005 collaboration was started with the Primary Care Unit of the faculty and disability became part of the master of public health course on "Children and society". In the academic year 2005-2006 a one semester course on "Aging with disability" was started as part of the master of science program in gerontology in our collaboration with the Center for Multidisciplinary Research in Aging. In 2010 collaborations with the Division of Pediatrics, Hadassah Medical Center, Hebrew University, Jerusalem, Israel.

## Research activities

The affiliated staff has over the years published work from projects and research activities in this national and international collaboration. In the year 2000 the International Journal of Adolescent Medicine and Health and in 2005 the International Journal on Disability and Human development of De Gruyter Publishing House (Berlin and New York), in the year 2003 the TSW-Child Health and Human Development and in 2006 the TSW-Holistic Health and Medicine of the Scientific World Journal (New York and Kirkkonummi, Finland), all peer-reviewed international journals were affiliated with the National Institute of Child Health and Human Development. From 2008 also the International Journal of Child Health and Human Development (Nova Science, New York), the International Journal of Child and Adolescent Health (Nova Science) and the Journal of Pain Management (Nova Science) affiliated and from 2009 the International Public Health Journal (Nova Science) and Journal of Alternative Medicine Research (Nova Science).

## National collaborations

Nationally the NICHD works in collaboration with the Faculty of Health Sciences, Ben Gurion University of the Negev; Department of Physical Therapy, Sackler School of Medicine, Tel Aviv University; Autism Center, Assaf HaRofeh Medical Center; National Rett and PKU Centers at Chaim Sheba Medical Center, Tel HaShomer; Department of Physiotherapy, Haifa University; Department of Education, Bar Ilan University, Ramat Gan, Faculty of Social Sciences and Health Sciences; College of Judea and Samaria in Ariel and in 2011 affiliation with Center for Pediatric Chronic Diseases and Center for Down Syndrome, Department of Pediatrics, Hadassah-Hebrew University Medical Center, Mount Scopus Campus, Jerusalem.

## International collaborations

Internationally with the Department of Disability and Human Development, College of Applied Health Sciences, University of Illinois at Chicago; Strong Center for Developmental Disabilities, Golisano Children's Hospital at Strong, University of Rochester School of Medicine and Dentistry, New York; Centre on Intellectual Disabilities, University of Albany, New York; Centre for Chronic Disease Prevention and Control, Health Canada, Ottawa;

Chandler Medical Center and Children's Hospital, Kentucky Children's Hospital, Section of Adolescent Medicine, University of Kentucky, Lexington; Chronic Disease Prevention and Control Research Center, Baylor College of Medicine, Houston, Texas; Division of Neuroscience, Department of Psychiatry, Columbia University, New York; Institute for the Study of Disadvantage and Disability, Atlanta; Center for Autism and Related Disorders, Department Psychiatry, Children's Hospital Boston, Boston; Department of Paediatrics, Child Health and Adolescent Medicine, Children's Hospital at Westmead, Westmead, Australia; International Centre for the Study of Occupational and Mental Health, Düsseldorf, Germany; Centre for Advanced Studies in Nursing, Department of General Practice and Primary Care, University of Aberdeen, Aberdeen, United Kingdom; Quality of Life Research Center, Copenhagen, Denmark; Nordic School of Public Health, Gottenburg, Sweden, Scandinavian Institute of Quality of Working Life, Oslo, Norway; Centre for Quality of Life of the Hong Kong Institute of Asia-Pacific Studies and School of Social Work, Chinese University, Hong Kong.

## Targets

Our focus is on research, international collaborations, clinical work, teaching and policy in health, disability and human development and to establish the NICHD as a permanent institute at one of the residential care centers for persons with intellectual disability in Israel in order to conduct model research and together with the four university schools of public health/medicine in Israel establish a national master and doctoral program in disability and human development at the institute to secure the next generation of professionals working in this often non-prestigious/low-status field of work.

### Contact

Joav Merrick, MD, DMSc
Professor of Pediatrics, Child Health and Human Development
Medical Director, Health Services,
Division for Intellectual and Developmental Disabilities,
Ministry of Social Affairs and Social Services, POB 1260, IL-91012 Jerusalem, Israel.
E-mail: jmerrick@zahav.net.il

# Section 3. Index

# Index

## B



## C

## D

## G



## H

## I



## J



## K



## L

## M

## N



## O



## P

## Q



## R

## T